Dieter Huhn (Ed.)

New Diagnostic Methods in Oncology and Hematology

Springer-Verlag Berlin Heidelberg GmbH

Preface

Since Paul Ehrlich introduced aniline dyes to the staining procedures for hematological smears in the second half of the last century, morphological techniques have been at the center of developments in clinical diagnostics and research in hematology for about 100 years. The results of morphologic and cytochemical methods in the diagnostics of hematological disease have been compiled in several excellent monographs. During the 1960s our understanding of cellular structure and function was consolidated by the introduction of electron microscopy. With few exceptions (e.g. dyserythropoietic anemia), knowledge of the ultrastructure of the cells made no essential contributions to practical clinical diagnostics.

During the past 25 years our understanding of the pathogenesis of hematological and oncological disease as well as practical clinical diagnostics of these diseases has been revolutionized by the introduction of new methods. This new era in hematology initially began with the introduction of polyclonal antibodies to demonstrate membrane antigens on hematological cells and tumor cells. With the application of monoclonal antibodies in conjunction with immunocytochemistry and flow cytometry, diagnostics became more sophisticated. These developments are not yet complete. New antibodies are giving rise to new qualitative evidence while multiparameter flow cytometry is accelerating the discovery of quantitative evidence.

Parallel to the development of immunophenotyping, new methods have been introduced to clinical cytogenetics. The first conventional staining methods improved the identification of the chromosomes; then diagnosis of chromosomal aberrations was refined by combining morphological and immunological methods and finally by in situ hybridization.

In the early 1980s new frontiers were discovered with further developments in molecular biology. Molecular biology has given us new perspectives for understanding the genesis of systemic disease. It has refined the clinical diagnostics of systemic disease, metabolic disturbances and infections; molecular genetics is in the process of changing classical serologic tissue typing to a more precise and better reproducible molecular genetic typing.

Even in "classical" immunohematology our understanding of the cause of disease and clinical diagnostics has progressed. The same applies for coagulation research, which has integrated new biochemical, immunological and molecular genetic methods to discover the cause of diseases and new methods for their diagnosis.

Today's practicing physicians have hardly had the opportunity to follow these developments during medical school or during their professional life. This is even true for clinically active hematologists and oncologists, who can no longer deal with all of the different facets of modern diagnostic methods in hematology and oncology today. Ignorance of modern immunological and molecular genetic methods is often such that even the nomenclatures of these special methods are not known. This impedes the comprehension of the numerous important papers, which require a large knowledge of immunological and molecular genetic methods and findings. A great discrepancy exists between the requirements regarding special laboratory methods demanded by the professional associations and those that are in fact required in later professional life. It is a fact that numerous modern methods, a knowledge and understanding of which is indispensable, are insufficiently covered in the textbooks and handbooks available today.

The editors and authors of this book on "New Diagnostic Methods in Hematology and Oncology" therefore saw an important task in conveying these modern methods to students and physicians in the way described above. Essentially the individual chapters are structured such that first the principle of the method, then the more important clinical applications and finally the practical procedure are described concisely. The greatest value was placed upon avoiding overlap with present monographs covering hematological laboratory diagnostics. Cytology and cytochemistry were also dispensed with. On the other hand, great emphasis was placed on portraying the important "modern" methods comprehensively, to give even nonspecialists the understanding or, if necessary, the support needed to establish or apply these methods in their own laboratories.

Berlin, June 1998 D. HUHN

Dieter Huhn (Ed.)

New Diagnostic Methods in Oncology and Hematology

With Contributions by
R. Blasczyk, C. Fonatsch, D. Huhn, O. Meyer,
S. Nagel, A. Neubauer, J. Oertel, A. Salama, S. Serke,
B. Streubel, and C. Thiede

With 82 Figures

Springer

Professor Dr. med. DIETER HUHN

Universitätsklinikum Charité
Medizinische Fakultät
der Humboldt-Universität zu Berlin
Augustenburger Platz 1
D-13353 Berlin
Germany

ISBN 978-3-642-63739-1

Library of Congress Cataloging-in-Publication Data

New diagnostic methods in oncology and hematology / D. Huhn (ed.).
p. cm.
Includes bibliographical references and index.
ISBN 978-3-642-63739-1 ISBN 978-3-642-58803-7 (eBook)
DOI 10.1007/978-3-642-58803-7

1. Blood--Diseases--Diagnosis. 2. Cancer--Diagnosis.
3. Diagnosis, Molecular. 4. Immunohematology. 5. Human chromosome abnormalities--Diagnosis. I. Huhn, Dieter.
[DNLM: 1. Neoplasms--diagnosis. 2. Hematologic Neoplasms--diagnosis. 3. Immunohistochemistry. 4. Molecular Biology--methods. QZ 241 N5288 1998]
RB45.N47 1998
616.1'5075--dc21
DNLM/DLC

Originally published by Springer-Verlag Berlin Heidelberg New York in 1998

Typesetting: Data conversion by Springer-Verlag, Heidelberg
Cover Design: Design & Production, Heidelberg
SPIN 10565866 09/3137 - 5 4 3 2 1 0 - Printed on acid-free paper

Contents

Contributors

Priv.-Doz. Dr. Rainer Blasczyk
Universitätsklinikum Charité, Medizinische Klinik mit Schwerpunkt Hämatologie und Onkologie, Campus Virchow-Klinikum, Blutbank, Augustenburger Platz 1, D-13353 Berlin, Germany

Prof. Dr. Christa Fonatsch
Institut für Medizinische Biologie der Medizinischen Fakultät der Universität, Währinger Straße 10, A-1090 Vienna, Austria

Prof. Dr. Dieter Huhn
Universitätsklinikum Charité, Medizinische Klinik mit Schwerpunkt Hämatologie und Onkologie, Campus Virchow-Klinikum Augustenburger Platz 1, D-13353 Berlin, Germany

Dr. Oliver Meyer
Universitätsklinikum Charité, Medizinische Klinik mit Schwerpunkt Hämatologie und Onkologie, Campus Virchow-Klinikum Augustenburger Platz 1, D-13353 Berlin, Germany

Dr. Stefan Nagel
Universitätsklinikum Charité, Medizinische Klinik mit Schwerpunkt Hämatologie und Onkologie, Campus Virchow-Klinikum Augustenburger Platz 1, D-13353 Berlin, Germany

Prof. Dr. Andreas Neubauer
Medizinische Klinik und Poliklinik I, Hämatolgie/Onkologie, Universitätsklinikum Carl Gustav Carus, Technische Universität Dresden, Fetscherstraße 74, D-01307 Dresden, Germany

Prof. Dr. Joachim Oertel
Universitätsklinikum Charité, Medizinische Klinik mit Schwerpunkt Hämatologie und Onkologie, Campus Virchow-Klinikum Augustenburger Platz 1, D-13353 Berlin, Germany

Prof. Dr. Abdulgabar Salama
Universitätsklinikum Charité, Medizinische Klinik mit Schwerpunkt Hämatologie und Onkologie, Campus Virchow-Klinikum, Blutbank, Augustenburger Platz 1, D-13353 Berlin, Germany

Priv.-Doz. Dr. Stefan Serke
Universitätsklinikum Charité, Medizinische Klinik mit Schwerpunkt Hämatologie und Onkologie, Campus Virchow-Klinikum Augustenburger Platz 1, D-13353 Berlin, Germany

Dr. Berthold Streubel
Institut für Medizinische Biologie der Medizinischen Fakultät der Universität, Währinger Straße 10, A-1090 Vienna, Austria

Dr. Christian Thiede
Medizinische Klinik und Poliklinik I, Universitätsklinikum Carl Gustav Carus, Technische Universität Dresden, Fetscherstrasse 74, D-01307 Dresden, Germany

1 Immunocytochemistry

J. Oertel · D. Huhn

1.1 Principles of Immunocytochemistry

The application of immunocytological methods has enhanced the diagnostic accuracy in hematology. Immunocytology is the study of cells by the use of techniques involving antigen-antibody reactions. Investigation of cells can be carried out either by immunofluorescence (using unfixed cells and cell suspensions in most cases) or by immunocytochemistry (using fixed cells and slides). In all these techniques the antibody is allowed to react with its specific antigen. This reaction is identified by a marker, which is linked to the antibody. This marker is a fluorochrome in immunofluorescence and an enzyme in immunocytochemistry. A review about immunocytochemistry was published by Hayhoe [1].

1.1.1 Specimens

Peripheral blood smears and cytospins are often more suitable than bone marrrow cells because bone marrow cells are very sensitive to damage by aspiration and immunostaining. However, the indication for immunocytochemical investigation of bone marrow is given in case of isolated bone marrow involvement. Cytospin preparations are well suited to investigate body cavity effusions, cerebrospinal fluid and bronchoalveolar lavage. Cytospin centrifugation is also applied to fine-needle aspirates of lymph nodes and other organs. Air dried unstained specimens can be kept up to 2 days at room temperature without loss of immunoreactivity. It is possible to preserve immunoreactivity for many years by storing air-dried preparations wrapped in foil at –20∞C.

1.1.2 Fixation

Many methods of fixation are used in immunocytochemistry. An ideal fixative should be convenient to use and produce optimal preservation of cytomorphology and immunoreactivity with a low level of background staining [2]. The staining results are influenced by the cell preparation and immunostaining procedures. For fixation most investigators apply 100% acetone (10 min) or 100% ethanol (10 min). Analysis of 23 fixation protocols showed that fixation in 0.1% formol saline overnight at room temperature followed by 10 min fixation in 100% ethanol produces the optimal preser vation of immunoreactivity which can be further enhanced by microwave treatment for epitope retrieval. Blocking of endogenous peroxidase is not necessary.

Bone marrow cells are quite sensitive to damage by aspiration and immunostaining. We observed acceptable immunostaining (immunoperoxidase) after 5 min fixation in May-Grünwald solution [3].

1.1.3 Controls

Negative controls are set up by replacing the primary antibody with a nonimmune antibody of the same isotype. Preparations of normal blood and bone marrow are used as positive controls in most cases. Special preparations are necessary for cytokeratin, TdT and estrogen receptor antibodies.

1.2 Methods for Immunostaining

1.2.1 Immunoalkaline Phosphatase Anti-alkaline Phosphatase (APAAP) Method (Fig. 1.1)

After fixation cytocentrifuge preparations or smears are placed in a humid chamber or in coverplates (Shandon) and incubated with the primary monoclonal antibody (in most cases from the mouse) which is bound to the correspondent antigen [4, 5]. Addition of human AB serum (except in cases of im-

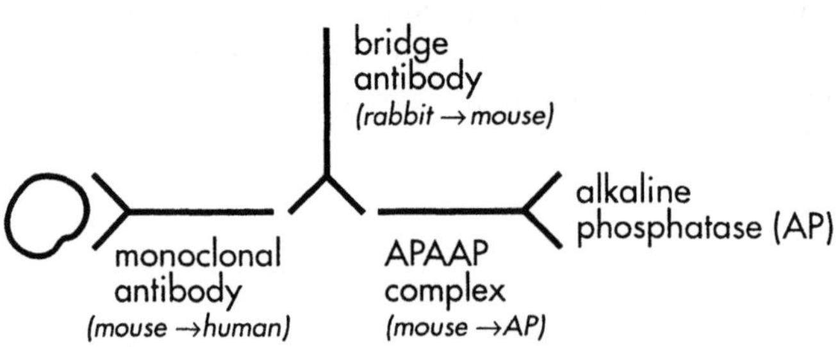

Fig. 1.1. APAAP method

munoglobulin detection) to the fixed cells or to the primary antibody prevents unspecific binding. In a second incubation step the bridge antibody (in most cases rabbit anti-mouse) is applied. The slides are washed again and incubated with immunoalkaline phosphatase anti-alkaline phosphatase (APAAP) complexes. Immunostaining is increased by repeated incubation with rabbit anti-mouse immunoglobulin and APAAP complexes. The use of primary rabbit anti-human antibodies requires an extra incubation step with mouse anti-rabbit-immunoglobulin.

Following a new wash the slides are incubated with a solution for cytochemical detection of alkaline phosphatase and after further washing the slides are counterstained with a nuclear stain. For analysis of stained cells an ordinary light microscope is all that is necessary. Positive cells show red or blue staining in the cytoplasm and/or on the cell surface. Various cell types exhibit endogenous alkaline phosphatase. Levamisole (added to the chromogen) inhibits most of the activity of endogenous alkaline phosphatase, whereas tracer alkaline phosphatase and intestinal alkaline phosphatase are not affected. Therefore the APAAP method with levamisole cannot be recommended for investigation of intestinal cells.

1.2.2 Peroxidase-Anti-peroxidase (PAP) Method (Fig. 1.2)

After fixation cytospins or smears are incubated in a humid chamber or in coverplates (Shandon) with the primary monoclonal antibody and, after washing, with a rabbit anti-mouse immunoglobulin [6]. The slides are washed again and incubated with immune complexes of peroxidase and mouse antibodies to this peroxidase (PAP complex). Following a new wash the slides are incubated with the solution for the cytochemical detection of peroxidase and after washing they are counterstained with a nuclear stain. For use of primary polyclonal rabbit antibodies a swine anti-rabbit immunoglobulin and a rabbit PAP complex are necessary.

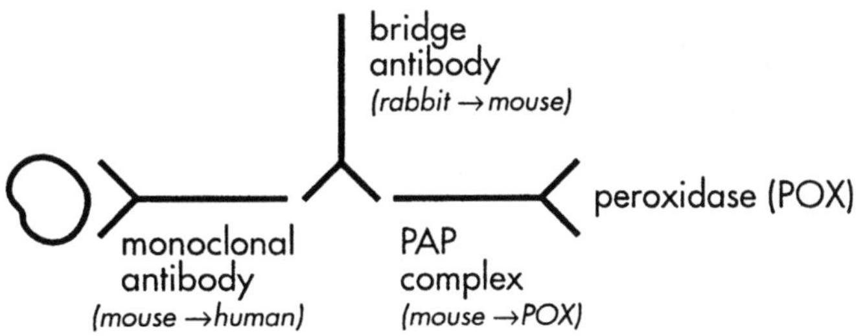

Fig. 1.2. PAP method

1.2.3 Immunoperoxidase (Fig. 1.3)

After fixation cytospins or smears are incubated in a humid chamber or in coverplates (Shandon) with the primary monoclonal antibody. After washing the specimens are incubated with a rabbit anti-mouse immunoglobulin (peroxidase-conjugated) and then a swine anti-rabbit immunoglobulin (peroxidase-conjugated) [7]. Peroxidase is developed with diaminobenzidine and H_2O_2.

The slides are counterstained. In positive cells the cytoplasm and/or the cell surface are stained yellow.

Several methods (1%–3% H_2O_2 or 0.1% sodium azide in 0.3% H_2O_2) have been proposed to inhibit endogenous peroxidase. However, many antigens are destroyed by this treatment. We found endogenous peroxidase activity only in eosinophils following addition of 10% fetal calf serum to the wash solution (phosphate buffered saline). The eosinophils are distinguished from other cells by their characteristic morphological picture with large intensely peroxidase-positive granules [3].

1.2.4 Enhanced Polymer One-Step (EPOS) Staining (Fig. 1.4)

This is a one-step immunostaining procedure. The EPOS antibody consists of high molecular weight polymers (dextran), on which a number of molecules of specific antibody and peroxidase is bound covalently [8, 9]. The main advantage in the use of these conjugates in immunostaining is the reduction of assay time as it enabled us to immunostain in one step. Its sensitivity equals that of the three step techniques. A drawback of this method is that the range of commercially available EPOS reagents is restricted.

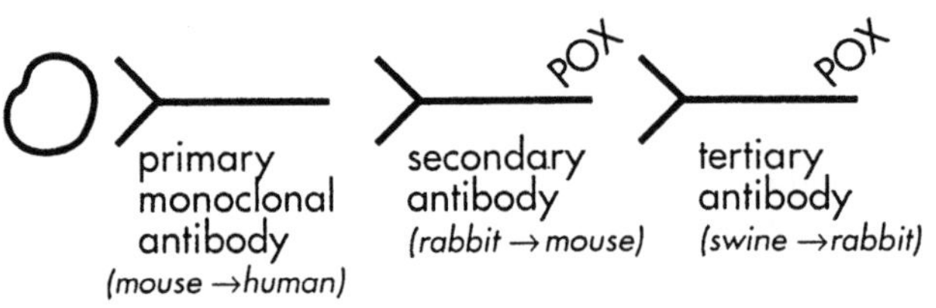

Fig. 1.3. Immunoperoxidase

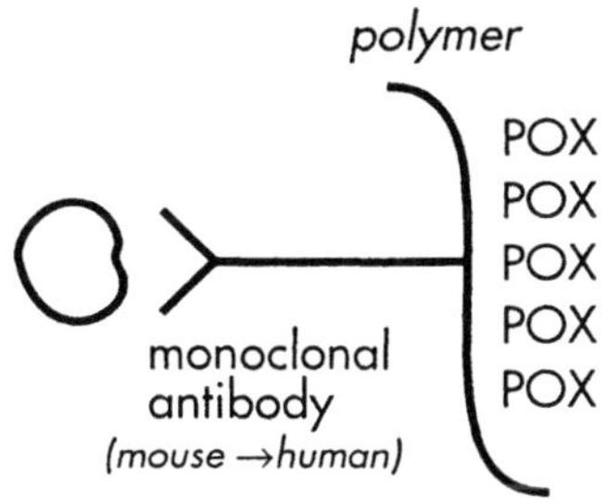

Fig. 1.4. EPOS antibody staining

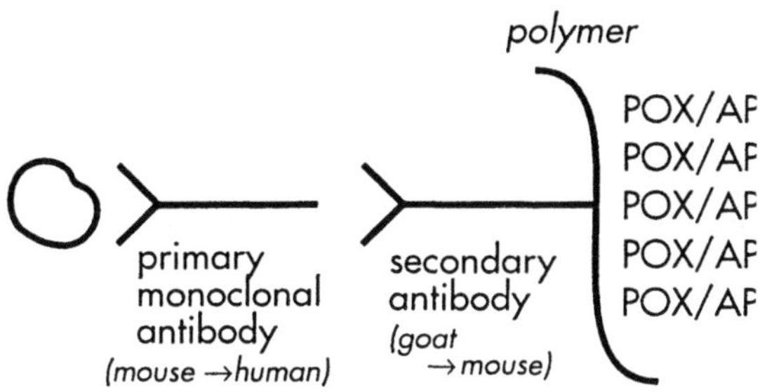

Fig. 1.5. Enhanced labelled-polymer system

1.2.5 Enhanced Labeled-Polymer System (ELPS, EnVision-DAKO) (Fig. 1.5)

This is a highly sensitive two-step immunostaining procedure. A goat anti-mouse antibody is conjugated to peroxidase or alkaline phosphatase labeled polymer [10]. After incubation of cytospins or smears with the primary specific antibody this secondary antibody is used. The peroxidase or alkaline phosphatase is developed with the corresponding chromogen. This method is better than a three-step staining procedure (immunoperoxidase, streptavidin-biotin method) in regard to sensitivity, and the assay time as well as background staining are reduced. It is a non-avidin-biotin system circumventing the problem of endogenous biotin.

1.2.6 Avidin-Biotin Systems (Fig. 1.6)

Avidin is an egg-white derived glycoprotein with a high affinity for biotin. Several biotin-avidin methods have been developed. The most widely used technique is the ABC method [11]. Incubation with the primary antibody is the first step. After washing a biotin-labeled secondary antibody is added. The third step is the addition of an avidin-biotinylated enzyme complex (ABC). Formation of the complex is achieved by mixing avidin and biotinylated enzyme prior to use. The enzymes are peroxidase or alkaline

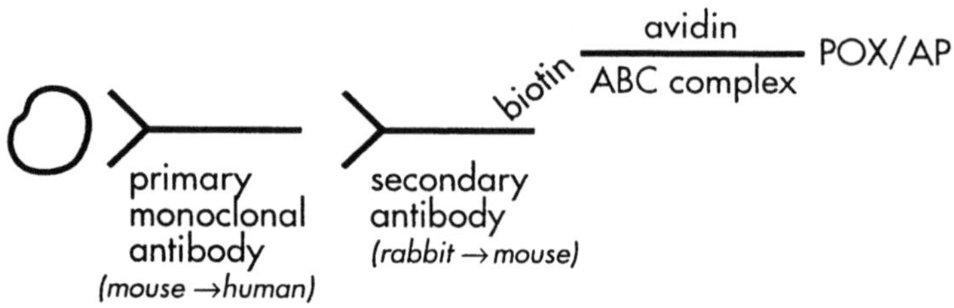

Fig. 1.6. Avidin-biotin system

phosphatase, which are developed by incubation with a substrate. Some tissues (liver, kidney, intestinal organs) may contain endogenous biotin that gives rise to unwanted staining. Streptavidin is a protein resembling egg-white derived avidin. Its affinity for biotin is lower. In most applications streptavidin and avidin are interchangeable.

1.2.7 Tyramide Enhanced Immunostaining [Catalyzed Signal Amplification (CSA) System] (Fig. 1.7)

This method is based on the avidin-biotin technique. The first step is incubation with a specific primary antibody. This is followed by incubation with a biotinylated secondary antibody and a streptavidin biotinylated peroxidase complex. After this conventional streptavidin-biotin technique, staining enhancement is achieved by incubation with biotinylated tyramide which binds to peroxidase [12, 13]. The biotin binds additional peroxidase labeled streptavidin. This procedure increases the sensitivity of immunostaining without loss of specificity. A further 30 min are required for addition of the tyramide step to this procedure.

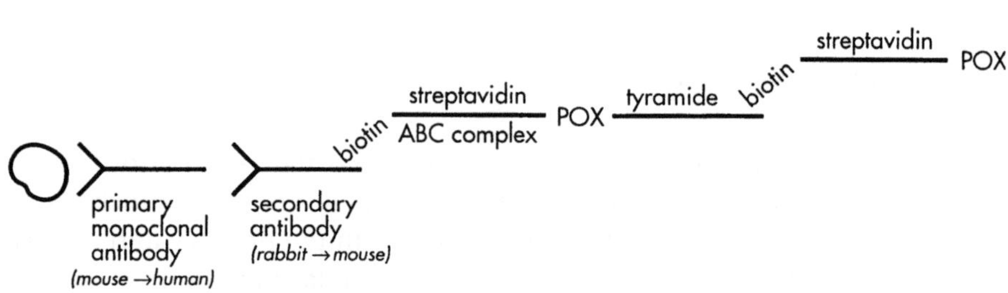

Fig. 1.7. Tyramide enhanced immunostaining (CSA system)

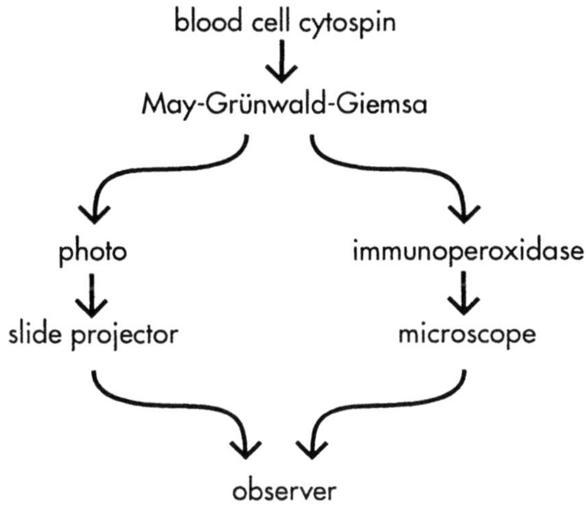

Fig. 1.8. Morphological-immunocytochemical technique

1.2.8
Sequential Morphological-Immunocytochemical Technique (Fig. 1.8)

The diagnostic potential of immunocytochemistry has not been fully utilized due to difficulties in morphological identification of immunostained cells. We apply an immunoperoxidase technique following May-Grünwald-Giemsa staining for successive morphological and immunocytochemical analysis [3]. The fixed cells are stained with May-Grünwald-Giemsa and photographed. Immunoperoxidase is performed afterwards on the same preparation. With this method it is possible to immunotype small morphologically identified cell populations.

1.2.9
Comparison of Immunocytochemistry and Immunofluorescence

Cells have been studied in cell suspensions by immunofluorescence microscopy. This method is invaluable in the study of blood cells. However, there are some disadvantages to this method. Only limited information concerning the morphology of the labeled cells is supplied by this method and investigation of heterogeneous samples with immunofluorescence microscopy is often difficult. Moreover, the preparations are not permanent and a fluorescence microscope is required. Studies of cell suspensions allow identification of cell surface antigens, but not of intracytoplasmic or intranuclear antigens, which can be detected on smears and cytospin preparations. However, gentle permeabilization of cells in suspension allows detection of cytoplasmic and nuclear antigens [14]. In contrast to immunocytochemistry immunofluorescence supplies information regarding the density of antigen expression on the cells. This is important when investigating the expression of immunoglobulins in patients with chronic lymphoid leukemia. Immunofluorescence allows simultaneous or sequential staining for more than one antigen in the same specimen using directly labeled antibodies with different fluorochromes.

Flow cytometry is a powerful tool for the investigation of blood cells with immunofluorescence. Its ability to investigate a large number of cells and multiple parameters on individual cells at high speed is ideal for the study of blood cells. However, this method has the same drawbacks as immunofluorescence microscopy.

The use of one or the other method will depend on the facilities in each laboratory [15, 16].

1.2.10 Double Immunoenzymatic Staining

The availability of double immunoenzymatic methods is not widespread. The opinion regarding this technique is controversial. However, the development of new double staining methods can be considered a step forward in diagnostics [17]. A successful double staining depends on the presence of two differently colored precipitates after development of the enzymes. It is recommended to develop alkaline phosphatase in blue (naphthol-AS-MX-phosphate/fast blue BB) and peroxidase in red (H_2O_2/aminoethyl carbazole). The mixed color (purple) is well distinguishable from both basic colors. It is necessary to develop alkaline phosphatase first.

1.2.10.1 *Sequential Methods*

Two immunolabeling sequences are performed sequentially using two antibodies from the same animal species. Double immunostaining was first performed using an indirect immunoperoxidase method with elution of the antibody of the first stage before proceeding to the second stage [18]. Sternberger and Joseph [19] used two peroxidase anti-peroxidase systems sequentially, the two labels being marked with different peroxidase substrates. The diaminobenzidine reaction product masks the antibodies of the first labeling system and avoids the risk of cross-reactivity. However, other authors found cross-reactivity and suggested that its intensity is related to the strength of the diaminobenzidine product.

Another technique involves performance of an indirect immunoperoxidase method followed by an APAAP method [20]. This technique is useful for identification of antigens in different cell populations or at different sites in the same cell.

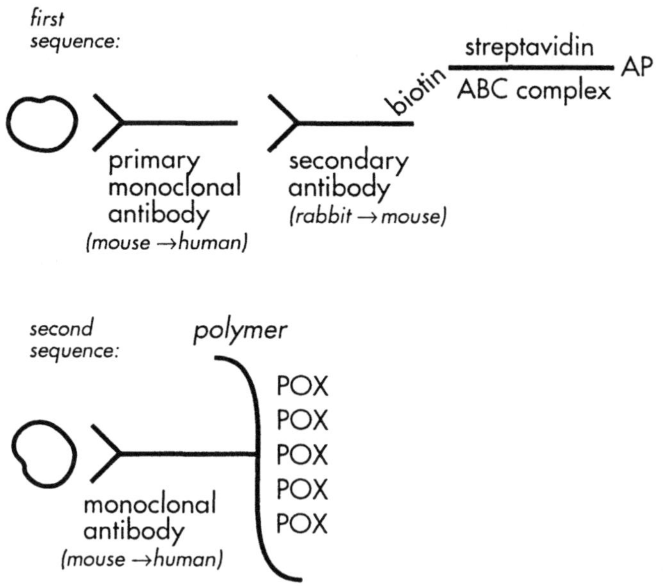

Fig. 1.9. Double immunoenzymatic staining with EPOS antibodies

Another sequential protocol involves the use of an unlabeled primary monoclonal antibody in conjunction with an indirect immunoenzymatic staining procedure and a second monoclonal antibody labeled with fluorescein isothiocyanate (FITC). Detection of FITC binding is possible with a rabbit anti-FITC and goat anti-rabbit immunoglobulin conjugated with a different enzyme [21]. There is no risk of cross-reactivity between these immunoenzymatic sequences. However, application of commercially available FITC-labeled monoclonal antibodies in immunocytochemistry is limited.

The newly developed EPOS antibodies were used together with an unlabeled primary antibody for immunoenzymatic double staining (Fig. 1.9) [22]. The first sequence was a biotin-streptavidin (alkaline-phosphatase labeled) combination followed by the peroxidase labeled EPOS antibody. The enzymes were developed with different colors. This method results in clear and distinct staining of two antigens either at separate sites or the same site. A drawback of this technique is that the range of commercially available EPOS antibodies is restricted.

1.2.10.2
Simultaneous Methods

The duration of these procedures is short because the incubation of the primary and secondary antibody are performed in a cocktail. These immunoenzymatic staining methods involve no risk of cross-reactivity between one another.

Two Primary Antibodies from Different Animal Species [23, 24]. This technique is performed simultaneously using primary antibody pairs of unrelated species in conjunction with two indirect immunostaining methods. The availability of such antibodies, however, is limited.

Two Antibodies of Different Isotype [25]. This method is a simultaneous technique using two primary antibodies of different isotype and two enzyme-labeled secondary antibodies raised against these immunoglobulin subclasses.

Two Primary Antibodies Available as Conjugates [26]. The primary antibodies are conjugated with enzymes, biotin, FITC, etc. A drawback of this technique is that the number of primary conjugated antibodies is limited.

1.2.11 Antibodies

Antibodies are either polyclonal or monoclonal. Polyclonal antibodies are produced in an appropriate host with a biochemically purified antigen followed by multiple absorptions. Monoclonal antibodies are produced by the hybridoma technique. Antibody-producing B cells are fused with myeloma cells to yield a hybrid cell. Individual antibodies may have several different names. This problem has been circumvented by the adoption of cluster designations for antibodies based on the recognized antigen. The clusters of differentiation (CD) have been derived from six international workshops on human leukocyte differentiation antigens; 162 antigens have been clustered up to now (Table 1.1). Clusters of interest in immunophenotyping, characterization of antigens and cell types positive for certain clusters are given in Chap. 2, "Flow Cytometry."

Table 1.1. International workshops on human leukocyte differentiation antigens

Workshop	Held in	Year	CD numbers
First	Paris	1982	1–15
Second	Boston	1984	16–26
Third	Oxford	1986	27–45
Fourth	Vienna	1989	46–78
Fifth	Boston	1993	79–130
Sixth	Kobe	1996	131–162

1.2.12
Reproducibility

It is important that the laboratories produce data using immunocytochemistry that are comparable between different laboratories. Blood and bone marrow from patients with acute leukemia, mature lymphatic diseases and multiple myeloma were investigated with an indirect immunoperoxidase technique and immunofluorescence [27]. A large interlaboratory variation was seen in the percentage of positive cells for each marker. This variation, however, did not influence the general agreement in immunological diagnosis very much.

1.3
Immunocytochemistry in the Diagnosis of Special Hematological and Other Disorders

Immunophenotyping has become a very important method in defining the distribution of leukocyte (especially lymphocyte) subpopulations. Methods for quantification of lymphocyte and other blood cell subpopulations will not be described in this chapter but in the chapter on flow cytometry.

On the other hand immunocytochemistry is an important tool for recognizing morphology and immunophenotype of hematological and lymphatic cells as well as tumor cells in the blood and bone marrow and in other cytological preparations. Immunocytochemistry may enable us to:

1. Define a certain cell line
2. Define the degree of maturation/differentiation
3. Define monoclonality in lymphoproliferative disorders of B-cell type

In the following some special hematological and lymphoproliferative malignancies will be discussed briefly. The immunological characteristics (the immune phenotype) of these disorders are summarized in Chap. 2 on Flow Cytometry.

1.3.1
Acute Lymphatic and Myeloid Leukemias (ALL, AML)

The classification of acute leukemias is based on a combined morphological, cytochemical and immunological investigation. The International Council for Standardization in Hematology (ICSH) proposed a three step investigation [16]: The first step is cytochemistry, the second intracellular phenotyping and the third membrane immunophenotyping. Myeloperoxidase (MPO) and alpha-naphthyl acetate esterase are able to delineate a significant proportion of the acute leukemias (FAB-M1, M2, M3, M4, M5). For cases of acute leukemia where myeloperoxidase and esterase cytochemistry is uninformative the ICSH recommends, as a second step, investigation of cytoplasmic B lineage-specific CD22 and T-lineage-specific CD3, cytoplasmic myeloperoxidase with antibodies to myeloperoxidase, nuclear TdT and cytoplasmic CD 13. Most B-lineage ALL will express cytoplasmic CD22 and most T-ALL are positive for cytoplasmic CD3. TdT expression will be seen in most cases of ALL. Coexpression of TdT, however, was found in 15%–20% of AML cases, too. Immunocytochemical detection of myeloperoxidase is diagnostic for AML and more sensitive than the cytochemical peroxidase assay. Cytoplasmic and nuclear antigens can be demonstrated by immunocytochemical methods and by immunofluorescence on fixed cells, by flow cytometry, however, only after permeabilization of the cells [14]. This is an important limitation of flow cytometry, as several of the antigens are primarily expressed in the cytoplasm.

The combination of membrane and intracellular immunophenotyping is especially relevant in the sub-classification of ALL, AML-M0, and AML-M7 [15]. The leukemic blasts in these subtypes do not express peroxidase and esterase activity in the cytochemical assay. Immunocytochemical detection of TdT supports the lymphatic character of the blasts. However, a minority of AML cases may be TdT positive, and B-ALL is TdT negative. The lymphatic character of blasts is verified by analysis of B and T cell markers, like the B cell associated markers CD19 and cytoplasmic CD22 and the T cell associated cytoplasmic CD3 and CD7. A second panel of antibodies can be used to characterize the B lineage ALL subtypes: pre-pre-B-ALL (=pro-B-ALL, early B lineage ALL, null-ALL) (CD10–), c-ALL (CD10+ and cytoplasmic μ–), pre-B-ALL (CD10+ and cytoplasmic μ+) and B-ALL (monoclonal immunoglobulins+ and TdT–).

Negativity of B and T cell markers suggests a myeloid character of blasts. The AML-M0 (undifferentiated myeloblastic leukemia) cases have blasts with undifferentiated morphology, lack of cytochemical peroxidase and esterase activity, lack of T and B cell markers and expression of myeloid associated markers CD13 (cytoplasmic) and/or CD33 and/or CD65. Immunocytochemical demonstration of myeloperoxidase is also useful. It must be noted that 20% of AML cases are CD7 and/or TdT positive. AML-M7 is characterized by expression of CD41/61 in blasts without cytochemical peroxidase activity.

There is no useful marker for identification of monoblasts. CD14 and CD68 are expressed only in a minority of AML-M5 A cases. Cytochemical detection of esterase is useful in these patients.

The coexpression of myeloid and lymphatic (B or T) markers on the leukemic blasts is described as biphenotypic acute leukemia. Most biphenotypic acute leukemias have a mixture of myeloid and lymphatic markers. In a scoring system CD22 (cytoplasmic) for B lineage, CD3 for T lineage and cytochemical peroxidase activity or anti-peroxidase have a high ranking [28] as specific markers. Typical ALL or AML with coexpression of CD13 or CD33 in ALL and CD7 and/or TdT in AML represent minimal deviations of no prognostic importance in adults.

Complete remission of acute leukemia is achieved when bone marrow contains <5% blasts identifiable by morphological analysis. The precision of this investigaton is limited and may be improved by immunocytochemistry [29].

The multidrug resistant (MDR) gene product is known as P-glycoprotein. It is expressed in hemopoietic stem cells and extrudes anticancer drugs (anthracyclines, vinca alkaloids, epipodophyllotoxins, Taxus compounds). Immunocytochemical detection of MDR phenotype demonstrated positivity in 22%–70% of patients with AML. The better remission rates for MDR1 phenotype negative patients proved to be better than the positive ones. In patients with multiple myeloma there is an increase of MDR phenotype positivity with disease progression and anthracycline treatment [30].

Meningeal involvement is observed in many patients with acute lymphatic leukemia. The lymphoblasts are small or medium size cells with fine chromatin without clumping. Detection of TdT in these cells is an important finding. Cells expressing nuclear TdT or CD34 are not normally found in the cerebrospinal fluid. An exception is represented by CSF with blood contamination. The blasts are of identical immunotype as the leukemic blasts in blood and bone marrow [31].

Blast Transformation of Chronic Myeloid Leukemia. Immunocytochemistry plays no role in the chronic phase of this leukemia. There is a high probability of blast crisis in this disorder, which is lymphoblastic in about one third of cases [32]. Remission is more likely in lymphoblastic crisis. Several studies confirmed a 20%–25% incidence of pure lymphoid phenotypes with a high percentage of TdT and CD10 positive blasts.

Myelodysplasia. Myelodysplastic syndromes comprise a group of hematological disorders characterized by blood cytopenias and dyserythropoiesis, dysgranulopoiesis and dysmegakaryopoiesis of bone marrow cells [33]. The FAB classification recognizes three groups of patients, according to bone marrow blasts less than 5% (refractory anemia, refractory anemia with ring sideroblasts), 5%–20% (refractory anemia with excess of blasts = RAEB), 21%–30% (RAEB in transformation = RAEB-T). The percentage of blasts in chronic myelomonocytic leukemia (CMML) is variable. Immunological investigation of myelodysplastic syndromes were performed using flow cytometry [34] and immunocytochemistry [35, 36]. The last authors used a combined morphological-immunocytochemical technique and found that the increase of bone marrow blasts in RAEB patients is related to CD34 negative type II and III blasts. A clone of undifferentiated CD34 positive blasts is characteristic for RAEB-T and acute leukemia evolving from myelodysplasia.

1.3.2 Lymphoproliferative Disorders

Consensus classification for lymphoid neoplasms was proposed by the International Lymphoma Study Group [37]. This revision of current or prior European and American lymphoma classifications is called the "revised European-American classification of lymphoid neoplasms" (REAL). Results of immunophenotyping of lymphoma entities classified according to the REAL classification will be described briefly in the following. The REAL classification does not distinguish between lymphomas of low and high malignancy. This classification prefers the determination of the growth fraction with the antibody Ki67. The FAB group published an excellent review about the morphological and immunocytological picture of the leukemic phase of these disorders [38]. There are three major categories of lymphoid malignancies, namely B-cell neoplasms, T/NK-cell neoplasms and Hodgkin's disease.

1.3.2.1 *B-Lymphoproliferative Disorders*

Over 95% of malignant lymphoproliferations are derived from B cells. Immunocytochemistry of fixed cells show increased percentages of cells expressing B cell markers (CD19, CD20, CD22, CD79a) (Fig. 1.12). Light chain restriction is able to demonstrate the monoclonal character of the cells. That means that all cells of this population have the same light chain type (lambda or kappa). This is also a powerful technique for demonstrating monoclonality in small B cell populations of patients with a normal white cell differential. Not all monoclonal antibodies directed at light chains are useful [39]. Most investigators prefer polyclonal antibodies for this analysis. In cases in which light chain restriction is not detectable by flow cytometry an immunocytochemical method is useful for detecting monoclonality. Bone marrow is a frequent site of infiltration in B-non-Hodgkin's lymphomas of low malignancy. The examination of trephine biopsies represents the gold-standard in evaluating bone marrow involvement. In addition to cytomorphology immunostaining improves the diagnostic sensitivity for detecting bone marrow infiltration by low grade non-Hodgkin's lymphomas in aspirates [40]. Immunocytochemistry of bone marrow aspirates from healthy persons with the APAAP technique showed 4.1±2.8% CD19 positive B cells. Erythropoietic cells were not included. The mean B cell count in patients with low grade non-Hodgkin's lymphomas was 38±23%. A B cell percentage of less than 20% was considered as negative bone marrow infiltration in the absence of morphological atypias of lymphocytes. Detection of light chain restriction in bone marrow is more difficult than in peripheral blood. Preparation of cytospins from bone marrow cells is necessary.

It has been shown that histological classification of lymphomas infiltrating the bone marrow is possible by trephine biopsy and reveals congruent results with lymph node histology [41] in the majority of cases. Other results indicate that, with the exception of hairy cell leukemia, the diagnostic relevance of immunocytochemistry in bone marrow aspirates for lymphoma typing is of limited value [42].

1.3.2.1.1
Chronic Lymphocytic Leukemia (B-CLL) (Figs. 1.10, 1.11)

The predominant cell is a small lymphocyte with a round nucleus, dense chromatin and an inconspicuous nucleolus. Larger lymphoid cells (pro-lymphocytes and paraimmunoblasts) are always present.

Immunocytochemistry demonstrates the B cell character (CD19, CD20; CD22; CD79a) of these lymphocytes and the light chain restriction as in all B lymphoproliferative disorders. The cells of B-CLL carry only a small amount of surface immunoglobulins. This explains the weak immunofluorescence when analysing immunoglobulins in cell suspensions. All other chronic lymphoid leukemias show moderate or strong immunofluorescence upon analysis of the surface immunoglobulins. IgM is the most prevalent heavy chain type followed by IgM and IgD or IgD only. Cytoplasmic immunoglobulins are detectable on fixed cells in most cases with this disorder. One or two percent of B-CLL patients did not show cytoplasmic immunoglobulins [43, 44].

Immunocytochemistry demonstrates expression of CD5 and CD23 positivity in most B-CLL patients. CD5 positivity is also observed in mantle cell lymphoma, however CD23 is not detectable in most cases of this lymphoma. Weak positivity was found with CD11c and CD25 in 20% and 50% of the B-CLL patients. A small number of patients with B-CLL show an evolution to prolymphocytic transformation with an increased percentage of pro-lymphocytes. This term should be reserved for cases with a history of previously diagnosed B-CLL.

1.3.2.1.2
B-Prolymphocytic Leukemia (B-PLL)

The prolymphocytes (>55% of the lymphocytes) are characterized by their size (>2 erythrocytes), ample cytoplasm, a round nucleus with a prominent

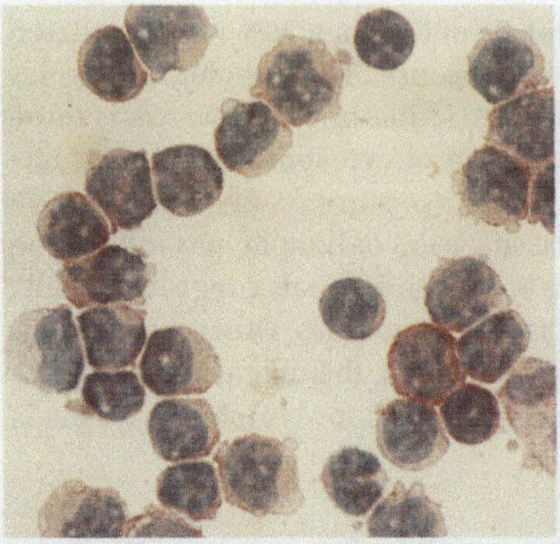

1.10

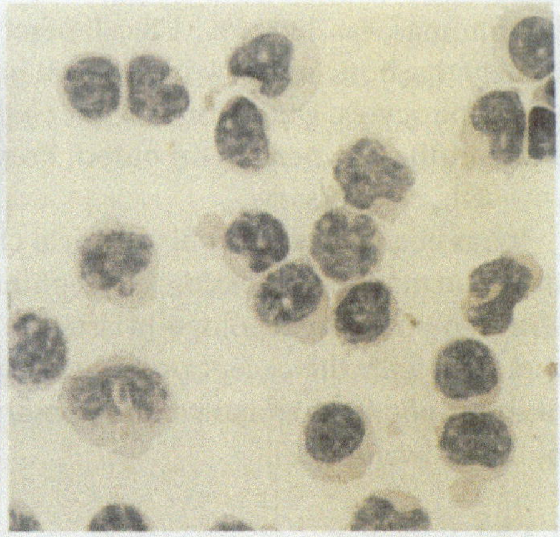

1.11

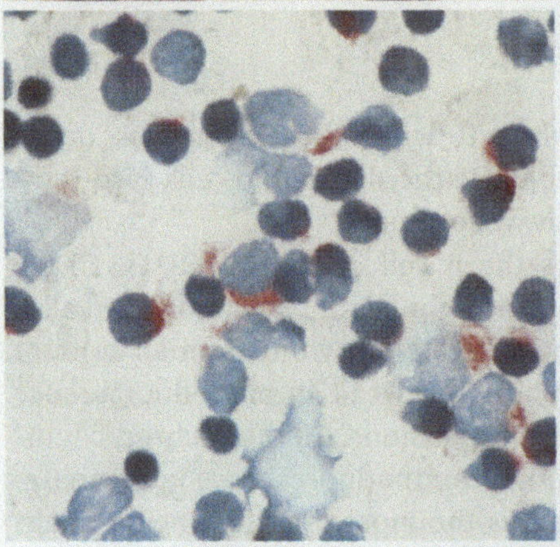

1.12

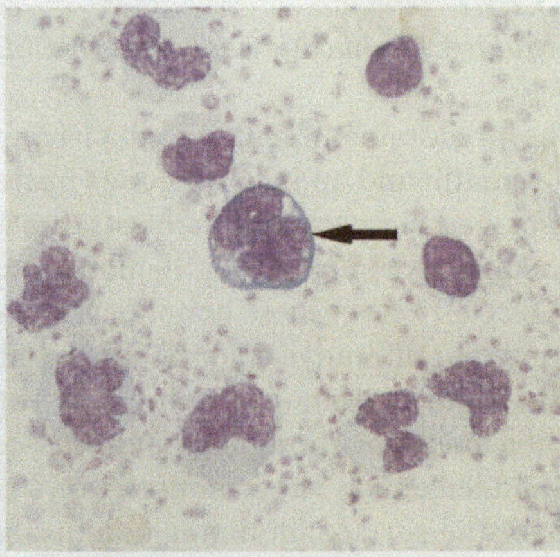

1.13

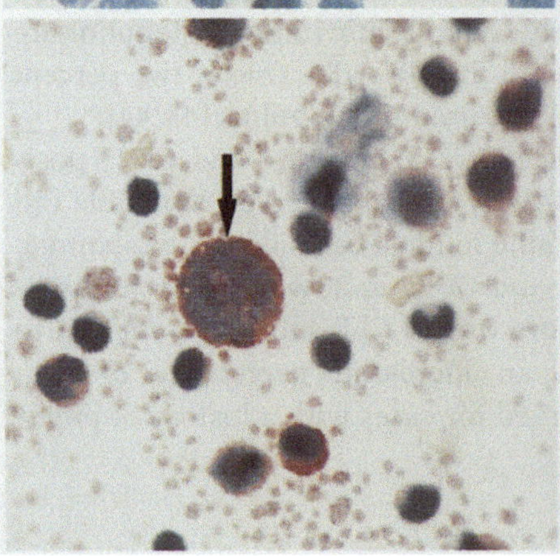

1.14

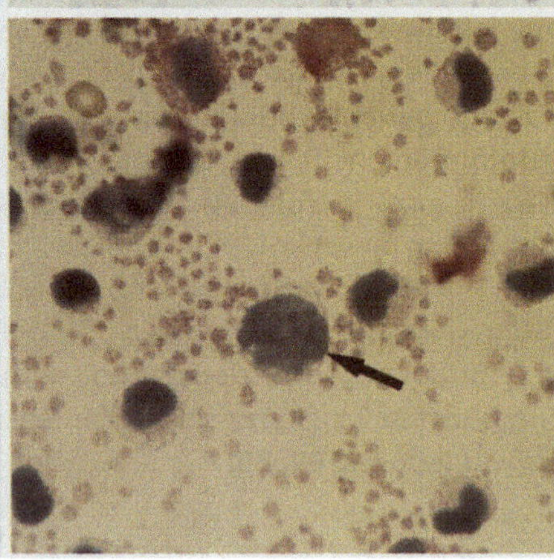

1.15

Figs. 1.10 - 1.15

nucleolus and clumped chromatin. This morphological picture is the basis for the diagnosis.

Immunocytochemistry is necessary only for demonstration of the B cell character. There is no immunological marker specific for this disorder. Investigation of cell suspensions with immunofluorescence shows in contrast to B-CLL a strong immunofluorescence upon analysis of the immunoglobulins and expression of FMC7. Immunocytochemistry detecting surface and cytoplasmic immunoglobulins demonstrates identical expression of immunoglobulins in B-CLL cells and B-PLL cells. Light chain restriction is detectable in all patients. The antibody FMC7 is not useful in immunocytochemistry.

1.3.2.1.3
Lymphoplasmacytoid Lymphoma (Immunocytoma)

This is a very rare subtype of indolent lymphoma comprising less than 5% of non-Hodgkin's lymphomas. The cells of this entity are similar to B-CLL cells. Cytoplasmic Ig (usually of IgM type) can be demonstrated in at least some of the lymphoma cells by immunohistochemical investigation of a lymph node, and expression of CD5 is absent. The REAL classification of malignant lymphomas proposed to restrict the term lymphoplasmacytoid lymphoma/immunocytoma in most cases to Waldenström's macroglobulinemia with monoclonal serum paraprotein of IgM type. Morphologic investigation of the blood smear do not allow to distinguish between B-CLL and lymphoplasmacytoid lymphoma.

1.3.2.1.4
Hairy Cell Leukemia

Most patients have a low leukocyte count and only few patients have an increased white cell count. The characteristic hairy cells show fine cytoplasmic villi. The oval or kidney-shaped nucleus has finely dispersed chromatin with-

Fig. 1.10. APAAP immunostaining (anti-kappa) of a cytospin (mononuclear blood cells) from a patient with B-CLL

Fig. 1.11. APAAP immunostaining (anti-lambda) of a cytospin from the same patient as in Fig. 1.10

Fig. 1.12. APAAP immunostaining (anti-CD19) of a bone marrow smear from a patients with marrow infiltration by a small cell B-non-Hodgkin's lymphoma

Fig. 1.13. May-Grünwald-Giemsa staining of mononuclear blood cells from a patient with large cell B-lymphoma; → centroblast

Fig. 1.14. APAAP immunostaining (anti-kappa); same patient as in Fig. 1.13

Fig. 1.15. APAAP immunostaining (anti-lambda); same patient as in Fig. 1.13

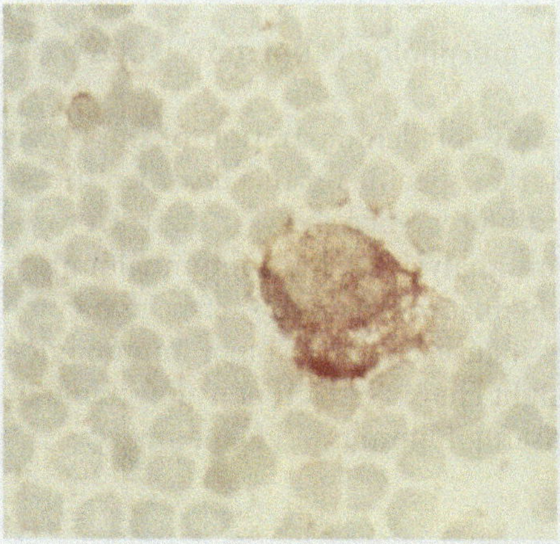

1.16

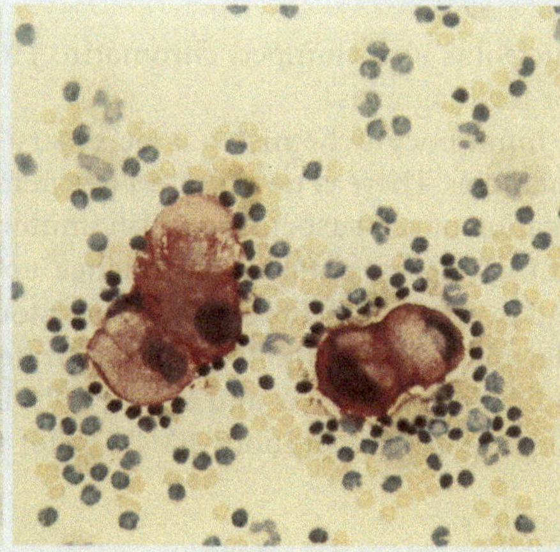

1.17

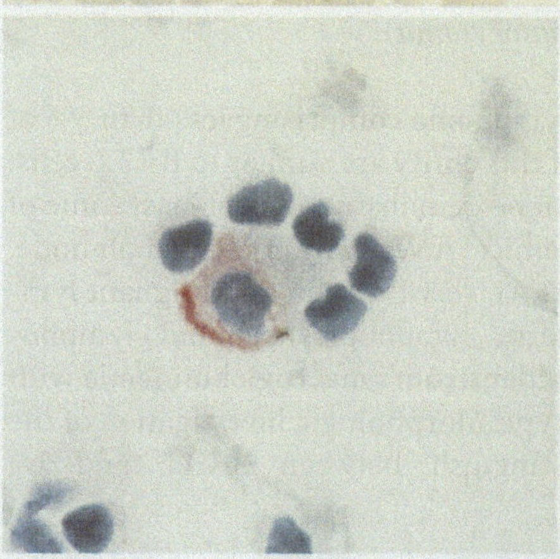

1.18

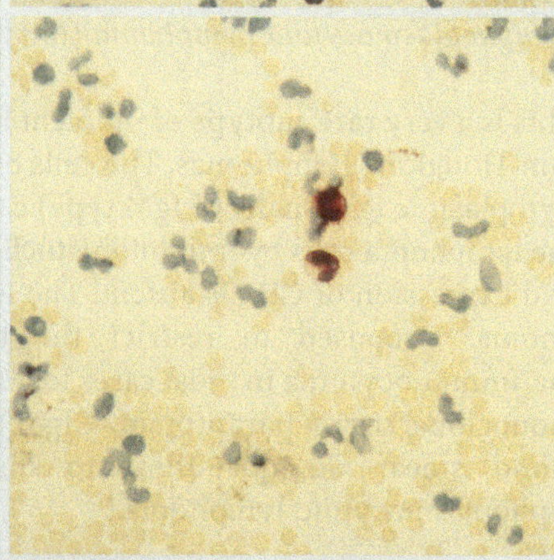

1.19

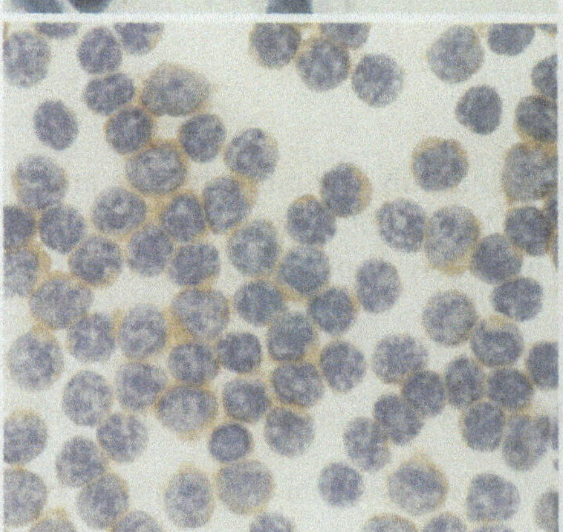

1.20

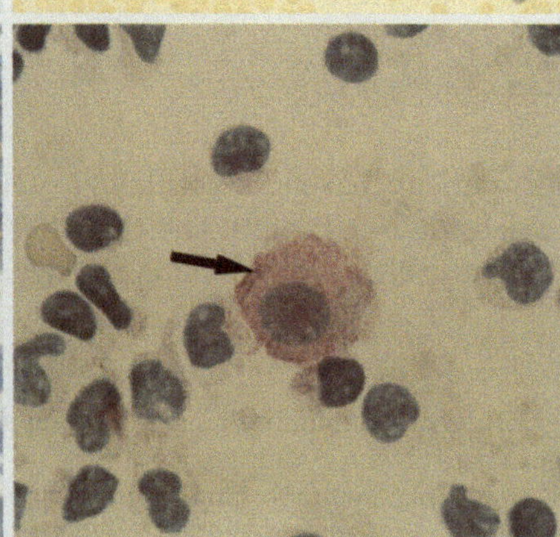

1.21

Figs. 1.16 - 1.21

out a nucleolus and is eccentrically placed. Often there are only a few hairy cells in the blood smear. Immunocytochemistry of blood leukocytes can support the diagnosis. B cell markers CD19, CD20, CD22 and CD79 a and light chain restriction are demonstrable. The expression of the marker CD103 is important (Fig. 1.21). However, a minority of cases with SLVL also express this marker [45]. Most patients with hairy cell leukemia show expression of CD11c and CD25. These markers, however, are not specific for this disorder.

Hairy cell leukemia variant is a very rare lymphoproliferative disorder. The morphological feature is intermediate between prolymphocytes and hairy cells. The nucleolus is more prominent than in SLVL. The hairy cell marker CD103 is positive in some cases. There is no marker profile characteristic for this disorder.

1.3.2.1.5
Marginal Zone Lymphoma

The entity may be nodal or extranodal (lymphoma of mucosa associated lymphatic tissues). Marginal zone lymphoma may be of indolent (small cell) or aggressive (large cell) type. Tumor cells are characterized by the expression of monoclonal immunoglobulins. B-cell associated antigens are expressed, and the lymphoma cells are CD5–, CD10–, CD23–.

There is overlap between this lymphoma and chronic B-lymphocytic leukemia, called splenic lymphoma with villous lymphocytes (SLVL). Splenomegaly is usually present and the leukocyte count is moderately increased in this disorder. The lymphocytes are larger than normal lymphocytes and have round or oval nuclei with clumped chromatin. The cytoplasm is marked by short villi often with a polar distribution. Distinct small nucleoli are noted in some of these cells. All patients express the B cell markers CD19, CD20, CD22 and CD79a. Light chain restriction and IgM or IgM and IgD are demonstra-

Fig. 1.16. APAAP immunostaining (anti-CD30) of a lymph node aspirate from a patient with Hodgkin's disease showing a CD30 positive Hodgkin's cell

Fig. 1.17. APAAP immunostaining (anti-EP4) of a pleural effusion from a patient with adenocarcinoma of the ovary

Fig. 1.18. APAAP immunostaining (anti-cytokeratin 8/18) of a tumor cell in peripheral blood from a patient with non-seminomatous carcinoma isolated with the magnetic labeling system

Fig. 1.19. APAAP immunostaining (anti-cytomegalovirus early antigen) of a cytospin (blood leukocytes) from a patient after liver transplantation

Fig. 1.20. Immunoperoxidase staining (anti-cyclin D1) of a lymph node aspirate from a patient with mantle cell lymphoma

Fig. 1.21. APAAP immunostaining (anti-CD103) of mononuclear blood cells from a patient with hairy cell leukemia

ble. The hairy cell marker CD103 is positive in 15%, the markers CD25, CD10, CD5 and CD23 in a minority of cases [46].

1.3.2.1.6 Follicle Center Lymphoma

According to morphological criteria three cytologic grades are distinguished: grade 1 (predominantly small cell); grade 2 (mixed small and large cell); grade 3 (predominantly large cell). The tumor is composed of centrocytes and centroblasts, the pattern is at least partially follicular. The characteristic blood cell is the centrocyte with scanty cytoplasm, densely condensed chromatin and deep clefts. In addition to centrocytes a small population of centroblasts with loose chromatin and multiple nucleoli are seen.

The malignant cells express the B cell markers CD19, CD20, CD22 and CD79a and monoclonal immunoglobulin (IgM or IgM and IgG or IgD). In the majority of patients the lymphoma cells do not express CD5 and CD23. However, occasional expression of CD5 is demonstrable. Analysis of FMC7 and CD10 is not possible with immunocytochemistry. Flow cytometry shows FMC7 and CD10 positivity in most cases.

Translocation t(14, 18) involving the rearrangement of the bcl-2 gene is present in 70%–95% of cases. The translocation in most cases is associated with high expression of the BCL-2 protein which permits immunohistochemical demonstration in neoplastic follicles [47]. However, this oncogen protein is also detectable in blood lymphocytes and in T-cell areas and mantle zone of lymph nodes of healthy persons. Therefore, it is not useful for immunocytochemical investigation of blood lymphocytes and lymph node aspirates in patients with follicle center lymphoma.

1.3.2.1.7 Mantle-Cell Lymphoma

The entity consists of small cleaved cells with dense chromatin and inconspicuous nucleoli. The tumor cells are IgM+, usually in combination with IgD+. B-cell associated antigens and CD5 are positive, CD23 negative. In most cases of this lymphoma entity translocation, t(11; 14), resulting in an overexpression of cyclin D1, can be observed. Immunocytochemical detection of cyclin D1 was shown in all cases of mantle cell lymphoma [48] and not in other lymphomas (Fig. 1.20). Further investigations are necessary to describe the importance of cyclin D1 for the diagnosis of mantle cell lymphoma. It appears that the histologic evaluation of a lymph node biopsy will remain fundamental for the diagnosis of mantle cell lymphoma.

1.3.2.1.8
Multiple Myeloma

The plasma cells in this disorder are negative for immunoglobulins when tested in suspension. Analysis of fixed cells with immunocytochemistry permits the demonstration of monoclonal cytoplasmic immunoglobulins IgG or IgA and light chains. B-cell marker are lacking. CD38 is detectable in these cells. However, this marker is not specific for plasma cells. Detection of a monoclonal peak in the serum supports the diagnosis multiple myeloma.

Plasma cell leukemia is the leukemic phase of this disorder. There are two morphological types of this disorder. Type one is characterized by mature plasma cells with deep basophilic cytoplasm, eccentric nucleus and clear Golgi zone. The cells of type two are blast-like cells interspersed with a few mature plasma cells.

1.3.2.1.9
Diffuse Large B-Cell Lymphoma

The entity is composed of large cells with basophilic cytoplasm, vesicular nuclei and prominent nucleoli. B-cell associated antigens are positive (CD19, 20, 22 79a). Positivity of the following markers may be demonstrated in some cases: monoclonal immunoglobulins +/–, CD45+/–, CD5 –/+, CD10 –/+. Large B-cell lymphomas are frequent and constitute 30%–40% of non-Hodgkin's-lymphomas, the spontaneous course is aggressive.

Leukemia is rare in large cell lymphomas [49]. The malignant cells of these lymphomas are large blasts. The differential diagnosis is acute leukemia, in particular acute monoblastic leukemia. Cytochemical stains (esterase and perioxidase) and immunocytochemistry are needed to make the distinction reliably. Useful is the detection of light chain restriction and B cell markers in B cell lymphomas (Figs. 1.13 - 1.15).

Most of the non-Hodgkin's lymphomas with cerebrospinal involvement are B-cell lymphomas of large cell type. The immunocytochemical evaluation of cerebrospinal fluid demonstrates light chain restriction in patients with higher cell count [31]. A minority of non-Hodgkin's lymphomas with cerebrospinal involvement is of T cell type. Most of these lymphomas are large cell lymphomas expressing the markers according to the immunotype of the lymphoma. Immunocytochemical analysis of CSF was improved by using poly-L-lysine coated multispot slides [50]. The authors were able to discriminate between benign cells and lymphoma cells in CSF with inconclusive cytomorphology.

1.3.2.1.10
Burkitt's Lymphoma

The cells are medium-sized with multiple prominent nucleoli and basophilic cytoplasm. Cytoplasmic lipid vacuoles are frequently evident. Most cases are characterized by the translocation of c-myc from chromosome 8 to the Ig heavy chain region on chromosome 14.

1.3.2.2
T/NK-Lymphoproliferative Disorders

T-cell lymphomas are divided into precursor T-cell lymphomas, that is T-lymphoblastic lymphoma/leukemia and peripheral T-cell neoplasms.

1.3.2.2.1
T-Lymphoblastic Leukemia/Lymphoma

T-lymphoblastic lymphoma/leukemia is typically positive for TdT and for the T-cell markers CD7 and CD3 (the latter at least cytoplasmic). The expression of additional T-cell associated antigens (CD2, 4, 5, 8) is variable. CD4, 8 may be both positive or both negative.

The delineation of lymphomas from T-lymphoblastic leukemia is arbitrary and depends on the percentage of lymphoblasts in the bone marrow.

1.3.2.2.2
Large Granular Lymphocyte (LGL) Leukemia [51, 52, 53]

Most patients with this disorder have pancytopenia. The number of large granular lymphocytes (LGL cells) is increased for over 6 months (in contrast to viral infection). These cells are large lymphocytes with several azurophilic granules. The nucleus is eccentric with clumped chromatin. Most cases have a CD2+CD3+CD8+CD4– CD16+CD56–CD57+/– immunotype (T-LGL leukemia). Double immunoenzymatic staining is helpful in identifying leukemic LGL cells as CD3+CD57+ or CD3+CD16+. Cells expressing these antigens are rare components of normal blood. Clonal disease is detected by T cell receptor clonal bands on Southern blot hybridization. In a minority of patients the LGL cells are CD3 and CD8 negative and have NK activity. The usual phenotype is CD3–CD4–CD8 –CD16+CD56+CD57+/–. Investigation of clonality in these patients is difficult. Newer techniques are useful to identify expansion of discrete LGL proliferations even in patients with a LGL count <2000/µl [54]. T cell receptor is explored using specific anti-TCRVβ region monoclonal antibodies. In T-LGL leukemia a dominant TCR Vβ region is demonstrable [54]. In NK-LGL leukemia monoclonal antibodies against p68 molecules are useful [55].

LGL cells in healthy persons comprise 10%–15% of blood mononuclear cells. Most of these cells are natural killer cells with expression of CD2, CD16 and CD56. Only a small fraction of LGL cells expresses CD2, CD3 and CD56.

1.3.2.2.3
T-Prolymphocytic Leukemia

There is frequently marked leukocytosis. The medium sized or large lymphocytes have a single prominent nucleolus. The nucleus is round in half of the cases and irregular with folded contours in the remainder (knobby type). In a minority of patients the nucleolus is apparent only on electron microscopy. Immunocytochemistry demonstrates the T cell character of these cells (most are CD3+CD2+CD5+CD7 positive). In the majority of cases the malignant cells express CD4 whereas CD8 is negative. The immunotypes CD4+/CD8+ were also observed.

1.3.2.2.4
Sezary Syndrome

Patients with this rare disorder have generalized erythroderma. Lymphadenopathy occurs in half of the cases. The Sezary cells are small or large with a convoluted cerebriform nucleus. Immunocytochemistry demonstrates a helper T cell phenotype (CD3+CD4+CD8–).

1.3.2.2.5
Adult T Cell Leukemia

This uncommon disorder is characterized by leukemic cells with marked lobulation of the nuclei (flower cells). Immunological investigation shows a helper T cell type (CD3+CD4+CD8–) with expression of CD25. There is positive serology for HTLV-1. Most cases occur in Japan, but an endemic focus is found in the Caribbean and sporadic cases are found in the USA and other countries.

1.3.2.2.6
Peripheral T-Cell Lymphomas

Peripheral T-cell lymphomas contain a mixed population of small and large atypical lymphocytes. The large cells may resemble immunoblasts. The expression of T-cell antigens (CD3, CD2, CD5, CD7) is variable. Lack of cytoplasmic CD3 expression has been described. The small cell variants of these lymphomas are very difficult to distinguish from reactive lymphadenopathy in fine needle aspirates. The large cell variants are easy to diagnose in fine needle aspiration. Specific variants of this lymphoma type are angioimmunoblastic T-cell lymphoma and angiocentric lymphoma. The anaplastic large cell lymphoma (T- or null cell type) is composed of large pleomorphic blasts with multinucleated cells resembling Reed-Sternberg cells. The lymphoma cells are CD30 positive and larger than the cells of the diffuse large cell lymphoma. A minority of these lymphomas lack CD45.

1.3.2.3 *Hodgkin's Disease*

This malignant lymphoma is a disease of the lymph nodes. The aspirates in most cases contain lymphocytes (T cells with polyclonal B cells) with a small number of macrophages, eosinophils and neutrophils. The characteristic cell is the Hodgkin cell (mononuclear) and the Reed-Sternberg cell (polynuclear). These cells are CD30+, CD15+/– and CD45–. Immunocytochemistry supports the cytological analysis of lymph node aspirates (Fig. 1.16). Surgical biopsy is necessary in most cases for satisfying the diagnosis and subclassification in nodular sclerosis, mixed cellularity, lymphocyte depletion and lymphocyte-rich classical Hodgkin's disease. In Hodgkin's disease with lymphocyte predominance (paragranuloma) usually no Reed-Sternberg cells are found. The malignant cells are "popcorn" cells in a background of lymphocytes. The atypical cells express CD45 and B cell markers. CD30 is often positive.

1.3.3 Tumor Cells

Immunocytochemistry is important for classifying solid tumors and for delineation from hematological or lymphatic malignancies. Immunocytochemistry, furthermore, is used to recognize the state of differentiation and the function of tumor cells, such as proliferation, apoptosis and hormone receptors. Finally, immunocytochemistry is used to detect tumor cells in serous effusions, in the bone marrow and in the peripheral blood.

1.3.3.1 *Tumor Cells in Serous Effusions*

One of the most difficult diagnostic tasks in the cytologic investigation of serous effusions is the discrimination of malignant cells from reactive cells. Mesothelial cells and macrophages may mimic malignant cells. On the other hand, some metastatic cells do not show nuclear atypias and might be interpreted as reactive cells. Immunocytochemistry increases the accuracy of serous fluid cytology.

Benign effusions contain macrophages, mesothelial cells and some lymphocytes and granulocytes. Antibodies against cytokeratin stain epithelial and mesothelial cells. Some benign macrophages also exhibit occasional staining in their cytoplasmic vacuoles. This is probably a result of phagocytosis. Hematopoietic cells are not stained by cytokeratin antibodies. Cytokeratin antibodies are of no diagnostic benefit because carcinoma and reactive cells both express these intermediate filaments.

Antibodies against epithelial membrane antigen (EMA) have a strong affinity to epithelial cells and occasionally plasma cells. However, mild to moderate EMA staining may be seen in mesothelial cells [56]. Most or all carcinomas show EMA positivity. In conclusion, strong EMA positivity is not completely reliable. Antibodies against human milk fat globule (HMFG) are reactive with epithelial cells and some macrophages [56]. HFMG positivity was found in most carcinomas but also in several benign effusions. Therefore, this antibody is not useful for detecting malignant cells in effusions. Anti-CEA is highly specific for adenocarcinoma, but its sensitivity for carcinomas is only 60% [56]. False positive cases were rarely observed. The antibody B72.3 recognizes a tumor-associated globulin (TAG) in the majority of epithelial tumors [56]. But the antibody is not exclusively expressed by malignant cells. Mesothelial cells were found to be positive in some cases.

The antibody Ber EP4, which is reactive with many epithelial tumors and non-malignant epithelial cells, is most useful (Fig.1.17). The antibody does not label mesothelial cells and hepatocytes [57, 58, 59]. In rare cases a diffuse granular cytoplasmic staining, presumably in macrophages, can be observed. The antibody does not react with lymphomas, sarcomas, melanomas or mesothelioma cells. It has been concluded that BerEP4 positivity excluded the diagnosis of malignant mesothelioma. However, this analysis was not confirmed by other authors. The reactivity of BerEP4 resembles that of HEA 125. Both antibodies show identical results in sequential immunoprecipitates. For the detection of lymphoma cells in serous effusions the antibodies CD45 (against common leukocyte antigen), CD19 (against B cells) and anti-lambda/kappa for analysis of light chain restriction are very useful.

1.3.3.2
Tumor Cells in Bone Marrow

The bone marrow is a frequent site of metastases for malignant tumors, particularly carcinoma of the breast, lung, kidney and prostate as well as small cell tumors. Metastatic bone marrow infiltration is easily diagnosed in aspirates when the disorder is advanced. Immunocytochemical investigation of bone marrow aspirates should be used in cases of carcinoma whenever conventional examination yields negative results. Anti-cytokeratin antibodies were found to be the most valuable reagent. Normal bone marrow cells are consistently unreactive. In a significant proportion of metastatic carcinoma it was only possible to detect malignant cells with immunocytochemistry [60]. Immunocytochemical assays based on monoclonal antibodies to cytokeratins were used to detect epithelial cells (micrometastases) in bone marrow of patients free from metastases. Clinical investigations have indicated the prognostic significance of these cells in breast, colorectal, gastric and lung cancer [61–68]. Another series of investigations in breast cancer failed to demonstrate such relevance [69–73]. The considerable variability in results is probably due to differences in methodology. Studies differ not only in the immunological methods applied, but also the type of antibodies and controls used. The monoclonal antibodies against epithelial membrane antigen and human milk fat globulin (directed at mucin-like epithelial membrane proteins) cross-react with hematopoietic cells in 30%–40% of patients without malignant disease. Analysis with the monoclonal antibodies CK2 (against cytokeratin 18) and A45-BB3 (pancytokeratin) revealed one or two positive cells in 4/75 (5.3%) patients without malignant disease [74]. Other authors found in 9/72 patients with non-metastatic breast cancer K1-1-positive cells in bone marrow. However, these cells remained positive even when the primary antibody was replaced by the IgG isotype. It is suggested that literature results can be overestimated owing to antibody non-specificity (75].

A comparison of flow cytometric and immunocytochemical technique in detecting tumor cells in bone marrow demonstrated that the immunocytochemical method was the most sensitive [76].

1.3.3.3 *Tumor Cells in Blood*

There are reports demonstrating the presence of circulating tumor cells in children with neuroblastoma, in patients with metastatic breast cancer [77, 78] and in patients with metastatic ovarian cancer [79]. These investigations used immunocytochemical methods with cytokeratin antibodies for detection of tumor cells in peripheral blood or blood stem cell collections. The sensitivity of detection of tumor cells is one tumor cell in 100–500,000 mononuclear leukocytes. Only a low percentage of these patients with metastatic cancer showed tumor cells in peripheral blood. These methods require tedious labor-intensive slide screening. Most authors concluded that blood stem cell collections contain fewer tumor cells than paired bone marrow specimens.

A tumor cell clonogenic assay provides evidence that tumor cells in blood stem cell collections are viable and capable of in vitro clonogenic growth. The tumor colony growth in vitro correlated significantly with immunocytochemical investigations [77]. Other authors investigated patients with metastatic breast cancer and advanced lung cancer [78]. It was found that mobilization of tumor cells after chemotherapy/granulocyte colony-stimulating factors induced recruitment of blood stem cells.

Recently, a magnetic labeling system for enrichment of epithelial tumor cells from blood was established (Miltenyi Biotec, Bergisch Gladbach). The enrichment of tumor cells is performed by positive selection of cytokeratin 8/18 positive cells. The mononuclear blood cells are permeabilized and incubated with paramagnetic microbeads conjugated with the monoclonal antibody against cytokeratin. The magnetically labeled cells are enriched on a selection column in a magnetic field. After removing the column from the magnetic field the retained cells are eluted and cytospins are prepared. Immuncytochemical staining of tumor cells is performed with the antibody against cytokeratin. Only 10–20 ml blood are necessary for this analysis. The sensitivity is one tumor cell in 10^7–10^8 leukocytes. Using this analysis system we found cytokeratin positive cells in peripheral blood of patients with metastatic cancer (Fig. 1.18).

1.3.3.4
Malignant Tumors in Fine Needle Aspirates

Fine needle aspiration of lymph nodes and other tumors is a rapid and simple method. The most obvious advantages are that it is quickly performed, not very painful and easily repeatable. The cytological details are much better than in surgical biopsy sections. The immunocytochemistry provides a means of combining cytological and immunological markers [80–82]. In most cases two aspirations from the same lymph node are performed. One aspirate is used to make air-dried smears. The cells of the other aspirate are suspended in phosphate-buffered saline. Several cytospins are made and stained by an immunocytochemical procedure.

The diagnosis of metastatic carcinomas or sarcomas on lymph node aspirates is no problem in most cases. However, it is difficult to distinguish large cell malignant lymphomas from poorly differentiated carcinomas. Immunocytochemistry demonstrates CD45 expression in malignant lymphomas and cytokeratin positivity in most carcinomas. A lack of CD45 expression was observed in patients with large cell anaplastic lymphoma showing strong positivity for CD30. There are very few markers that are specific for different subsets of carcinomas. Metastatic prostatic carcinomas are frequently positive for prostate-specific antigen and demonstration of thyroglobulin establishes the thyroid origin in differentiated thyroid carcinomas. β-HCG or AFP is detected in metastatic nonseminomatous germ cell tumors and α-fetoprotein in hepatocellular carcinoma. Neuron-specific enolase is observed in neuroendocrine tumors. Evaluation of the receptor status (estrogen and progesterone receptor) is well established in breast cancer.

p53 is a tumor-suppressor gene. The most frequent mechanism by which the wild-type p53 is inactivated in malignancies is point mutation. The wild-type p53 protein has a very short half life, whereas the mutated p53 protein is stable and accumulates in tumor cells. Normally, p53 protein is undetectable by immunocytochemistry. However, mutant p53 leads to immunocytochemical overexpression. A caveat for immunocytochemical detection is that not all p53 mutations result in protein overexpression [83]. In several series examining node-negative breast cancer, p53 was found to be a prognostic factor for relapse and survival. Other studies demonstrated a lack of prognostic relevance.

Despite the immunocytochemical information obtained from the lymph node aspirates this method is incapable of replacing surgical lymph node biopsy. However, lymph node aspirates with immunocytochemistry can be very useful under certain circumstances. On the basis of anamnesis and palpation of the lymph nodes, where malignancy is suspected, lymph node aspiration and surgical biopsy can be performed simultaneously. The lymph node aspiration supplies a preliminary result in only a few hours and staging investigations can be carried out without delay. As soon as the biopsy result is available the diagnosis can be confirmed or in certain cases revised. In cases of lymphadenopathy where the aspirate suggests a reactive process, a surgical biopsy may sometimes be avoidable. A strict follow-up of such patients is, however, necessary. The analysis of lymph node aspirates is useful for detection of recurrent malignant tumor.

1.3.4 Infectious Disorders

Immunochemistry is an important tool for diagnosis of several infectious disorders such as cytomegalovirus (CMV) infection. Traditionally, infectious agents were identified in the microbiology laboratory by culture and serological technique. However, some infectious agents can be difficult to culture and serology results can be difficult to interpret from patients with immunodeficiency. Immunocytochemistry has become a method for the identification of a wide variety of infectious agents. Many commercially available antibodies are useful for these immunocytochemical investigations [84] (*Linscotts's Directory of Immunological Reagents*). In immunocompromised patients (AIDS, organ transplantation, immunosuppressive medication) immunocytochemistry demonstrates pneumocystis carinii in bronchoalvelolar lavage. Polyclonal antibodies raised against strains of mycobacteria are used to detect the organism in tissue sections [85]. Rapid identification of infectious agents is possible because fragmented organisms are also stained. *Aspergillus* species can cause pulmonary infections in immunocompromised patients. A definite diagnosis can be made only by demonstration of tissue invasion by fungal mycelia and positive culture. Histological examination alone is not reliable because numerous fungi cannot be differentiated from aspergillus by routine fungi stains. Immunoperoxidase staining using a monoclonal antibody against *Aspergillus* permits identification of *Aspergillus* in tissue sections [86].

Cytomegalovirus (CMV) is a cause of mortality after bone marrow transplantation subsequent to virus reactivation or primary infection. The virus culture assay is time consuming. Detection of CMV antigen in blood granulocytes with the APAAP technique is a very useful aid for the decision to start antiviral treatment in these patients [87] (Fig. 1.19).

1.4 Protocols for Immunostaining

1.4.1 Protocol I: Immunoalkaline Phosphatase Anti-alkaline Phosphatase (APAAP) Method [4]

Specimens: cytospins from blood, bone marrow, serous effusions, cerebrospinal fluid, fine needle aspirates, bronchoalveolar lavage, smears from blood, bone marrow or fine needle aspirates
Performance: in coverplates (Shandon) or in a humid chamber or in an automatic staining procedure.

Immunostaining:		Dilution
Fixation with acetone (100%)	10 min	
Primary antibody (mouse anti-human)[b]	60 min	titration
Wash with TBS[a]		
Rabbit anti-mouse Ig antiserum[b] (e.g., DAKO Z 259)	30 min	1:50
Wash with TBS		
APAAP complex[c] (e.g., DAKO D 651)	30 min	1:50
Wash with TBS		
Alkaline phosphatase detection[d]	15 min	
Wash with TBS and then with water		

Nuclear staining (hemalum, Merck No. 9249)	5 min (30 s for TdT or Ki67)
Mount in an aqueous mounting medium (e.g., Glycergel)	

[a]TBS=TRIS buffered saline (dilute stock solution 0.5 M TRIS/HCl with pH 7.6, 1/10 with 0.15 M isotonic saline)
[b]Dilution with TBS with 20% human AB serum (inactivated not for immunoglobulin detection)
[c]The intensity of staining can be enhanced by repeating incubation with rabbit-anti-mouse Ig antiserum (10 min) and APAAP complex (10 min)
[d]Dissolve 2 mg naphthol AS-MX phosphate (Sigma No. 4875) in 0.2 ml dimethylformamide in a glass tube and dilute to 10 ml with 0.1 M TRIS buffer pH 8.2 Add 10 µl 1 M levamisole. Immediately before staining dissolve 10 mg Fast-Red TR salt (Sigma No. F 1500).

1.4.2 Protocol II: Immunoperoxidase [7]

Specimens: cytospins from blood, bone marrow, serous effusions, cerebrospinal fluid, fine needle aspirates, bronchoalveolar lavage; smears from blood, bone marrow or fine needle aspirates
Performance: in coverplates (Shandon), in a humid chamber or in an automatic procedure

Immunostaining:		Dilution[a]
Fixation with May-Grünwald (Merck-Nr. 1.01424)	3 min	
Wash with PBS		
Primary antibody (mouse-anti-human)[b]	60 min	titration 1:10–1000
Wash with PBS		
Rabbit anti-mouse Ig antiserum (peroxidase conjugated; DAKO P260)	30 min	1:50
Wash with PBS		
Swine anti-rabbit Ig antiserum (peroxidase conjugated; DAKO 217)	30 min	1:50
Wash with PBS		
Peroxidase detection (50 mg diaminobenzidine hydrochloride +10 µl H_2O_2 +100 ml PBS)	5 min	
Wash with PBS		
Nuclear staining (hemalum, Merck No. 9249)	5 min (30 s for TdT or Ki67)	

[a]Dilution buffer: PBS +10% fetal calf serum +10% bovine serum albumin +10% human Ab serum (not for immunoglobulin detection)

[b]An extra incubation step is required by using an rabbit anti-human antibody. After washing, the cells are incubated for 20 min with mouse anti-rabbit Ig antiserum.

1.4.3
Protocol III: Avidin-Biotin Technique [11]

Specimens: cytospins from blood, bone marrow, serous effusions, cerebrospinal fluid, fine needle aspirates, bronchoalveolar lavage; smears from blood, bone marrow or fine needle aspirates

Performance: in coverplates (Shandon) or in a humid chamber or in an automatic staining procedure

Immunostaining:		Dilution
Fixation with acetone (100%)	10 min	
Primary antibody (mouse-anti-human)	60 min	titration 1:10–1000
Wash with TBS[a]		
Biotinylated rabbit anti-mouse Ig antiserum	30 min	
Wash with TBS		
Avidin-biotin-peroxidase complex[b]	30 min	
Wash with TBS		
Peroxidase detection (50 mg diaminobenzidine hydrochloride +10 µl H_2O_2 +100 ml TBS)	5 min	
Wash with TBS		
Nuclear staining (hemalum, Merck Nr. 9249)	5 min (30 s for TdT or Ki67)	

[a]TBS=TRIS buffered saline (dilute stock solution 0.5 M TRIS/HCl with pH 7.6 1/10 with 0.3 M NaCl)

[b]Prepare this complex at least 30 min prior to use by mixing avidin and biotin conjugated horseradish peroxidase according to recommendations of the manufacturer.

1.4.4
Protocol IV: Enhanced Polymer One-Step (EPOS) Staining [8, 9]

Specimens: cytospins from blood, bone marrow, serous effusions, cerebrospinal fluid, fine needle aspirates, bronchoalveolar lavage; smears from blood, bone marrow or fine needle aspirates

Performance: in coverplates (Shandon) or in a humid chamber or in an automated staining procedure

Immunostaining:	
Fixation with May-Grünwald (Merck No. 1.01424)	3 min
Wash with PBS	
EPOS antibody[a] (DAKO; ready to use)	60 min
Wash with PBS	
Peroxidase detection (50 mg diaminobenzidine hydrochloride +10 µl H_2O_2 +100 ml PBS)	5 min
Wash with PBS	
Nuclear staining (hemalum, Merck No. 9249)	5 min

[a]EPOS antibodies are available against actin, calcitonin, CD3, CD20, CD45RO, CD68, chromogranin, cytokeratin, cytokeratin 10, 19, desmin, EMA, kappa, lambda, Ki67, CD45, melanoma, NSE, neutrophilic elastase, proliferating cell nuclear antigen (PCNA) PSA, S100, synaptophysin, thyreoglobulin, vimentin and von Willebrand factor.

1.4.5
Protocol V: Enhanced Labeled-Polymer System (ELPS, Envision) [10]

Specimens: cytospins from blood, bone marrow, serous effusions, cerebrospinal fluid, fine needle aspirates, bronchoalveolar lavage; smears from blood, bone marrow or fine needle aspirates
Performance: in coverplates (Shandon), in a humid chamber or in an automatic staining procedure

Immunostaining:		Dilution
Fixation with acetone (100%)	10 min	
Primary antibody(mouse/rabbit anti-human)[b]	30–60 min	titration 1:10–1000
Wash with TBS[a]		
Polymer conjugated with goat anti-mouse/rabbit antibody andalkaline phosphatase (DAKO K4017)	15–30 min	ready to use
Wash with TBS		
Alkaline phosphatase detection[c]	15 min	
Wash with TBS and then with water		
Nuclear staining (hemalum, Merck No. 9249)	5 min (30 s for TdT and Ki67)	
Mount in an aqueous mounting medium (e.g., Glycergel)		

[a]TBS=TRIS buffered saline (dilute stock solution 0.5 M TRIS/HCl pH 7.6, 1/10 with 0.15 M isotonic saline)
[b]Dilution with TBS with 20% human AB serum (not for immunoglobulin detection)
[c]Dissolve 2 mg naphthol AS-MX phosphate (Sigma No. 4875) in 0.2 ml dimethylformamide in a glass tube and dilute to 10 ml with 0.1 M TRIS buffer pH 8.2. Add 10 µl levamisole. Immediately before staining dissolve 10 mg Fast-Red TR salt (Sigma No. F 1500).

1.4.6
Protocol VI: Morphological-Immunocytochemical Technique [3]

Specimens: cytospins from blood and bone marrow
Performance: in coverplates (Shandon), in a humid chamber or in an automated staining procedure

Procedure:	
May-Grünwald (Merck No. 1.01424)	3 min
Giemsa (Merck No. 9204; 1/10 diluted with 0.01 M phosphate buffer pH 7.2)	20 min
Cells were photographed (going out from the margin of the cytospin)	
Removal of oil with Paraclear (Earth safe industries, BB 1494)	
Immunostaining (immunoperoxidase protocol II)	
Analysis of the photographed cells using a slide projector and simultaneously on the immunostained cytospins	

1.4.7
Protocol VII: EPOS Staining for Immunoenzymatic Double-Labeling

Specimens: cytospins from blood or bone marrow or other cytological preparations
Performance: in coverplates (Shandon) or in a humid chamber

Immunostaining:		Dilution
Fixation with acetone (100%)	10 min	
Primary antibody (mouse anti-human)[b]	30–60 min	1:10–1000
Wash with TBS[a]		
Rabbit anti-mouse Ig antiserum[b] (DAKO Z 259)	30 min	1:50
Wash with TBS		
APAAP complex (DAKO D 651)	30 min	1:50
Wash with TBS		

EPOS antibody (DAKO; ready to use)	60 min
Wash with PBS	
Alkaline phosphatase detection[c]	15 min
Wash with TBS	
Peroxidase detection (50 mg diaminobenzidine hydrochloride +10 µl H_2O_2 +100 ml PBS)	5 min
Nuclear staining (hemalum, Merck No. 9249)	5 min
Mount in an aqueous mounting medium (e.g., Glycergel)	

[a]TBS-TRIS buffered saline (dilute stock solution 0.5 M TRIS/HCl pH 7.6, 1/10 with 0.15 M isotonic saline)

[b]Dilution with TBS with 20% human AB serum (inactivated; not for immunoglobulin analysis)

[c]Dissolve 2 mg naphthol AS-MX phosphate (Sigma No. 4857) in 0.2 ml dimethylformamide in a glass tube and dilute to 10 ml with 0.1 M TRIS buffer pH 8.1. Add 10 µl 1 M levamisole. Immediately before staining dissolve 10 mg fast red TR salt (Sigma No. F 1500).

References

1. Hayhoe FGJ, Quaglino D (1994) Haematological cytochemistry. Churchill Livingstone, Edinburgh
2. Suthipintawong C, Leong A Sy (1996) Immunostaining of cell preparations: A comparative evaluation of common fixatives and protocols. Diag Cytopathol 15:167–174
3. Oertel J, Oertel B, Schleicher J, Huhn D (1996) Immunotyping of blasts in human bone marrow. Ann Haematol 72:125–129
4. Cordell JL, Falini B, Erber WN et al. (1984) Immunoenzymatic labeling of monoclonal antibodies using immune complexes of alkaline phosphatase and monoclonal anti-alkaline phosphatase (APAAP) complexes. J Histochem Cytochem 32:219–229
5. Erber WN, Pinching AJ, Mason DY (1984) Immunocytochemical detection of T and B cell populations in routine blood smears. Lancet 1:1042–1046
6. Mason DY, Cordell JL, Abdulaziz Z et al. (1982) Preparation of PAP complexes for immunohistological labelling of monoclonal antibodies. J Histochem Cytochem 30:1114–21
7. Woods JC, Harris H, Springs AI et al. (1982) A new marker for human cancer cells. 3. Immunocytochemical detection of malignant cells in serous fluids with the Ca1 antibody. Lancet 1:512–515
8. Bisgaard K, Lihme A, Rolsted H et al. (1993) Polymeric conjugates for enhanced signal generation in enzyme immunoassays. Abstract Scand Soc Immunol, XXIV Annual Meeting University of Aarhus Denmark May 22–26, 1993
9. Tsutsumi Y, Senizawa A, Kawai K (1995) Enhanced polymer one-step staining (EPOS) for proliferating cell nuclear antigen (PCNA) and Ki-67 antigen: application to intraoperative frozen diagnosis. Pathology International 45:108–115

10. Heras A, Roach CM, Key ME (1995) Enhanced labelled-polymer system for immunohistochemistriy. Abstract XV European Congress of Pathology, Copenhagen, Denmark, September 3–8
11. Hsu SM, Raine L, Fanger H (1981) Use of avidin-biotin-peroxidase complexes (ABC) in immunoperoxidase technique: a comparison between ABC and unlabeled antibody (PAP) procedures. J Histochem Cytochem 29:577–580
12. Bobrow MN, Litt GJ, Shaughnessy KJ et al (1992) The use of catalyzed reporter deposition as a means of signal amplification in a variety of formats. J Immunol Methods 150:45–49
13. Merz H, Malisius R, Mannweiler S et al. (1995) Methods in laboratory investigation: Immunomax. A maximized immunohistological method for the retrieval and enhancement of hidden antigens. Lab Invest 73:149–156
14. Farahat N van der Plas D, Praxedes M et al (1994) Demonstration of cytoplasmic and nuclear antigens in acute leukaemia using flow cytometry. J Clin Pathol 47:843–849
15. General Hematology Task Force of BCSH (1994) Immunophenotyping in the diagnosis of acute leukaemias: J Clin Pathol 47:777–781
16. Scott CS, den Ottolander GJ, Swirsky D et al. (1993) Recommended procedures for the classification of acute leukaemias. Leukemia and Lymphoma 11:37–49
17. van der Loos CM, Becker AE, van den Oord JJ (1993) Practical suggestions for successful immunoenzyme double-staining experiments. Histochem J 25:1–13
18. Nakane PK (1968) Simultaneous localization of multiple tissue antigens using the peroxidase-labelled antibody method: a study on pituitary glands of the rat. J Histochem 16:557–559
19. Sternberger LA, Joseph SA (1979) The unlabeled antibody method, contrasting color staining of paired pituitary hormones without antibody removal. J Histochem Cytochem 27:1424–1429
20. Falini B, Abdulaziz Z, Gerdes J et al. (1986) Description of a sequential staining procedure for double immunoenzymatic staining of pairs of antigens using monoclonal antibodies. J Immunol Meth 93:265–273
21. van der Loos CM, Das PK, van den Oord JJ et al. (1989) Multiple immunoenzyme staining techniques. J Immunol Meth 117:45–52
22. van der Loos CM, Naruko T, Becker AE (1996) The use of enhanced polymer one step staining reagents for immunoenzyme double-labelling. Histochem J 28:709–714
23. Campbell CT, Bhatnager AS (1976) Simultaneous visualization by light microscopy of two pituitary hormones in a single tissue section using a combination of indirect immunohistochemical methods. J Histochem Cytochem 24:448–452
24. Mason DY, Sammons R (1978) Alkaline phosphatase and peroxidase for double immunoenzymatic labelling of cellular constituents. J Clin Path 31:454–460
25. Tidman N, Janossy G, Bodger M et al. (1981) Delineation of human thymocyte differentiation pathways utilizing double-staining techniques with monoclonal techniques with monoclonal antibodies. Clin Exp Imm 454:457–467
26. Boorsma DM (1984) Direct immunoenzyme double staining applicable for monoclonal antibodies. Histochemistry 80:103–106
27. van t Veer MB, Kluin-Nelemans JC, van der Schoot CE et al. (1992) Quality assessment of immunological marker analysis and the immunological diagnosis in leukaemia and lymphoma: a multicentre study. Br J Haematol 80:458–465
28. Catovsky D, Matutes E, Bucceri V et al. (1991) A classification of acute leukaemia for the 1990s. Ann Haematol 62:16–21
29. Campana D, Coustan-Smith E, Behm FG (1991) The definition of remission in acute leukemia with immunological techniques. Bone Marrow Transplant 8:429–437

30. Hegewisch-Becker S, Hossfeld DK (1996) The MDR phenotype in hematologic malignancies: prognostic relevance and future perspectives. Ann Hematol 72:105–117
31. Tani E, Costa I, Svedmyr E et al. (1995) Diagnosis of lymphoma, leukemia and metastatic involvement of the cerebrospinal fluid by cytology and immunocytochemistry. Diagn Cytopathol 12:14–22
32. San Miguel IF, Tavares de Castro I, Matutes E et al. (1985) Characterization of blast cells in chronic granulocytic leukaemia in transformation, acute myelofibrosis and undifferentiated leukaemia. Br J Haematol 59:297–309
33. Bennett JM, Catovsky D, Daniel MT et al. (1982) Proposals for the classification of the myelodysplastic syndromes. Br J Haematol 51:189–199
34. Guyotat D, Campos L, Thomas Y et al. (1990) Myelodysplastic syndromes: a study of surface markers and in vitro growth pattern. Am J Hematol 34:26–31
35. List AS, Spier CM, Cline A et al. (1991) Expression of the multidrug resistance gene product (P-glycoprotein) in myelodysplasia is associated with a stem cell phenotype. Br J Haematol 78:28–34
36. Oertel J, Oertel B, Beyer J, Huhn D (1994) CD34 immunotyping of blasts in myelodysplasia. Ann Hematol 68:77–80
37. Harris NL, Jaffe ES, Stein H et al. (1994) A revised European American classification of lymphoid neoplasms. Blood 84:1361–1392
38. Benett JM, Catovsky D, Daniel MT et al.(1989) Proposals for the classification of chronic (mature) B and T lymphoid leukaemias. J Clin Pathol 42:567–584
39. Oertel J, Lipski S, Lobeck H, Huhn D (1991) Detection of light chain restriction in chronic B-lymphoid leukaemia and B-non-Hodgkin's lymphoma. Clin lab Haemat 13:33–40
40. Schwonzen M, Pohl C, Steinmetz T et al. (1992) Bone marrow involvement in non-Hodgkin's lymphoma: increased diagnostic sensitivity by combination of immunocytology, cytomorphology and trephine histology. Br J Haematol 81:362–369
41. Bartl R, Hansman ML, Frisch B et al. (1988) Comparative histology of malignant lymphomas in lymph node and bone marrow. Br J Haematol 69:229–237
42. Schwonzen M, Pohl C, Steinmetz T et al. (1993) Immunophenotyping of low-grade B-cell lymphoma in blood and bone marrow: poor correlation between immunophenotype and cytological/histological classification. Br J Haematol 83:232–239
43. Pianezze G, Gentilini I, Casini M et al. (1987) Cytoplasmic immunoglobulins in chronic lymphocytic leukaemia B cell. Blood 69:1011–1014
44. Han T, Ozer H, Bloom M et al. (1982) The presence of monoclonal cytoplasmic immunoglobulins in leukaemic B cells from patients with chronic lymphocytic leukemia. Blood 59:435–438
45. Matutes E, Morilla R, Owusu-Ankomah K et al. (1994) The immunophenotype of splenic lymphoma with villous lymphocytes and its relevance to the differential diagnosis with other B-cell disorders. Blood 83:1558–1562
46. Troussard X, Valensi F, Duchayne E et al. (1996) Splenic lymphoma with villous lymphocytes: clinical presentation, biology and prognostic factors in a series of 100 patients. Br J Haematol 93:731–736
47. Pezzella F, Tse AGD et al. (1990) Expression of the bcl-2 oncogene protein is not specific for the 14; 18 chromosomal translocation. Am J Pathol 137:225–232
48. Yang WI, Zuckerberg LR, Motokura T et al. (1994) Cyclin D1 (Bcl–1, PRAD1) protein expression in low-grade B-cell lymphoma and reactive hyperplasia. Am J Pathol 145:86–96
49. Bain B, Matutes E, Robinson D et al. (1991)Leukaemia as a manifestation of large cell lymphoma. Br J Haematol 77:391–410

50. Kranz BR, Thiel E, Thierfelder S (1989) Immunocytochemical identification of meningeal leukemia and lymphoma: poly-L-lysine-coated slides permit multimarker analysis even with minute cerebrospinal fluid cell specimens. Blood 73:1942–1950
51. Loughran TP (1993) Clonal diseases of large granular lymphocytes. Blood 82:1–14
52. Dhodapkar MV, Li Cv, Lust JA, et al. (1994) Clinical spectrum of clonal proliferations of T-large granular lymphocytes: a T-cell clonopathy of undetermined significance. Blood 84:1620–1627
53. Semenzato G, Zambello R, Starkebaum G et al. (1997) The lymphoproliferative disease of granular lymphocytes: updated criteria of diagnosis. Blood 89:256–260
54. Kaneko T, Mizoguchi H, Oshimi K (1993) Expression of T-cell receptor Vβ regions in granular lymphocyte-proliferative disorders. Blood 81:3482–3483
55. Zambello R, Trentin L, Ciccone E et al. (1993) Phenotypic diversity of natural killer populations in patients with NK-type lymphoproliferative disease of granular lymphocytes. Blood 81:2381–2388
56. Esteban JM, Yokora S, Husain S et al. (1990) Immunocytochemical profile of benign and carcinomatous effusions. Am J Clin Pathol 94:698–705
57. Latza U, Niedobitek G, Schwarting R et al. (1990) Ber-EP4:new monoclonal antibody which distinguish epithelia from mesothelia. J Clin Pathol 43:213–219
58. Matter-Walstra KW, Kraft R (1996) Atypical cells in effusions. Diagn Cytopathol 15:263–269
59. Jensen ML, Johansen P (1996) Immunocytochemical staining of smears and corresponding cell blocks from serous effusions: a follow-up and comparative investigation. Diagn Cytopathol 15:33–36
60. Ghosh AK, Erber WN, Hatton CSR et al. (1985) Detection of metastatic tumour cells in routine bone marrow smears by immunoalkaline phophatase labeling with monoclonal antibodies. Br J Haematol 61:21–30
61. Cote RJ, Rosen PP, Lesser ML (1991) Prediction of early relapse in patients with operable breast cancer by detection of occult bone marrow micrometastases. J Clin Oncol 9:1749–1756
62. Harbeck N, Untch M, Pache L et al. (1994) Tumour cell detection in the bone marrow of breast cancer patients at primary therapy: results of a 3-year median follow-up. Br J Cancer 69:566–571
63. Schlimok G, Lindemann F, Holzmann K et al. (1992) Prognostic significance of disseminated tumour cells detected in bone marrow of patients with breast and colorectal cancer: a multi-variant analysis. Proc Am Soc Clin Oncol 11:102
64. Diel U, Kaufmann M, Goemer R et al. (1992) Detection of tumour cells in bone marrow of patients with primary breast cancer: A prognostic factor for distant metastasis. J Clin Oncol 10:1534–1539
65. Lindemann F, Schlimok G, Dirschedl P et al. (1992) Prognostic significance of micrometastatic tumour cells in bone marrow of colorectal cancer patients. Lancet 340:685–689
66. Jauch KW, Heiss MM, Gruetzner U et al. (1996) Prognostic significance of bone marrow micrometastasis in patient with gastric cancer. J Clin Oncol 14:1810–1817
67. Schlimok G, Funke I, Pantel K et al. (1991) Micrometastatic tumor cells in bone marrow of patients with gastric cancer: Eur J Cancer 27:1461–1465
68. Pantel K, Ibzbicki J, Passlick B et al. (1996) Frequency and prognostic significance of isolated tumour cells in bone marrow of patients with non-small-cell lung cancer without overt metastases. Lancet 347:649–653
69. Mathieu MC, Friedman S, Bosq J et al. (1990) Immunohistochemical staining of bone marrow biopsies for detection of occult metastasis breast cancer. Breast Cancer Res 15:21–26

70. Kirk SJ, Cooper GG, Hoper M et al. (1990) The prognostic significance of marrow micrometastases in women with early breast cancer. Eur J Surg Oncol 16:481–485
71. Giai M, Natoli C, Sismondi P et al. (1990) Bone marrow micrometastases detected by a monoclonal antibody in patients with breast cancer. Anticancer Res 10:119–121
72. Courtemanche DJ, Worth AJ, Coupland RW et al. (1991) Monoclonal antibody LICR-LON-M8 does not predict the outcome of operable breast cancer. Can J Surg 34:21–26
73. Pecorini F, Veneziano M, Framarino Dei Malatesta ML et al. (1993) Considerations on the prognostic significance of bone marrow micrometastases in breast cancer. Eur J Gynec Oncol 14:501–505
74. Pantel K, Schlimok G, Angstwurm M et al. (1994) Methodological analysis of immunocytochemical screening for disseminated epithelial tumor cells in bone marrow. J Hematother 3:165–173
75. Lagrange M, Ferrero JM, Lagrange JI et al. (1997) Non-specific labelled cells that simulate bone marrow metastases in patients with non-metastatic breast cancer. J Clin Pathol 50:206–211
76. Molino A, Colombatti M, Bonetti F et al. (1991) A comparative analysis of three different techniques for the detection of breast cancer cells in bone marrow. Cancer 67:1033–1036
77. Ross AA, Cooper BW, Lazarus HM et al (1993) Detection and viability of tumor cells in peripheral blood stem cell collections from breast cancer patients using immunocytochemical and clonogenic assay techniques. Blood 82:2605–2610
78. Brugger W, Bross K, Glatt M et al.(1994) Mobilization of tumor cells and hematopoietic progenitor cells into peripheral blood of patients with solid tumors. Blood 83:636–640
79. Ross AA, Miller GW, Moss TJ et al (1995) Immunocytochemical detection of tumor cells on bone marrow and peripheral blood stem cell collections from patients with ovarian cancer. Bone Marrow Transplantat 15:929–933
80. Oertel J, Oertel B, Kastner M, Huhn D (1988) The value of immunocytochemical staining of lymph node aspirates in diagnostic cytology. Br J Haematol 70:307–316
81. Sneige N, Dekmezian RH, Katz RL et al. (1990) Morphologic and immunocytochemical evaluation of 220 fine needle aspirates of malignant lymphoma and lymphoid hyperplasia. Acta Cytol 34:311–322
82. Brown DC, Gatter KC, Mason DY (1990) Immunocytochemical analysis of lymphoid lesions using fine needle aspiration biopsy. Leukaemia and Lymphoma. 2:323–333
83. Fung CY, Fisher DE (1995) p53: from molecular mechanisms to prognosis in cancer. J Clin Oncol 13:808–811
84. Cartun RW (1995) Immunohistochemistry of infectious diseases. The J Histotechn 18:195–202
85. Wiley EL, Mulhollan TJ, Beck B et al. (1990) Polyclonal antibodies raised against Bacillus Calmette-Guerin, Mycobacterium duvalii and Mycobacterium paratuberculosis used to detect mycobacteria in tissue with the use of immunohistochemical techniques. Am J Clin Pathol 94:307–312
86. Verweij PE, Smedts F, Poot T et al. (1996) Immunoperoxidase staining for identification of Aspergillus species in routinely processed tissue sections. J Clin Pathol 49:798–801
87. Schmidt CA, Oettle H, Wilborn F et al.(1994) Demonstration of cytomegalovirus after bone marrow transplantation by polymerase chain reaction, virus culture and antigen detection in buffy coat leukocytes. Bone Marrow Transplant 13:71–75

2 Multiparameter Flow Cytometry

S. Serke

In a flow cytometer, cells in suspension are forced by hydrodynamic focussing to pass multiple detectors. At one given point of time, only one single cell is passing these detectors. There are detectors capable of registering changes in the impedance of the suspension as an indirect measure of the volume of the cells. Other detectors are capable of registering light signals emitted by the cells. Each signal generated by each single cell on any of these detectors is transformed into one single numerical value. Finally, each numerical value is subject to analysis by a software program, correlating each registered value to any defined cellular feature. Currently, all routine hematological counters are flow cytometers. Fixed, manufacturer-defined conditions are active for sample-processing within the device, fixed algorithms process the cell signals, and fixed analysis software produces the definite analysis.

In contrast to these dedicated single-application manufacturer-defined flow cytometers essentially designed exclusively for the complete blood cell count, operator-defined multiparameter flow cytometry is highly flexible. This flexibility is present in the choice of which sample to measure, how to process the sample prior to measurement, which parameters to measure, and finally how to process the measured data. For this high flexibility, this technique is used in many fields of current cell-based laboratory hematology. In this section, current applications of diagnostic operator-defined multiparameter flow cytometry are presented.

2.1 Essentials of Operator-Defined Multiparameter Flow Cytometry

2.1.1 The Flow Cytometer

A variety of different flow cytometers are currently marketed for routine applications, but there are no essential differences among all these devices. In particular, it is common to all devices that a 488 nm laser generates the signals and only light signals are registered. Typically, 100 µl of a sample with at least 1000 leukocytes/µl are required for one single measurement. The sample is aspirated out of a 4-ml tube, and by a sheath fluid the cells are forced to pass a laser beam as a single cell suspension at a frequency ranging from less than 10 cells/s to more than 1000 cells/s, with only one single cell at one given point of time exposed to the laser beam, and with only one single cell at one point of time sending its light emissions to the detectors. The light emissions are produced by features inherent to each cell, such as diameter and internal texture (often referred to as granularity), and they are produced by fluorochromes binding to cellular components (DNA and RNA dyes) or by fluorochromes coupled to ligands detecting cellular components. These ligands mostly are monoclonal antibodies coupled to a fluorochrome. The light emissions pass through a variety of blocking lenses, focussing the signal to an optimum emission range for each single fluorochrome. Upon being registered by the light detector, this emission will generate a signal proportional to the energy absorbed from the emitted light signal. There is, however, not a continuum of registration of energy. Rather, the energy is registered according to defined heights of energy, and each height of energy relates to one channel of the scale of the light detector. Typically, the operator can set the registration to a 256-channel or to a 1024-channel resolution. The 1024-channel resolution allows for the detection of minor differences of light emissions, and obviously the 256-channel resolution offers a less discrete resolution. In view of the different range of variability of light emissions among the different fluorochromes, reflecting the variability of the cellular ligands, this signal generated in the light detector will be processed by either linear or logarithmic amplification. In cell-cycle analysis, the maximum difference in the light signal generated by propidium iodide bound to deoxynucleic acid is by a factor of 2, e.g. G0/G1 cells versus G2/M cells. In this setting, and also in analysis of ploidity, a linear amplification is used. The light signals generated by cell-inherent features, granularity and diameter, are also processed by linear amplification. In contrast, a logarithmic amplification is used when the light signals will typically differ by more than a factor of 4. This holds true in the major field of operator-defined flow cytometry, the analysis of antigen expression by fluorochrome-labeled monoclonal antibodies. Once the light signal is measured and amplified, the concrete numerical value is recorded on-line. Typically, 5 different light signals are recorded from each cell, the diameter, the granularity, and the signals from three fluorochromes. From these five parameters, a list of concrete numerical values is generated for each single cell, and thus the data are stored on-line as a "list-mode data-file". This list-mode data file is processed finally using analysis software programs which allow for operator-defined settings of discriminators. Typically, from the list-mode data-file a two-dimensional depiction correlating two out of the five parameters stored is generated. In this depiction, one single dot represents one single cell. The software allows for mutual correlation of all five parameters, thus allowing for an extremely complex analysis of the list-mode data-file. With regard to each correlation of the parameters, the discriminators can be set as rectangular, ellipsoid, or amorphous regions with the cells of interest clustering into these regions. After the discriminators have been placed, a statistic is calculated on the whole list-mode data-file, generating the percentage of each cell subset identified by the respective region and the fluorescence intensity of each cell subset. In view of the major impact of multiparametric analysis, the classical single parameter analysis presented as a histogram is currently performed only in the setting of DNA analysis (cell cycle and ploidity).

2.1.2
Reagents Used for the Detection of Cellular Components

Since the availability of monoclonal antibodies, an immense number of these antibodies have been introduced into cell analysis. According to similar or identical reactivity with a panel of reference cells and/or biochemical characterization, monoclonal antibodies have been grouped into clusters of differentiation, e.g. CD, through the various workshops held since 1984 (Bernard et al. 1984). There are, however, drastic differences of reactivity among the antibodies grouped into one single CD when working with clinical samples, and these differences reflect the different epitopes detected (see Sect. 2.4.4) by the various single-CD monoclonal antibodies. These differences in reactivity among the various antibodies of one single CD allow for only very limited comparability of results as determined working with different antibodies. The current list of CD monoclonal antibodies is shown in Table 2.1. Rarely, polyclonal antibodies are used. In fact, nowadays these reagents are limited in their use as second layer antibodies to detect primary monoclonal antibodies in indirect immunofluorescence, and as primary antibodies detecting human immunoglobulins.

2.1.3
Fluorochromes

The flow cytometers used in the routine laboratories are typically equipped with one single argon-laser, emitting light at 488 nm. This allows for the proper excitation of a variety of suitable fluorochromes: FITC, PE, PE/Cy5, and propidium iodide (Table 2.2). Whereas FITC, PE, and PE/Cy5 are labels for monoclonal (and for polyclonal) antibodies, propidium iodide is used as a DNA staining dye. Only recently, two-laser devices allowing for the excitation and measurement of a fourth label-fluorochrome, allophycocyanin being one example, have been introduced. In view of partially spectral overlap of the emissions of some of the fluorochromes, proper compensation when measuring samples stained with more than one of these fluorochromes is essential.

Table 2.1. List of currently defined "clusters of differentiation" (=CD), defining the cellular specificity of monoclonal antibodies (data extracted from Barclay et al. 1997)

CD	Cells expressing this antigen	Diagnostic application
CD1a	Cortical thymocytes	L/Ly
CD2	T-lymphocytes, activated B-lymphocytes, NK cells	L/Ly
CD3	T-lymphocytes	IM, L/Ly
CD4	T-helper lymphocytes, monocytes	IM, L/Ly
CD5	T-lymphocytes, some B-lymphocytes	L/Ly
CD7	T-lymphocytes, NK cells, some myeloid leukemias	L/Ly
CD8	T-suppressor/cytotoxic lymphocytes, some NK cells	IM, L/Ly
CD10	B- and T-precursor lymphocytes, granulocytes	L/Ly
CD13	Granulocytes, monocytes, myeloid precursor cells	L/Ly, SPC
CD14	Monocytes, granulocytes, some B-lymphocytes	IM, L/Ly
CD15	Granulocytes, monocytes	L/Ly
CD16	Neutrophils, lymphocytes	IM, L/Ly, PNH
CD19	B-lymphocytes	IM, L/Ly
CD20	B-lymphocytes	L/Ly
CD21	B-lymphocytes	L/Ly
CD22	B-lymphocytes	L/Ly
CD23	B-lymphocytes; eosinophils; some NK cells and T-lymphocytes	L/Ly
CD24	B-lymphocytes, neutrophils, precursor cells	L/Ly, PNH
CD28	T-lymphocytes, plasma cells	IM, L/Ly
CD33	All mono-myeloid cells	L/Ly
CD34	Lympho-hemopoietic stem and progenitor cells, some AL	L/Ly
CD36	Platelets, monocytes, erythroid precursors	L/Ly, SPC
CD38	Lympho-hemopoietic stem and progenitor cells, plasma cells activated T-lymphocytes	IM, L/Ly, SPC
CD41a	Platelets, megakaryocytic progenitors	L/Ly
CD42b	Platelets, megakaryocytic progenitors	L/Ly
CD45	All leukocytes (at different levels)	IM, L/Ly, SPC
CD52	Lymphocytes, granulocytes, monocytes, not on plasma cells, not on stem and progenitor cells	PNH
CD56	NK cells, cytotoxic T-lymphocytes	IM, L/Ly
CD57	NK cells, cytotoxic T-lymphocytes	IM, L/Ly
CD61	Megakaryocytic progenitors, platelets, monocytes	L/Ly
CD65	Neutrophils	L/Ly
CD66b	Neutrophils	PNH
CD69	Neutrophils, eosinophils, activated T-lymphocytes	IM
CD71	Cycling cells (generally), erythroid precursors, reticulocytes	L/Ly, RetC
CD79	B-lymphocytes	L/Ly
CD90	Lympho-hemopoietic stem cells, activated T-lymphocytes	L/Ly, SPC,
PNH		
CD103	Some lymphocytes, hairy cell leukemia cells	L/Ly
CD117	Lympho-hemopoietic stem and progenitor cells, some AL	L/Ly, SPC
CD134	Activated T-lymphocytes	IM

Table 2.1. (Continued)

CD	Cells expressing this antigen	Diagnostic application
n.a.	(glycophorin-A) all erythroid cells	L/Ly
n.a.	(HLA-DR) B-lymphocytes, stem and progenitor cells, activated T-lymphocytes	IM, L/Ly, SPC
n.a.	(Myeloperoxidase) neutrophils, monocytes, some precursors	L/Ly, SPC
n.a.	(Terminal deoxynucleotidyl transferase,TdT), thymocytes some AL	L/Ly

AL, acute leukemia; IM, Immune-monitoring; L/Ly, leukemia/lymphoma immunphenotyping; n.a., not assigned to a defined CD; PNH, PIG anchor deficiency; RetC, reticulocyte counting; SPC, stem and progenitor cell analysis

Table 2.2. Fluorochrome, optimal excitation at maximum emission

FITC	495 nm	525 nm
PE	565 nm	575 nm
PE/Cy5	488 nm	670 nm
APC	650 nm	665 nm
PI	488 nm	670 nm
PerCP	488 nm	670 nm

This compensation is achieved by mathematical processing of the light emissions.

2.2 Sample-Processing

2.2.1 Direct Versus Indirect Immunofluorescence

The most widely currently used method is that of direct immunofluorescence. A monoclonal antibody labeled with one single fluorochrome is added to the sample. Typically, one species of monoclonal antibody will be coupled to FITC, and a simultaneously added species of monoclonal antibody will be coupled to PE. This allows for the simultaneous detection of different antigens, with different fluorochrome labels for different monoclonal antibodies. Using FITC, PE, and PE/Cy5 as labels for three different species of monoclonal antibodies, three different antigens can be measured simultaneously. The use of indirect immunofluorescence is limited to the work with monoclonal antibodies which are not fluorochrome labeled, and subsequent to incubating the cells with this primary antibody, a fluorochrome-labeled second antibody, detecting the primary antibody, is added for staining. The crucial advantages of direct over indirect immunofluorescence consist in the short time of staining, 30 min versus 90 min, the lower unspecific staining of cells, and the feasibility of staining without much effort one single sample with a variety of antibodies simultaneously. A further advantage of direct immunofluorescence is considered to be the extremely small lot-to-lot variability of fluorochrome-labeled monoclonal antibodies. This allows for extremely reliable comparisons working with different lots of one single reagent. Conventionally, samples are washed free off the monoclonal antibody after staining by centrifugation. This reduces background staining.

2.2.2 DNA Staining

There is no established value of DNA analysis in the routine clinical setting. Nonetheless, both ploidity and cell-cycle analyses are informative in the research setting. Although DAPI may be the more preferable DNA dye, PI is the dye most widely used. In contrast to DAPI, which needs an excitation at 350 nm, PI is easily and sufficiently excitated at 488 nm, the wavelength the lasers of the routine flow cytometers are emitting at. Cells must be permeabilized by fixation in 70% (v/v) ice-cold methanol or ethanol. In order to reduce background staining due to PI bound to RNA, samples should be treated with RNAse (Serke et al. 1991b; Siegert and Serke 1996). Figure 2.1 shows typical one-parameter histograms of PI-stained cells allowing for cell-cycle analysis, and in comparison the dual-parameter analysis in form of dot plots is shown.

2.2.3 Mononuclear Cell Preparation Versus "Whole Blood" Preparation

Traditionally, fluorescence-based microscopic immunophenotyping of leukocytes has been performed on cells separated from the native sample by means of density-gradient separation. Currently, there is no reason to perform diagnostic flow-cytometric measurements on density-gradient separated so-called mononuclear cells. Measuring density-gradient separated cells should be limited now to settings, in which these separated cells are the only cells of interest. As one typical example, measurements of lectin-stimulated lymphocytes may be quoted. There is strong evidence that the so-called mononuclear cells as separated by centrifugation do not equal to those cells classically defined by microscopy as mononuclear cells. Measuring leukocytes and determining by microscopy the mononuclear cells, then performing density-gradient separation and measuring these so-called mononuclear cells and de-

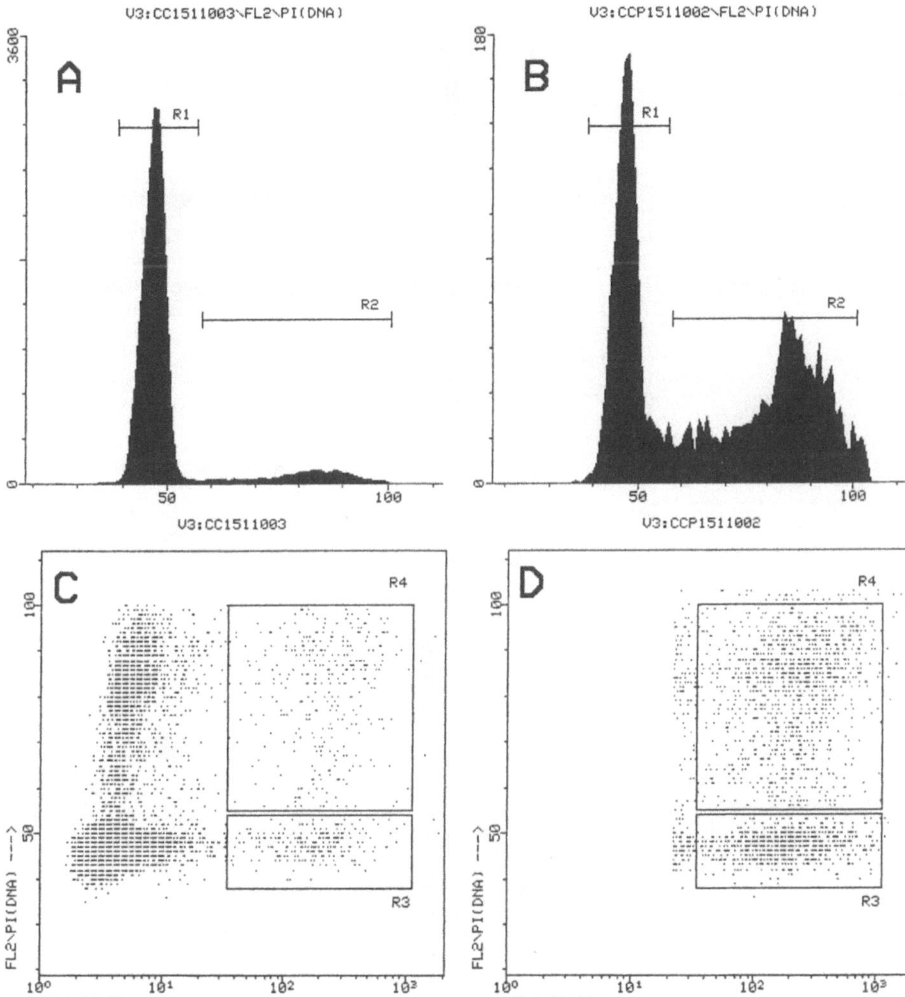

Fig. 2.1A–D. Cell-cycle analysis of bone marrow cells, staining with CD71 monoclonal antibody+rabbit-anti-mouse-IgG-FITC and with PI; in **A** and **C**, all bone marrow cells; in **B** and **D**, opto-electronically isolated ("gated") CD71-expressing cells. **A,B** One-parameter histograms, showing the numbers of cells (*y*-axis) and the intensity of PI staining (*x*-axis); the analysis region *R1* denotes the cells in G0/G1 phase, and *R2* denotes the cells in S/G2/M phase. **C,D** Two-parameter dot plots, correlating CD71 expression (*x*-axis) to PI staining (*y*-axis); each dot represents one single cell; the analysis region *R3* denotes cells in G0/G1 phase, and *R4* denotes the cells in S/G2/M phase. Of all bone marrow cells, about 8% are in S/G2/M phase (*R1* in **A**), and of all CD71-expressing cells, accounting for about 3.5% of all bone marrow cells, about 50% are in S/G2/M phase (*R2* in **B** and *R4* in **D**)

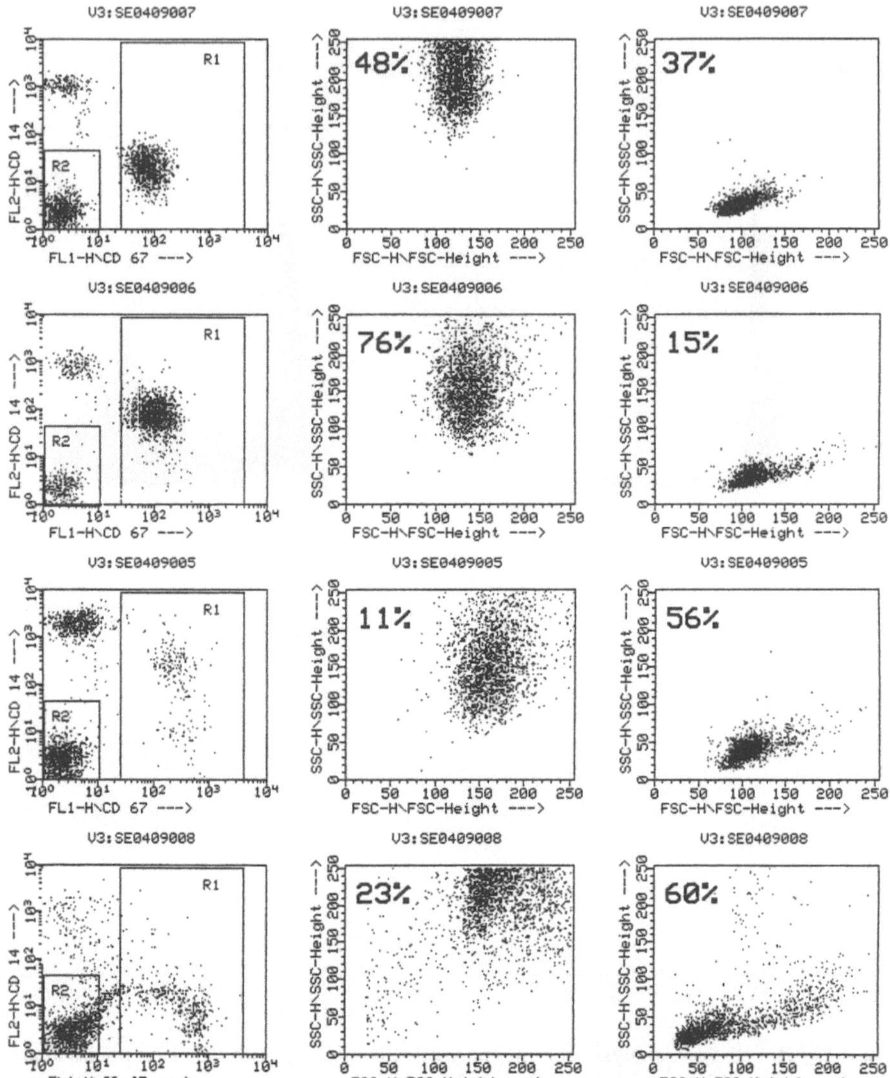

A

Fig. 2.2A,B. Depiction of the effects of density-gradient centrifugation on the composition of the cell sample in terms of distribution of the "mononuclear cells". A Uncentrifuged samples. *First row:* correlation of CD67 expression (currently referred to as CD66b) to CD14 expression; the analysis region *R1* denotes the neutrophils; *second and third row:* correlation of forward light scatter and sideward light scatter; *1st line:* steady-state blood, 48% neutrophils and 37% lymphocytes; *2nd line:* mobilized blood (chemotherapy + filgrastim), 76% neutrophils and 15% lymphocytes; *3rd line:* cytapheresis product, 11% neutrophils and 56% lymphocytes; *4th line:* bone marrow; 23% neutrophils and 60% lympho-

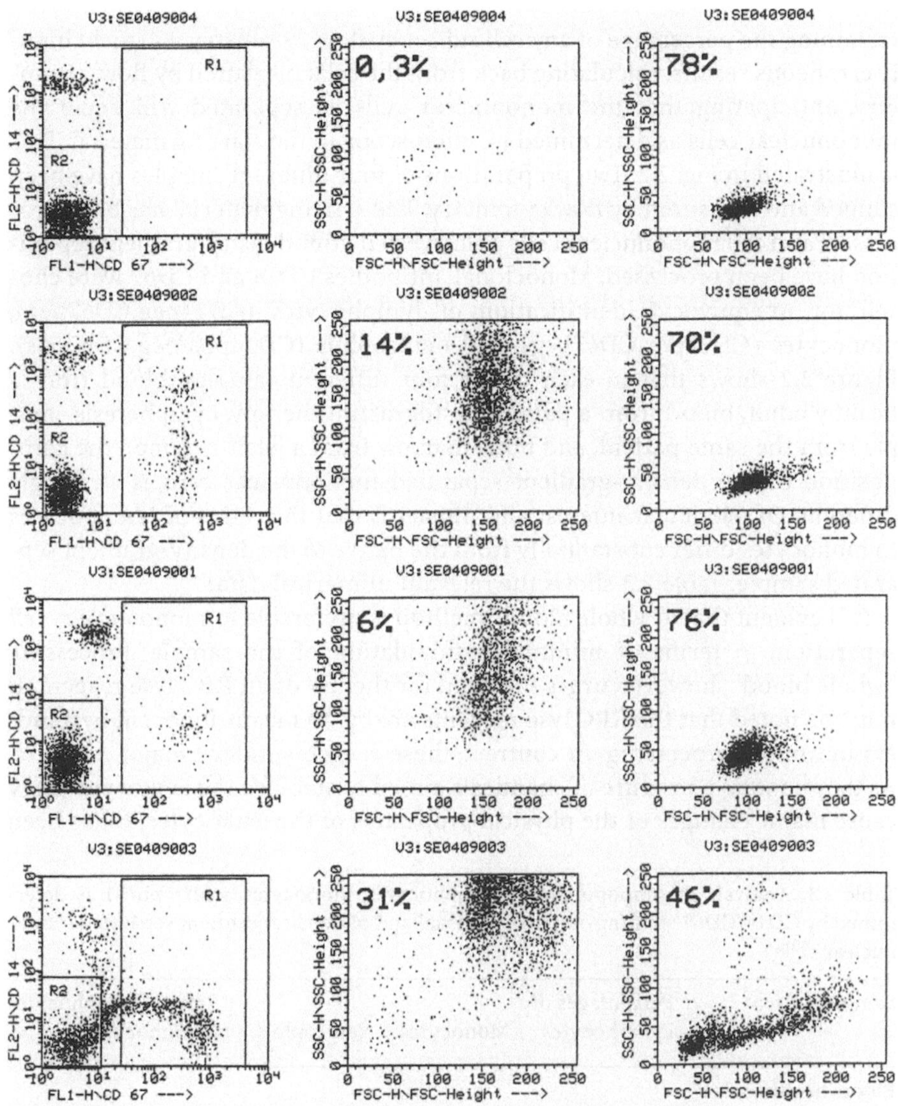

B

cytes (+ erythroblasts). **B** Samples subjected to density-gradient separation. *First row:* correlation of CD67 expression (currently referred to as CD66b) to CD14 expression; the analysis region *R1* denotes the neutrophils; *second and third row:* correlation of forward light scatter and sideward light scatter; *1st line:* steady-state blood, 0.3% neutrophils and 78% lymphocytes; *2nd line:* mobilized blood (chemotherapy + filgrastim), 14% neutrophils and 70% lymphocytes; *3rd line:* cytapheresis product, 6% neutrophils and 76% lymphocytes; *4th line:* bone marrow, 31% neutrophils and 46% lymphocytes (+ erythroblasts)

termining the percentage of any cell subset by flow cytometry will yield highly erroneous results, calculating back from the cells measured by flow cytometry, anticipating that the mononuclear cells as separated will equal the mononuclear cells as determined by microscopy in the starting material. This is illustrated in Fig. 2.2. Two preparations of four different samples have been stained and measured by flow cytometry. The starting material has been processed, and the mononuclear cells as harvested after density-gradient separation have been processed. Monoclonal antibodies CD14 and CD67 were chosen for unequivocal identification of lymphocytes (CD14neg,CD67neg), monocytes (CD14pos,CD67neg), and neutrophils (CD14pos/neg,CD67pos). Figure 2.2 shows that in each of the four different samples, blood from a healthy adult, blood from a patient on filgrastim therapy, cytapheresis sample from the same patient, and bone marrow from a healthy donor, the composition of the density-gradient separated mononuclear cells is strikingly different. Of particular interest and impact is that the ratios of lymphocytes to monocytes differ substantially from the native to the density-gradient separated sample. Table 2.3 shows the relevant numerical data.

It is evident that a "whole blood" method is preferable to mononuclear cell separation, in terms of minimal manipulation of the sample. Processing "whole blood", however, urges the need for the use of an RBC lyse reagent. It must be noted that the RBC lyse reagents are by no means innocent bystanders in sample processing. In contrast, these reagents induce major artifacts. As they contain a mixture of chemicals aimed to stabilize the leukocytes, they cause major changes of the physical properties of the leukocytes. It has been

Table 2.3. Analysis of subpopulations (lymphocytes, monocytes, neutrophils) as determined by CD14/CD67 staining of native material and of density-gradient separated mononuclear cells

Sample source	Percentages of Lymphocytes	Monocytes	Neutrophils	Ratio of lymphocytes to monocytes
Blood, healthy adult				
Native	37	15	48	2.47
Density gradient	78	21	0.3	3.71
Blood + filgrastim				
Native	15	9	76	1.66
Density gradient	70	16	14	4.37
Cytapheresis				
Native	56	33	11	1.69
Density gradient	76	18	6	4.22
Bone marrow				
Native	60	17	23	3.53
Density gradient	46	23	31	2.00

shown that one of these RBC lyse reagents causes a selective loss of lymphocytes upon centrifugation (Serke and Huhn 1993). It has also been shown that the partial fixation exerted by these reagents has pronounced effects on the staining intensity as a partial destruction of sensitive epitopes might be induced (Kreissig et al. 1994; Macey et al. 1997). As a recent development, the so-called "no-wash" method of sample-processing has been introduced (Serke and Huhn 1993). This method offers two distinct advantages over the conventional technique which includes at least one run of centrifugation. First, essentially all cells of the sample are available for the measurement, as no loss occurs due to centrifugation. Second, a direct counting of the absolute cell numbers is feasible. This is achieved by mixing equal volumes of the sample with the unknown concentration of cells, and of a suspension of polystyrene beads with a known concentration. Figure 2.3 shows such a bead-based determination. The absolute number of cells in the sample then can be calculated easily by the equation:

$$\frac{\text{Number of cells}}{\text{Number of beads}} \times \text{beads/ml} = \text{cells/ml}$$

The drawbacks of this "no-wash" method must be noted, too. First, due to the high dilution by the RBC lyse reagent, typically 2000 µl/100-µl sample, measurements of samples with low numbers of leukocytes are extremely time-consuming. Second, there are difficulties in proper titration of the monoclonal antibody. Whereas high-affinity antibodies can be used at extremely small amounts, low-affinity antibodies must be used at amounts not essen-

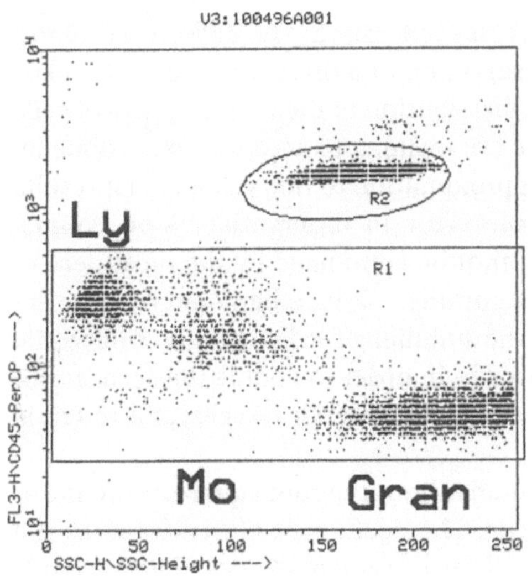

Fig. 2.3. Depiction of the flow cytometric direct absolute cell counting based on counting beads; blood sample stained with CD45-monoclonal antibody; counting beads with a concentration of 1040/µl added to the sample processed "no-wash"; in *R1*, all leukocytes (*n*=8200) as defined by CD45 expression and light scatter (*Ly* lymphocytes, *Mo* monocytes, *Gran* neutrophils + eosinophils); in *R2*, counting beads (*n*=1700); thus, the number of leukocytes can be calculated as:

$$\frac{8200}{1700} \times 1040/\mu l = 5016/\mu l$$

tially different from those used in processing conventionally. Therefore, substantial unspecific background-staining is present. Third, the costs per single measurement are substantial.

2.2.4
Staining of Intracellular Antigens

Intracellular antigens are of critical importance in the diagnosis of acute leukemia, and also the KI-67 antigen, the most widely used antigen to measure cellular proliferation, is an intracellular (nuclear) antigen. Therefore, intracellular staining has been established as a routine method. Staining of intracellular antigens urges the need for permeabilization of the cells. This is best accomplished by defined mixture of both permeabilizing and fixating reagents. These reagents are commercially available. The intracellular antigens with proven diagnostic value are: CD3, CD22, myeloperoxidase (MPO), and terminal deoxynucleotidyl transferase (TdT) (Serke 1995). An extensive critical appraisal of the available techniques and reagents for intracellular staining by monoclonal antibodies has been published recently (Groeneveld et al. 1996).

2.3
Counting Statistics

The interest in applied counting statistics with regard to cellular diagnostics can be traced back to the early thirties, when C. W. Barnett wrote in the *Journal of Clinical Investigation* a paper entitled "The unavoidable error in the differential count of the leukocytes in the blood" (Barnett 1933). More than of historical value are the reflections Barnett raised: "In differential blood counting, one attempts by careful observation of a limited number of leukocytes to obtain a picture of the actual distribution of the various types of cells in the blood stream. Many physicians are inclined to accept a count done by a competent person as a very close approximation to this value.... The results show that the completely unavoidable error in differential blood counts, which is due to chance, and which cannot be eliminated by the most perfect technique, may be of considerable magnitude.... It is to be noted that the error is inversely proportional not to the number of cells counted but to the square root of the number. In other words, in order to double the accuracy of a count it is necessary to count four times the number of cells, and to triple it, nine times."

Formally, the standard deviation equals about the root square of the mean of the effectively counted "target" cells. The coefficient of variation, as the measure of the inaccuracy of a series of measurements, is calculated according to the equation:

$$\text{Coefficient of variation} = \frac{\text{Standard Deviation}}{\text{Mean}} \times 100\%$$

Thus, in the setting of a typical 100-cell differential by microscopy, this equation reads for a given number of 10 lymphocytes effectively seen among 100 leukocytes:

$$\text{Coefficient of variation} = \frac{3.2}{10} \times 100\% = 32\%$$

The only way to increase the accuracy, or better stated, to decrease the inaccuracy, consists in simply increasing the numbers of effectively measured cells. There is no way to do so by a microscopic technique as it is not feasible to count 10,000 cells by microscopy, but flow cytometry has the advantage of being capable of including thousands of cells in one single measurement. It should be noted, however, that the definition of the numbers of cells to be measured depends on the cell population of interest. Thus, immunophenotyping lymphocytes measurements of 5000 lymphocytes will provide accurate data, e.g. data with an expected coefficient of variation of about 15%, on cell populations accounting for 1%, e.g. 50 cells per measurement. In contrast, measuring CD34-expressing hemopoietic cells in the setting of monitoring for cytapheresis, the cell population of interest may account for only 0.1% of all leukocytes, and hence measurements of at least 50,000 leukocytes are mandatory to work with an expected coefficient of variation of about 15%. Figure 2.4 shows that the impact of counting statistics has been clearly evidenced by us in the setting of determination of CD34-expressing hemopoietic cells and in vitro grown hemopoietic colonies (Serke et al. 1997). Things are getting more drastic when designing measurements for minimal residual disease, when the cell population of interest may account for less than 0.001%. A single one of these measurements, performed at a reasonable level of inaccuracy, then may contain up to several 100,000 of cells.

2.4 Quantitative Flow Cytometry

Flow cytometric measurements consistently do not allow only for the determination of a certain number of cells, in terms of percentage of a cell subset among all cells measured, but also allow for the characterization of cells in terms of quantitation of the fluorescence intensity of each cell detected by any given fluorochrome-labeled antibody. This capability, however, is little

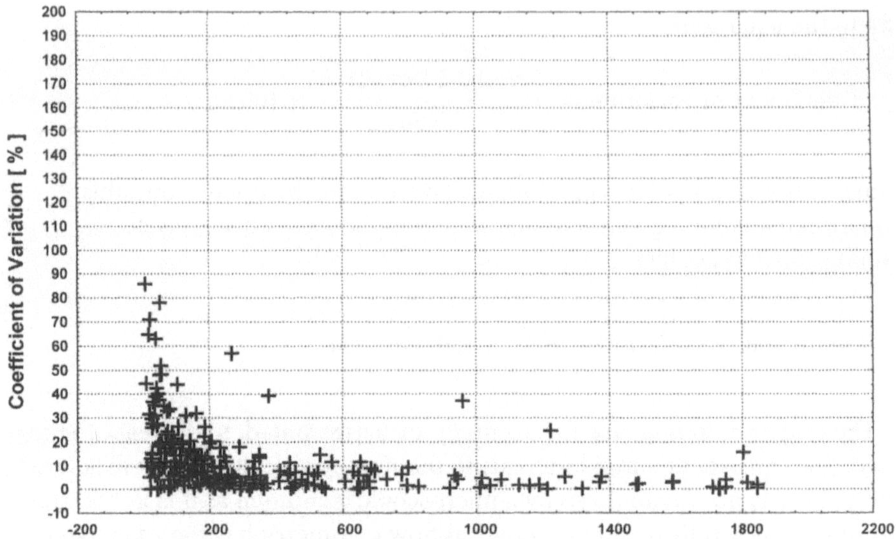

A Mean Number of CD34-Expressing Cells (from triplicates)

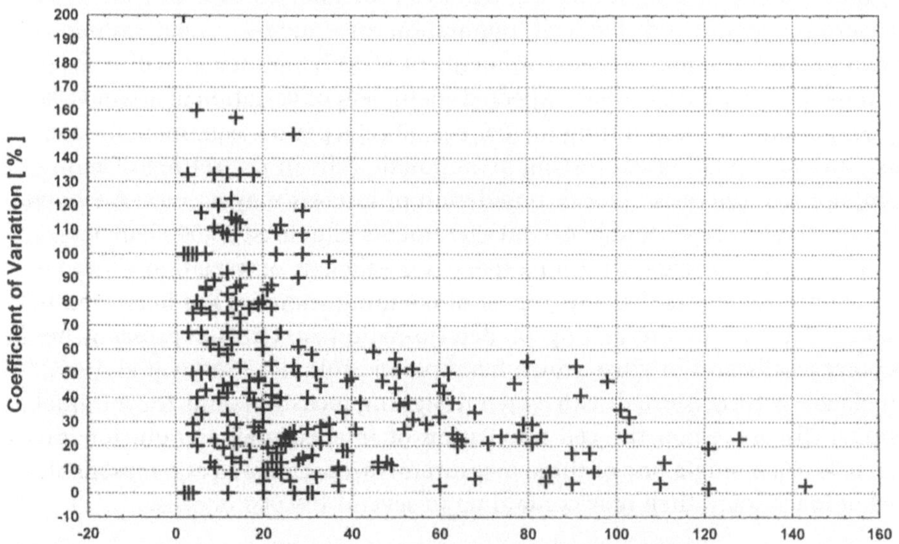

B Mean Number of CFU-GM colonies (from triplicates)

Fig. 2.4A,B. Correlation of the effectively measured numbers of CD34-expressing cells (by flow cytometry) and of the effectively measured CFU-GM colonies (by in vitro cultures) to the imprecision as measured by the coefficient of variation; data from triplicate determinations; data from one single institution; **A** CD34-expressing cells/coefficient of variation; 264 individual samples. **B** CFU-GM colonies/coefficient of variation; 238 individual samples. The more complete data, including 575 measurements of CD34-expressing cells and 1550 measurements of CFU-GM colonies, have been published previously. (Serke et al. 1997)

appreciated in current routine diagnostic flow cytometry. There are a number of reasons for the reluctance of flow cytometry users not to appreciate this feature of multiparameter flow cytometry. The reagents used for sample-processing are not standardized, and it has been shown that the different RBC lyse-reagents strongly influence the fluorescence signals. Second, there is strong evidence that the optics of the different flow cytometers are not equally sensitive (Chance et al. 1995). Third, the variability of the different fluorochrome conjugates, e.g. the variability of the fluorochrome/antibody ratio, is a further obstacle preventing standardized quantitative measurements. Fourth, the arbitrary units (channel numbers), which the measurement of the fluorescence intensity is transformed into, do not allow for any comparison of measurements at various sites and with various flow cytometer settings. Thus, typical descriptions of the fluorescence intensity of cells stained with fluorochrome-labeled antibodies will sound like "absent", "dim", "intermediate", and "bright".

Recently, however, calibration beads have been made available, which allow for a standardized quantitative determination of fluorescence intensity. There is one such bead assay available for indirect immunofluorescence, the QIFI assay, and another bead assay is available for direct immunofluorescence, the QSC assay. In the QIFI assay (Bikoue et al. 1996), 5 classes of beads, differing in the numbers of monoclonal antibodies per bead, are stained with rabbit-anti-mouse-IgG-FITC. The fluorescence intensity of each class of beads is determined, and a correlation curve of the known numbers of monoclonal antibodies per bead versus the determined channel number of fluorescence intensity is constructed. Measuring cells labeled with any monoclonal antibody and finally stained with the same rabbit-anti-mouse-IgG-FITC then allows for the determination of the approximate number of monoclonal antibodies bound to the cell by entering the channel-number of the stained cells into the calibration equation obtained by the measurement of the beads. In the QSC assay (Denny et al. 1996), 4 classes of beads, differing in the numbers of goat-anti-mouse-IgG per bead, are stained with any fluorochrome-labeled monoclonal mouse-IgG antibody. The fluorescence intensity of each class of beads is determined, and a correlation curve of numbers of binding sites (goat-anti-mouse-IgG) per bead to the monoclonal antibody versus channel number of fluorescence intensity is constructed. Measuring cells stained with the same fluorochrome-labeled monoclonal antibody then allows for the determination of the approximate number of binding sites to the monoclonal antibody on the cell by entering the channel number of the stained cells into the calibration equation obtained by the measurement of the beads.

From Fig. 2.5 it is evident that these determinations are subject to a number of artifacts. Obviously, there is a major discrepancy between direct and

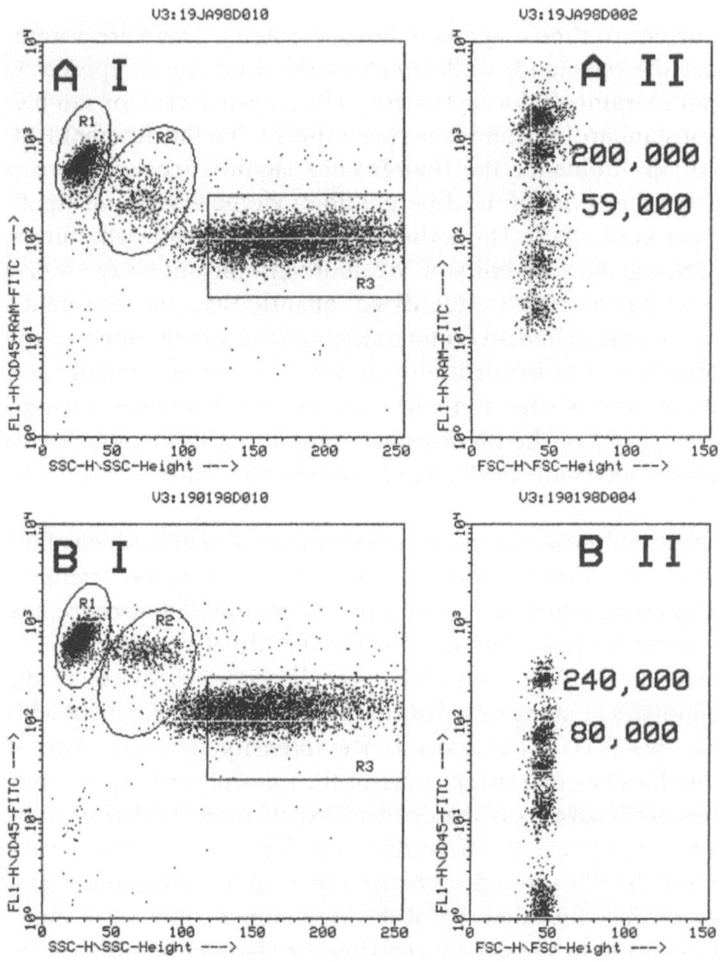

Fig. 2.5A,B. Depiction of the techniques to quantitate cellular binding sites to monoclonal antibodies by the use of beads with known numbers of binding sites to rabbit-anti-mouse-IgG-FITC (indirect immunofluorescence, QIFI technique) and by the use of beads with known numbers of binding sites to fluorochrome-labeled mouse monoclonal antibodies (direct immunofluorescence, QSC technique); **A** *I* Correlation of sideward light scatter (*x*-axis) to CD45 expression (*y*-axis) by indirect immunofluorescence staining with CD45 monoclonal antibody and rabbit-anti-mouse-IgG-FITC; the analysis regions denote lymphocytes (*R1*), monocytes (*R2*), and neutrophils (*R3*). **A** *II* Depiction of the QIFI beads stained with rabbit-anti-mouse-IgG-FITC; correlation of forward light scatter (*x*-axis) and FITC emission by rabbit-anti-mouse-IgG-FITC; the five classes of beads with different numbers of binding sites to rabbit-anti-mouse-IgG-FITC are evident; for two of these five classes, the numbers of binding sites as defined by the manufacturer are shown; by comparing to **A** *I*, it can be estimated that monocytes show staining with the CD45-monoclonal antibody equivalent to about 80,000 binding sites, whereas lymphocytes show about

indirect immunofluorescence with regard to the staining intensity with CD45-monoclonal antibody on monocytes. Whereas by direct immunofluorescence, monocytes have about the same fluorescence signal as have lymphocytes, this fluorescence signal on monocytes is substantially lower by indirect immunofluorescence. Consequently, the numbers of CD45 monoclonal antibodies bound per monocyte average 80,000 by indirect immunofluorescence, whereas the number of binding sites to the CD45-monoclonal antibody average 350,000 per monocyte by direct immunofluorescence. These discrepancies clearly warrant not accepting these quantitative determinations as a tool to determine absolute numbers of the respective CD-defined molecule per cell.

The value of these bead assays, however, and we are strongly recommending the QSC assay for direct immunofluorescence, is evident. Standardizing the reagents and the processing mode of the samples, absolute numbers of cellular binding sites to any given fluorochrome-labeled monoclonal antibody can be determined at different sites. Currently, there are few if any convincing data on the impact of the quantitation of antigen expression by flow cytometry, but this feature of flow cytometry is fully developing.

2.5 Diagnostic Tests

2.5.1 Cellular Immune Monitoring

This is the probably most widely performed diagnostic test in multiparameter flow cytometry. Taking this test as an example, the major limitations of multiparameter flow cytometry will be described herein. It is of historical interest that the introduction of multiparameter flow cytometers into the rou-

220,000 binding sites, and neutrophils show about 20,000 binding sites. **B** *I* Correlation of sideward light scatter (*x*-axis) to CD45-expression (*y*-axis) by direct immunofluorescence staining with CD45 monoclonal antibody coupled to FITC; the analysis regions denote lymphocytes (*R1*), monocytes (*R2*), and neutrophils (*R3*). **B** *II* Depiction of the QSC beads stained with CD45 monoclonal antibody coupled to FITC; correlation of forward light scatter (*x*-axis) and FITC emission by CD45 monoclonal antibody coupled to FITC; the four classes of beads with different numbers of binding sites to CD45 monoclonal antibody coupled to FITC are evident; for two of these four classes, the numbers of binding sites as defined by the manufacturer are shown; by comparing to B *I*, it can be estimated that monocytes show staining with the CD45-monoclonal antibody equivalent to about 350,000 binding sites, whereas lymphocytes show about 400,000 binding sites, and neutrophils show about 160,000 binding sites

tine diagnostic paralleled the gain of insight into the importance of the so-called T-helper lymphocytes in the course of the disease referred to in the early days as AIDS. Although recent data suggest that other lymphocyte subpopulations, the CD8+ CD38+ lymphocytes and the CD4+ CD28+ lymphocytes, may be prognostic factors as reliable as the numbers of T-helper lymphocytes (Liu et al. 1996; Effros et al. 1996), the accepted routine measurement focuses on the exact enumeration of the T-helper lymphocytes defined as CD3+ CD4+ lymphocytes. In view of the crucial importance of proper measurement of these cells, a consensus method has been defined recommending a validated strategy of how to perform this test (Centers for Disease Control and Prevention 1997). These recommendations state that the following combinations of antigens should be measured:

1. CD45–FITC+CD14–PE
   Cells to be detected: lymphocytes (CD45 bright, CD14 negative), monocytes (CD45 intermediate, CD14 bright), neutrophils (CD45 dim, CD14 dim)
2. CD3–FITC+CD19–PE
   Cells to be detected: T-lymphocytes (CD3 expressing), B-lymphocytes (CD19 expressing)
3. CD3–FITC+CD4–PE
   Cells to be detected: T-lymphocytes (CD3 expressing), T-helper lymphocytes (CD3 expressing and CD4 expressing)
4. CD3–FITC+CD8–PE
   Cells to be detected: T-lymphocytes (CD3 expressing), T-suppressor lymphocytes (CD3 expressing and CD8 expressing)
5. CD3–FITC+CD16–PE and/or CD56–PE
   Cells to be detected: T-lymphocytes (CD3 expressing), NK cells (CD16 and/or CD56 expressing, lacking coexpression of the CD3 antigen)

This recommended set of antigens illustrates some limitations of this test. Obviously, the numbers of CD19+ lymphocytes, B-lymphocytes, is of no defined diagnostic value in this setting. Likewise, the numbers of CD16+ and/or CD56+ cells without CD3 expression, NK cells, have no defined diagnostic value in this setting. The reason to include all these populations in the routine test is simply the need for an internal check in order to provide plausibility. This is required as there are a number of potential pitfalls in this test. First, the population of interest are the lymphocytes, but the test is performed on whole blood samples, with all leukocytes being stained and all leukocytes passing the detectors. In order to exclude all non-lymphocytes from the measurement, an opto-electronic focus is positioned on the cells regarded as lymphocytes. This is achieved by excluding all non-lymphocytes from the measurement by blocking all signals not compatible with signals generated by

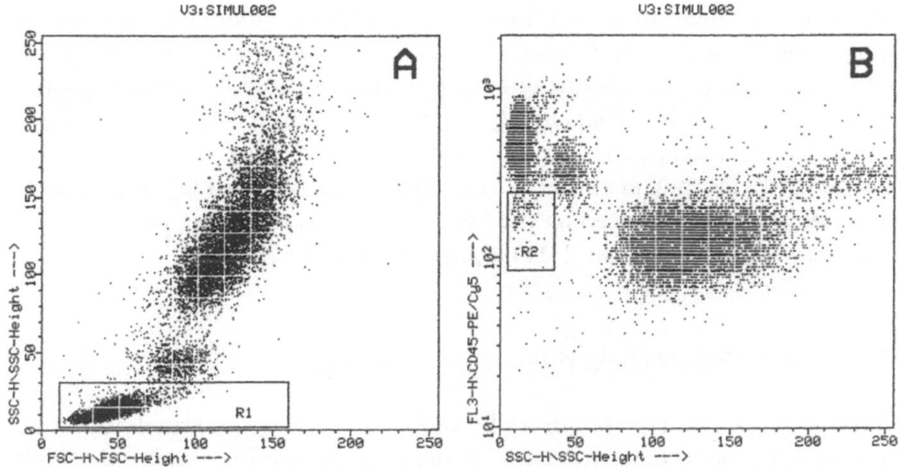

Fig. 2.6A,B. Depiction of two different approaches to lymphocyte gating; blood sample stained with CD45 monoclonal antibody-PE/Cy5. **A** Correlation of forward light scatter (*x*-axis) and sideward light scatter (*y*-axis). The analysis region *R1* denotes the lymphocytes. **B** Correlation of sideward light scatter (*x*-axis) and CD45 expression (*y*-axis); the analysis region *R2* denotes cells with a sideward light scatter equivalent to that of the lymphocytes (cells just above *R2*), but expressing the CD45 antigen to the same degree as do neutrophils (population of cells in the range of 75 arbitrary units to 180 arbitrary units in terms of sideward light scatter); these cells are basophils

lymphocytes. Traditionally, the parameters forward light scatter, reflecting the diameter of the cell, and sideward light scatter, reflecting the internal structure ("granularity") of the cell, are used. Figure 2.6A depicts this approach, positioning a so-called "gate" on lymphocytes based on the parameters sideward and forward light scatter. In Fig. 2.6B an alternative approach is shown, using the expression of the CD45 antigen. In this figure it can be seen that the population defined as lymphocytes in terms of light scatter features, effectively contains non-lymphocytes in terms of CD45 expression. These cells are basophils (Serke and Huhn 1993). It can be deduced from Fig. 2.6A,B that an analysis of lymphocyte subpopulations based on the cells positive with any monoclonal antibody will be highly erroneous given that non-lymphocytes are accounting for a substantial percentage of all cells regarded as lymphocytes in terms of light scatter features. This uncertainty is the base for the large number of different antigens to be analyzed in this setting. The numbers of T-lymphocytes (CD3+ lymphocytes), of B-lymphocytes (CD19+ lymphocytes), and of NK cells (CD3-negative CD16+ and/or CD56+ cells) should account for about 100% of all cells regarded as lymphocytes in terms of light scatter features. If this does not hold true, there is either a technical failure, incorrect pipetting being one example, or non-lymphocytes account for a major population among those cells regarded lymphocytes in terms of light scatter characteristics. Thus, all but one combinations of monoclonal antibodies used in this routine test merely serve as a tool for internal quality control. An alternative progressively more preferred is that of adding a CD45-PE/Cy5 monoclonal antibody to each test-tube and thus performing a 3-color test routinely (Mandy et al. 1997). The opto-electronic blocking of non-lymphocytes then can be based on the light scatter characteristics plus the typically high expression of the CD45 antigen on lymphocytes.

2.5.2 PIG (Phosphatidylinositolglycan) Anchor Deficiency

In this disease, also referred to traditionally as "PNH" (paroxsmal nocturnal hemoglobinuria), a point mutation in the gene coding for a molecule (PIG) serving as an anchor for a series of proteins causes the apparent loss, or marked reduction, of the expression of these PIG-anchored proteins. There is a large number of PIG-anchored proteins expressed on neutrophil granulocytes and on monocytes (CD14, CD16, CD24, CD55, CD59, CD62L), and also on erythrocytes (CD48, CD55, CD59). On lymphocytes, also expressing CD48 and CD59 via a PIG anchor, the CD16 antigen is not anchored on PIG, and thus the expression of CD16 is not affected by the PIG deficiency (Ostendorf et al. 1995). As the loss of the PIG anchor in PNH affects all these antigens to the same extent, the measurement of the expression of any of these antigens is informative. In fact, the flow cytometric analysis of erythrocytes and of leukocytes has provided major insights into the pathology of PNH. Notably, it has been shown that the PIG deficiency may be limited to the granulocytic and monocytic lineages, with no involvement of the erythrocytic lineage. The lymphatic lineage is generally affected, too, but in individual patients this lineage may be unaffected. In view of the capability of flow cytometry to detect even smallest populations of cells showing the PIG deficiency, this method can be regarded currently as the optimal method for the diagnosis of PIG deficiency. It should be emphasized that the classical test aimed for diagnosis of PNH, the Ham test, shows much less sensitivity, and obviously this test will be negative in patients with an unaffected erythroid lineage (Schubert and Schmidt 1992).

Figures 2.7 and 2.8 show typical depictions in a patient presenting with anemia, thrombocytopenia, and neutropenia, in whom a minor population of PIG-deficient leukocytes has been detected. Notably, in this patient it is evident that the B-lymphoid lineage is unaffected by the PIG deficiency. This can be deduced by the fact that all B-lymphocytes are CD24-expressing.

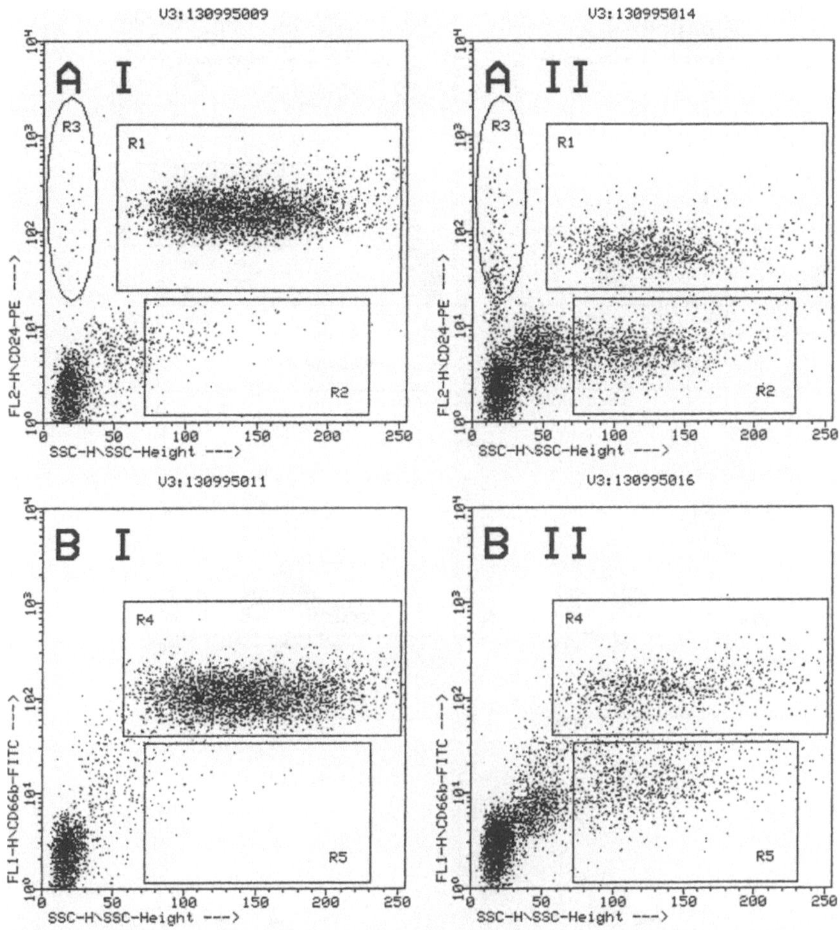

Fig. 2.7A,B. Depiction of the PIG deficiency by staining of blood leukocytes. *I*, healthy adult; *II*, patient with PIG deficiency. **A** Correlation of sideward light scatter (*x*-axis) and CD24 expression (*y*-axis). Analysis region *R1* denotes granulocytes with normal-level expression of the CD24 antigen; analysis region *R2* denotes granulocytes with PIG deficiency and as the consequence subnormal-level expression of the CD24 antigen; in **A** *II*, this PIG-deficient subpopulation accounts for about 40% of all granulocytes; analysis region *R3* denotes B-lymphocytes with normal expression of the CD24 antigen; additional staining (not shown) evidences that all B-lymphocytes of the patient with the PIG deficiency show normal CD24 expression, indicating that the B-lymphoid lineage is unaffected by the PIG deficiency. **B** Correlation of sideward light scatter (*x*-axis) and CD66b expression (*y*-axis); analysis region *R4* denotes granulocytes with normal-level expression of the CD66b antigen; analysis region *R4* denotes granulocytes with PIG deficiency and as a consequence subnormal-level expression of the CD66b antigen; in **B** *II*, this PIG-deficient subpopulation accounts for about 40% of all granulocytes

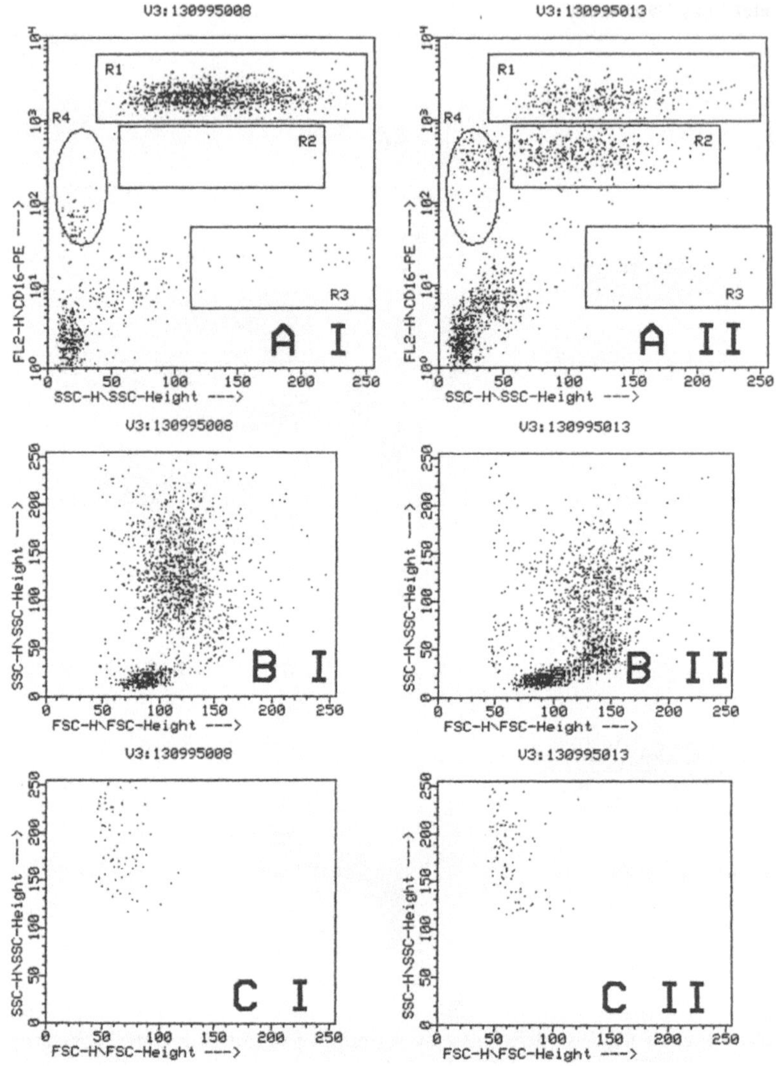

Fig. 2.8A–C. Depiction of the PIG deficiency by staining of blood leukocytes. *I*, healthy adult; *II*, patient with PIG deficiency. **A** Correlation of sideward light scatter (*x*-axis) and CD16 expression (*y*-axis). Analysis region *R1* denotes granulocytes with normal-level expression of the CD16 antigen; *R2* denotes granulocytes with subnormal level expression of the CD16 antigen; *R3* denotes granulocytes with absent expression of the CD16 antigen; these cells are present in the blood of the healthy subject (in A *I*) and of the patient with PIG deficiency (in **A II**); note: in R4 are shown the CD16-expressing lymphocytes; the population of CD16-expressing lymphocytes in the blood of the patient with the PIG deficiency must not be interpreted as the evidence of non-involvement of the T-cell lineage, as the expression of the CD16 antigen on T-lymphocytes is not PIG-dependent! The multiparametric analysis evidences that the cells defined by *R3* are eosinophils, physiologically lacking any expression of the CD16 antigen:**B, C** Correlation of forward light scatter (*x*-axis) and sideward light scatter (*y*-axis); in **B**, all blood leukocytes; in C, eosinophils as defined by *R3* in **A** *I* and in **A** *II*

2.5.3 Leukemia and Lymphoma

The classification of leukemias and lymphomas, by means of morphology and immunocytochemistry, is the main topic of another section in this book (J. Oertel). Flow cytometry is a technique alternative to immunocytochemistry, and this method is now routinely used for the classification of leukemias and lymphomas. All the particular strengths of flow cytometry play a major role in the growing acceptance of this method as the major tool to classify leukemias and lymphomas. The diagnosis can be established within 2 h, the parameters are objective (CD clustered monoclonal antibodies), and multiparametric analysis allows for the detection of even smallest populations of neoplastic cells. In particular the last feature enables flow cytometry to play an important role in the monitoring of patients in remission, with particular attention to the reappearance of neoplastic cells, indicative of relapse.

Much progress has been made concerning the standardization of the approach of how to perform flow cytometry in this setting. First, two European consensus protocols have been published in 1995 and 1996 (Bene et al. 1995; Rothe et al. 1996), and a series of publications have been published in 1997 defining a US-Canadian consensus protocol (Braylan et al. 1997; Stelzer et al. 1997; Stewart et al. 1997; Davis et al. 1997). The major aim of these consensus protocols has been to define the immunophenotype of the malignant cells in correlation to the classically defined neoplastic diseases. It should be emphasized here that current evidence does not support the view that flow cytometric immunophenotyping is a routinely necessary method for the diagnosis of myeloid leukemias. There are, however, three diseases in which the immunophenotyping is essential for making the correct diagnosis. AML FAB 0, FAB 6, and FAB 7 can be diagnosed only by means of immunological staining, and AML FAB 2 t(8;21) is diagnosed by the expression of the B-lineage associated antigen CD19 on these myeloid blasts (Porwit-MacDonald et al. 1996). Thus, in addition to the conventional immunophenotyping, classifying neoplastic cells according to the criterion "expression vs. non-expression" of any given antigen, multiparameter flow cytometry allows for more subtle description of neoplastic cells. Figure 2.9 shows that the intensity of the expression as measured by relative fluorescence intensity allows for the more concrete characterization of neoplastic cells. In Fig. 2.9 it is shown that the circulating neoplastic cells in a patient with histologically proven immunocytoma definitely are expressing the CD19 antigen at a much lower level than do the non-neoplastic B cells. Due to the capability of multiparameter flow cytometry to detect and to quantitate very rare cells, the flow cytometric determination of circulating myeloma cells has been established recently (Schneider et al. 1997). Figure 2.10 shows a representative analysis of circulating myeloma

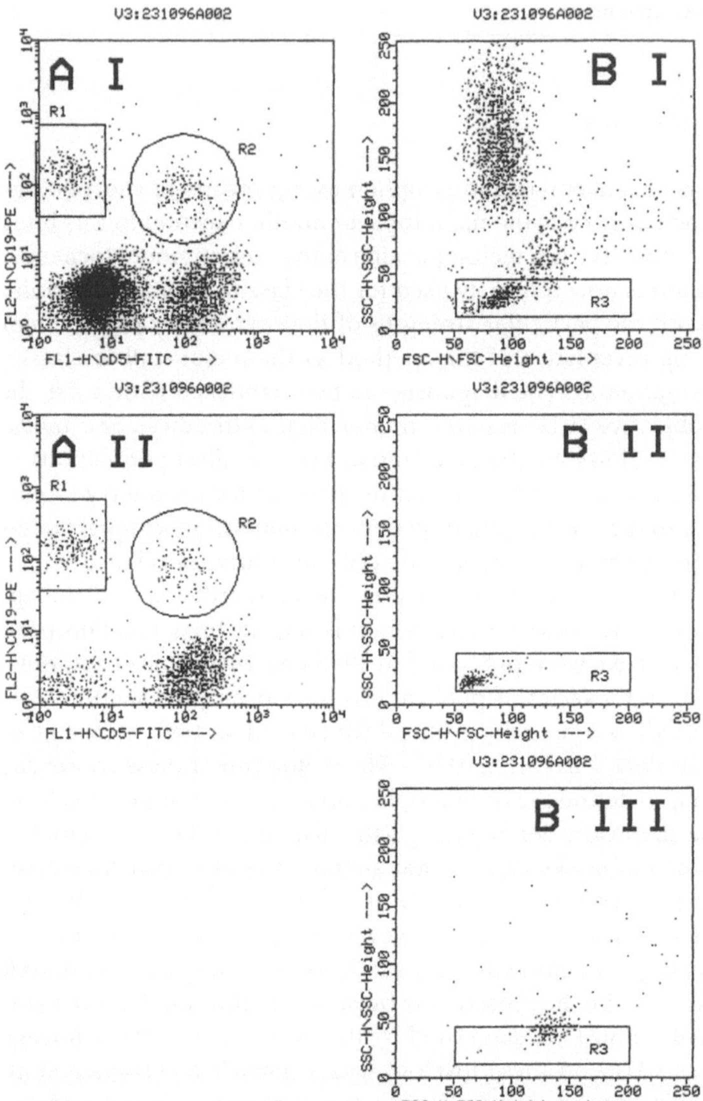

Fig. 2.9A,B. Depiction of the capability of flow cytometry to differentiate neoplastic cells in terms of abnormal degree of expression of one differentiation antigen and in terms of abnormal light scatter profile; blood, at diagnosis, from a patient with histologically proven immunocytoma. **A** Correlation of CD5 expression (*x*-axis) and CD19 expression (*y*-axis). **B** Correlation of forward light scatter (*x*-axis) and sideward light scatter (*y*-axis). **A** *I* All leukocytes; R1 denotes normal B-lymphocytes, and R2 denotes neoplastic B-lymphocytes characterized by abnormally low expression of the CD19 antigen and expression of the CD5 antigen. **A** *II* shows the same correlation as does **A** *I*, but on gated lymphocytes. **B** *I* All blood leukocytes; **B** *II* normal B-lymphocytes as defined by R1 in **A** *II*; **B** III neoplastic immunocytoma lymphocytes as defined by R2 in A *II*; note that by applying a "lymphocyte gate", as shown in **B** *I* (R3), the majority of immunocytoma cells would not be detected!

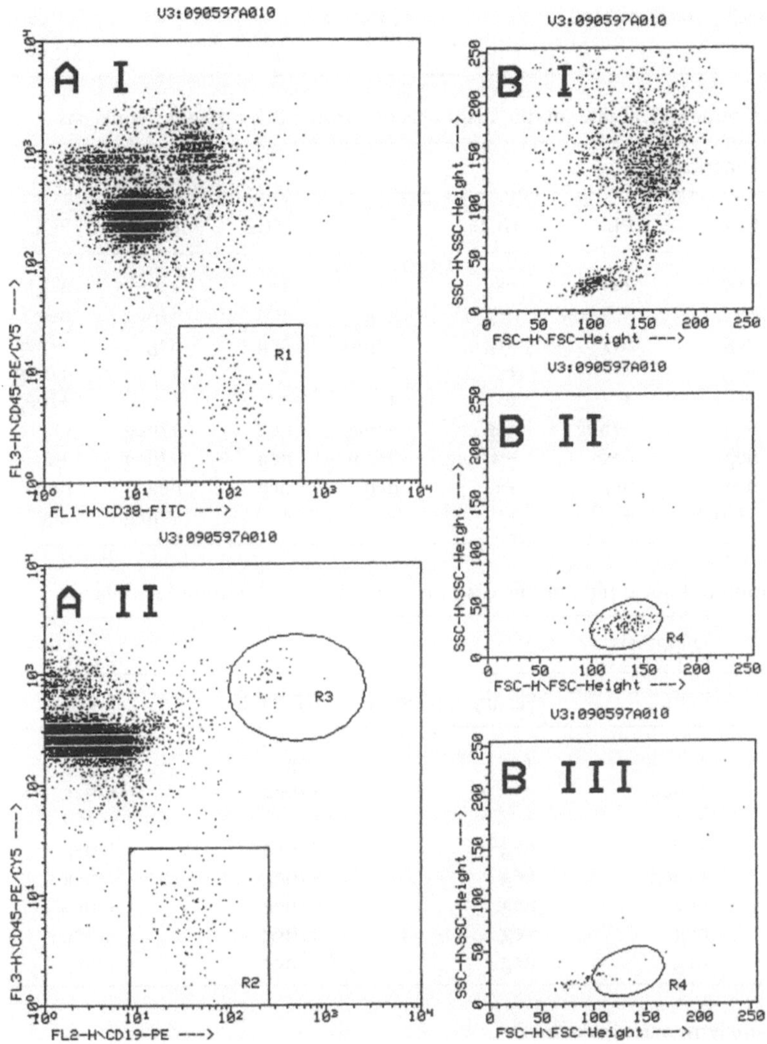

Fig. 2.10A,B. Depiction of the capability of flow cytometry to differentiate neoplastic cells in terms of abnormal degree of expression of two differentiation antigens and in terms of abnormal light scatter profile; blood, at diagnosis, from a patient with histologically proven multiple myeloma; 3-color staining with CD38-monoclonal antibody (FITC), CD19-monoclonal antibody (*PE*), and CD45-monoclonal antibody (*PE/Cy5*). **A** *I* Correlation of CD38 expression (*x*-axis) and CD45 expression (*y*-axis); the analysis region *R1* denotes myeloma cells, characterized by high expression of the CD38 antigen combined with low to absent expression of the CD45 antigen. **A** *II* Correlation of CD19 expression (*x*-axis) and CD45 expression (*y*-axis); the analysis region *R2* denotes myeloma cells, characterized by low to absent expression of the CD45 antigen combined with intermediate expression of the CD19 antigen; the analysis region *R3* denotes normal B-lymphocytes, characterized by high expression of both the CD45 antigen and the CD19 antigen. **B** Correlation of forward light scatter (*x*-axis) and sideward light scatter (*y*-axis). **B** *I*, all blood leukocytes; **B** *II*, myeloma cells as defined in **A** *I* (R1) and in **A** *II* (R2); the analysis region *R4* is drawn to encircle the myeloma cells. B *III*, normal B-lymphocytes as defined in **A** *II* (*R3*); by comparison to the myeloma cells shown in **B** *II*, it is evident that the normal B-lymphocytes show a substantially different light scatter profile

Table 2.4a. Immunological phenotypic diagnosis of chronic B-lymphoid neoplasias

Antigen	Diagnosis						
	CLL	PLL	HCL	FL	MCL	LP-IC	PCL
sIg	+w*	+s**	+s	+s	+s	+s	neg***
CD5	+	neg/+w	neg	neg	+	+/neg	neg
CD10	neg	neg	neg	+/neg	neg	neg	+/neg
CD19	+	+	+	+	+	+	+/neg
CD20	+	+	+	+	+	+	+/neg
CD23	+	+/neg	neg	+/neg	neg	+/neg	neg
CD38	neg	neg	+w/neg	+w/neg	neg	+/neg	+s
CD103	neg	neg	+s	neg	neg	neg	neg
FMC7	+w/neg	+	+	+	+	+/neg	neg

Table 2.4b. Immunological phenotypic diagnosis of chronic T-lymphoid neoplasias

Antigen	Diagnosis			
	T-PLL	Sezary syndrome	NK-LGL	T-LGL
CD3	+	+	neg	+
CD4	+/neg	+	+/neg	+/neg
CD5	+	+	+	+
CD7	+	neg	+/neg	+/neg
CD8	+/neg	neg	+/neg	+/neg
CD16	neg	neg	+/neg	+/neg
CD56	neg	neg	+/neg	+/neg
CD57	neg	neg	+/neg	+/neg

Table 2.5. Acute lymphatic leukemias

Antigen	Diagnosis						
	Pre-Pre-B-ALL	Common ALL	Pre-B-ALL	B-ALL	Early T-ALL	Cortical T-ALL	Mature T-ALL
TdT	+	+	+	neg	+	+	+/neg
CD34	+/neg	+/neg	+/neg	neg	+/neg	neg	neg
CD10	neg	+	+/neg	+/neg	+/neg	+/neg	neg
CD19	+	+	+	+	neg	neg	neg
cyIgM	neg	neg	+	neg	neg	neg	neg
sIg	neg	neg	neg	+	neg	neg	neg
CD1a	neg	neg	neg	neg	neg	+	neg
CD2	neg	neg	neg	neg	neg	+	+
cyCD3	neg	neg	neg	neg	+	+/neg	neg
CD3	neg	neg	neg	neg	neg	+/neg	+
CD7	neg	neg	neg	neg	+	+	+

cells in a patient with newly diagnosed myeloma. Of particular interest in this patient, the myeloma cells are coexpressing the CD19 antigen, albeit at much lower levels than do the non-neoplastic B cells.

The consensus protocols referred to (vide supra) suggest certain combinations of monoclonal antibodies as fixed panels which allow for the correct diagnosis of the various leukemias and lymphomas. These panels, together with the reactivity of the various leukemias and lymphomas, are shown in Table 2.4a (chronic B-lymphoid neoplasias), Table 2.4b (chronic T-lymphoid neoplasias), and Table 2.5 (acute lymphatic leukemias).

2.5.4 CD34-Expressing Hemopoietic Stem and Progenitor Cells

Traditionally, the hemopoietic potential of bone marrow or cytapheresis product harvested for transplantation/reinfusion has been estimated by means of in vitro cultures growing the committed granulocyte/macrophage progenitor cells, giving rise to hemopoietic colonies, since referred to as CFU-GM (colony forming unit–granulocyte/macrophage) (Metcalf 1977; Serke and Huhn 1991; Serke 1988). This assay has a number of inherent disadvantages. As an in vitro culture assay, it is cost- and manpower-intensive. The most outstanding drawback is that the read-out of this assay has a time-lag of about 14 days from initiation of cultures, as the progenitor cells need this time to produce the cells to be read out as a hemopoietic colony. Therefore, this assay is not a real-time test. In contrast, the flow cytometric test is a real-time test, and it can be performed applying a standard approach common to any other of the described flow cytometric tests. The test is based on the determination of hemopoietic stem and progenitor cells as identified as CD34-expressing cells (Krause et al. 1996). Serving as a guideline, a German/Austrian consensus protocol has been defined recently (Gutensohn and Serke 1996) and a worldwide consensus on this test is about to be defined (Marti et al. 1998).

The CD34 antigen is limited in its expression to the mitotic compartment of hemopoietic cells, including all stem and progenitor cells, and only a few morphologically recognizable blasts express the CD34 antigen (Civin et al. 1984). Thus, the expression of the CD34 antigen is extremely restricted. By biochemical definition, 3 distinct epitopes, class I, II, and III, of the CD34 antigen and the respectively binding monoclonal antibodies can be discriminated (Sutherland et al. 1992; Serke and Huhn 1996). As soon as the CD34 antibodies became available, the flow cytometric test for the characterization and the enumeration of hemopoietic CD34-expressing cells in hemopoietic transplantation emerged as a very versatile tool (Siena et al. 1989; Serke et al. 1991; Serke et al. 1991a). It should be emphasized that the flow cytometric determination of CD34-expressing cells is focussing on a cell population accounting for less than 0.1% of all blood leukocytes (Serke and Huhn 1992), and that the population of CD34-expressing cells rarely exceeds a percentage of 5 in clinical samples (Serke et al. 1996). Thus, the flow cytometric test for CD34-expressing cells must be regarded as the first routine hematological test focussing on the assessment of a rare population.

In fact, this test is routinely used for (1) monitoring patients during mobilization therapy with chemotherapy and/or cytokine, and (2) for estimation of the hemopoietic potential of cytapheresis product, as the numbers of transplanted/reinfused CD34-expressing cells are correlated fairly well to the time to hemopoietic recovery (Beyer et al. 1995). Thus, the test allows for proper timing of cytapheresis and it allows for the definition of the numbers of cytapheresis necessary in any individual patient or healthy donor. In fact, from the numbers of circulating CD34-expressing cells the volume of cytapheresis product to be harvested can be calculated (Serke et al. 1993; Schwella et al. 1996a,b).

The flow cytometric test for the determination of CD34-expressing cells explores all the advantages of state-of-the-art flow cytometry. Basically, at least two antigens are visualized. First, the CD45 antigen for the detection of all leukocytes is stained, and second, the CD34 antigen, preferably by the class III monoclonal antibodies 8G12 or 581.E8. The CD34-expressing cells express the CD45 antigen at the same density as do neutrophils, although rarely a few CD34-expressing cells may lack any expression of the CD45 antigen (Kreissig et al. 1994). The characteristic light scatter profile of the CD34-expressing cells greatly helps in identifying these rare cells. Typically, the CD34-expressing cells are clustering into the light scatter region of large lymphocytes to "low sideward light scatter" monocytes. We have introduced the term "extended lymphocyte/monocyte region" to describe this particular light scatter region (Serke et al. 1991a). A representative depiction of the analysis of CD34-expressing cells in a cytapheresis product is shown in Fig. 2.11. It should be emphasized at this point that the reliable determination of the CD34-expressing cells depends on the choice of the optimal reagents. The 3 different epitopes of the CD34 antigen are characterized by a pronounced, but variable sensitivity towards the actions of the different RBC lyse reagents. In fact, some of the epitopes are almost destroyed by the fixative-containing RBC lyse reagents. Figure 2.12 shows that while there are almost no effects of the fixative-containing RBC lyse reagents on the epitope detected by the reference class III monoclonal antibody (8G12), the epitopes detected by both the other class III CD34 monoclonal antibodies (581.E8 and Birma/K3) and the class II CD34 monoclonal antibody (QBEND/10) strongly suffer from the actions of the fixative-containing RBC lyse reagents.

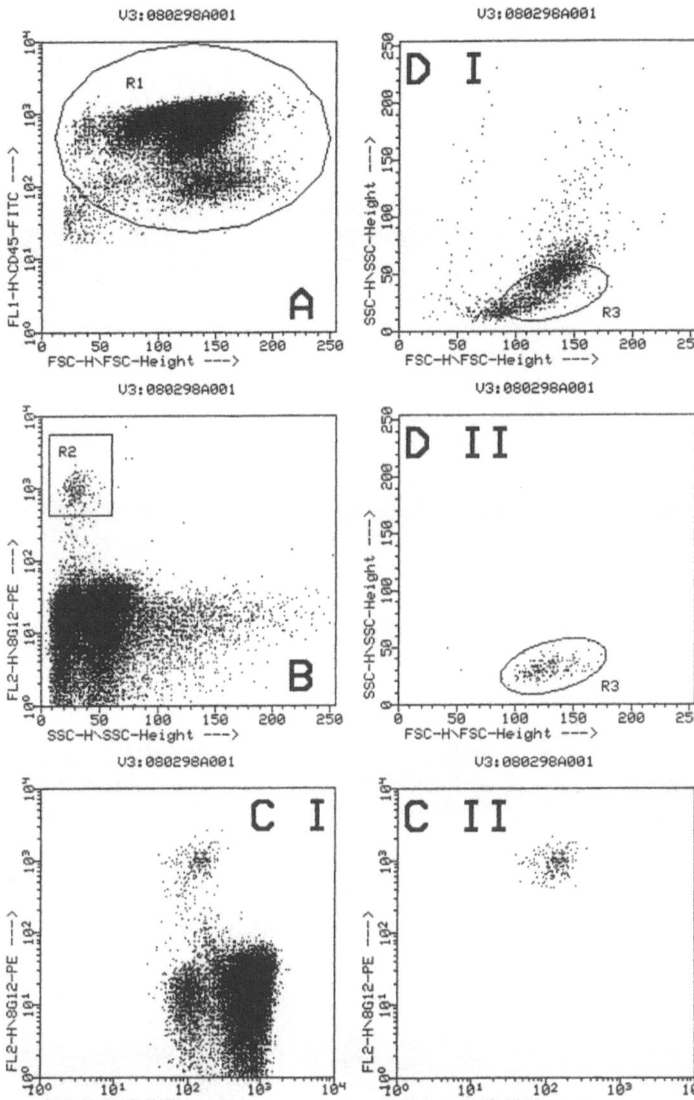

Fig. 2.11 A–D. Depiction of the basic technique to determine CD34-expressing cells; cytapheresis product stained with CD45-monoclonal antibody coupled to FITC and with CD34-monoclonal antibody coupled to PE; "no-wash" technique. **A** Correlation of forward light scatter (*x*-axis) and CD45 expression (*y*-axis); the analysis region *R1* encircles all counting events regarded as "cells". **B** Correlation of sideward light scatter (*x*-axis) and CD34 expression (*y*-axis); the analysis region *R2* denotes the cells regarded as CD34-expressing cells; data gated on *R1*. C *I* Correlation of CD45 expression (*x*-axis) and CD34 expression (*y*-axis); all cells as defined by *R1* in **A. D** *I* Correlation of forward light scatter (*x*-axis) and sideward light scatter (*y*-axis); all cells as defined by *R1* in **A. D** *II* Correlation of forward light scatter (*x*-axis) and sideward light scatter (*y*-axis); all CD34-expressing cells as defined by *R2* in **B**; the analysis region *R3* encircles these cells; comparing to all cells as shown in D *I*, the particular light scatter profile of the CD34-expressing cells is evident. C *II* Correlation of CD45 expression (*x*-axis) and CD34 expression (*y*-axis); all CD34-expressing cells as defined by *R2* in **B** and by *R3* in **D** II

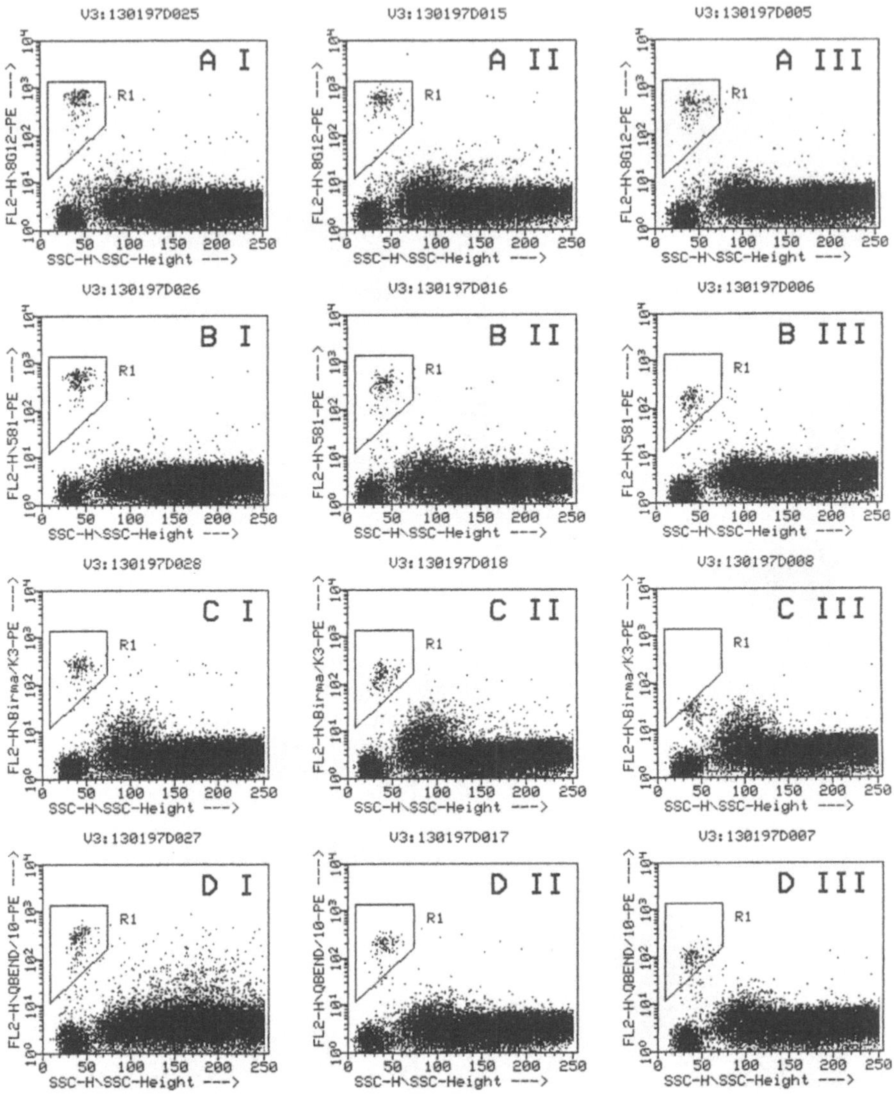

Fig. 2.12A–D. Depiction of the actions of the three most widely used RBC lyse reagents on the class III epitopes of the CD34 antigen as detected by the monoclonal antibodies 8G12, 581.E8, and Birma/K3 and the class II epitope of the CD34 antigen as detected by the monoclonal antibody QBEND/10; all monoclonal antibodies used as PE conjugates in saturating concentrations; blood sample; correlation of sideward light scatter (*x*-axis) and CD34 expression (*y*-axis); the analysis region *R1* denotes the CD34-expressing cells as determined applying the optimal technique (shown in **A** *I*). *I*, processing with the fixative-free ORTHOmune RBC lyse reagent; *II*, processing with the fixative-containing FACS-lyse RBC lyse reagent; *III*, processing with the fixative-containing ImmunoPrep RBC lyse reagent (*the numbers in brackets* show the mean of the fluorescence intensity of the CD34-expressing cells). **A** Staining with 8G12-PE: *I* (602), *II* (535), *III* (382). **B** Staining with 581.E8: *I* (449), *II* (321), *III* (141). **C** Staining with Birma/K3: *I* (235), *II* (153), *III* (25). **D** Staining with QBEND/10: *I* (274), *II* (186), *III* (92)

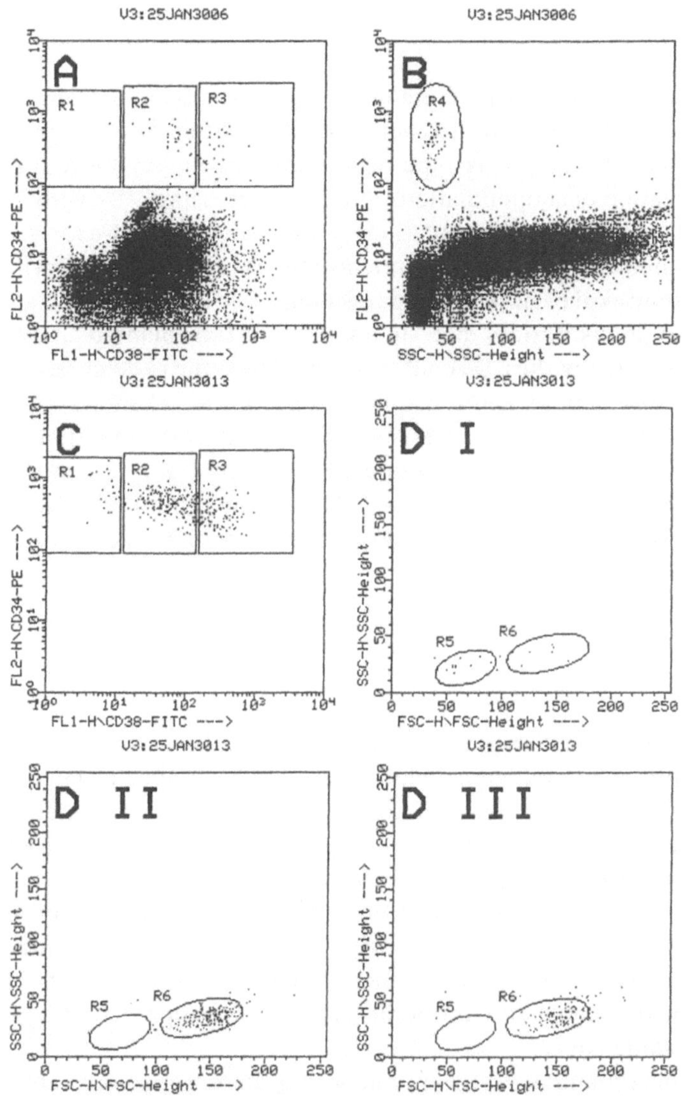

Fig. 2.13A–D. Depiction of the differential expression of the CD34 antigen and the CD38 antigen, and of the differential light scatter profiles, of subpopulations of CD34-expressing cells; blood sample from a patient on mobilization (chemotherapy + filgrastim). **A** Correlation of CD38 expression (*x*-axis) and CD34 expression (*y*-axis); all leukocytes; the analysis regions *R1*, *R2*, and *R3* denote different subpopulations of CD34-expressing cells according to the different intensities of the coexpression of the CD38 antigen. **B** Correlation of sideward light scatter (*x*-axis) and CD34 expression (*y*-axis); the analysis region *R4* encircles all CD34-expressing cells. **C** Correlation of CD38 expression (*x*-axis) and CD34 expression (*y*-axis); gated CD34-expressing cells; the analysis regions *R1*, *R2*, and *R3* denote different subpopulations of CD34-expressing cells according to the different intensities of the coexpression of the CD38 antigen. Note that with increasing expression intensity of the CD71 antigen (from *R1* through to *R3*), a decrease of the expression intensity of the CD34 antigen is associated! **D** Correlation of forward light scatter (*x*-axis) and sideward light scatter (*y*-axis). (Legend continued on page 32)

Recent interest has been created in the enumeration of subpopulations of CD34-expressing cells according to the coexpression of differentiation antigens (Dercksen et al. 1995a,b). This type of analysis allows for the multiparametric identification of subpopulations of CD34-expressing cells, with in vitro cultures of the respective subpopulations of flow-sorted CD34-expressing cells as the backbone supporting these phenotypic determinations (Bernstein et al. 1991; Udomsakdi et al. 1992). In particular, it has been demonstrated, albeit by one single institution, that the numbers of transplanted CD34-expressing cells coexpressing the CD41 antigen correlate to the platelet recovery following high-dose therapy and transplantation. Figure 2.13 shows a depiction of subpopulations of CD34-expressing cells according to the differential expression of the CD38 antigen. It is evident from this Fig. 2.13 that the distinct subpopulations of CD34-expressing cells not only differ with regard to the gradual coexpression of the CD38 antigen but also with regard to the differential light scatter profile.

2.6 Standardization

It has been evidenced that the parameters used in multiparameter flow cytometry are highly objective. Nonetheless, there are a number of factors which are prohibitive to generally standardized objective flow cytometric measurements. One of these factors, the different RBC lyse reagents and their effects on the CD34 epitopes, have been described (vide supra). Among the further factors the most outstanding ones contributing to heterogeneity of results among different laboratories, although working with identical samples and identical reagents, are: (1) the titration of monoclonal antibodies, (2) the incubation-time of sample and antibodies, and (3) the approach of how to analyze the list-mode data.

By convention, most manufacturers are marketing their monoclonal antibodies in "20 μl/100 μl blood" vials, e.g. 2000 μl/100 tests of 100 μl blood. Titrating any of these monoclonal antibodies, however, one finds that the recommended amount of monoclonal antibody is by far too high in terms of sufficient resolution of the stained populations. Therefore, it is preferable to add less monoclonal antibody per 100 μl blood, in order to save monoclonal

Fig. 2.13 (Continued) **D** *I* Primitive CD34-expressing cells ("stem cells") as defined by *R1* in C; the analysis region *R5* encircles the particular subpopulation of these cells with typically very low forward light scatter. **D** *II* Differentiated CD34-expressing cells (committed progenitor cells) as defined in *R2* in **C**; the analysis region *R6* encircles this main population of the mobilized CD34-expressing cells. **D** *III* Terminally differentiated CD34-expressing cells (erythroid progenitor cells) as defined in *R3* in **C**; notably, these cells show both larger forward and sideward light scatter than do the cells defined by *R2* in **C**

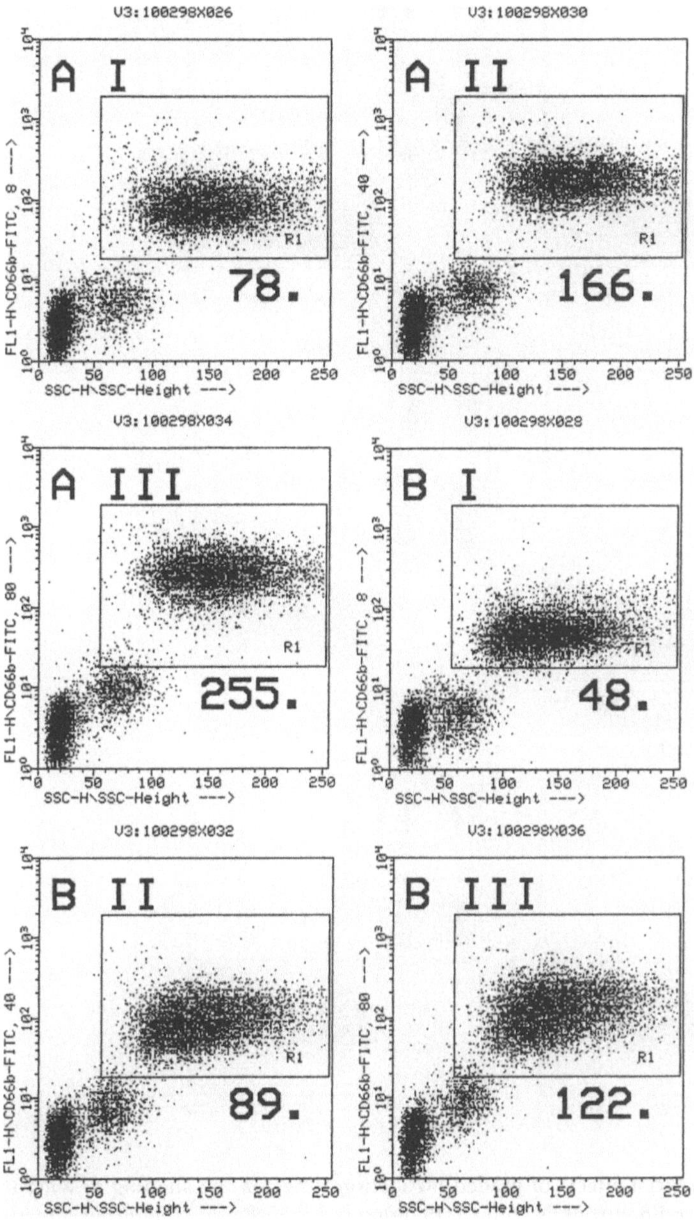

Fig. 2.14A,B. Effects of staining two blood samples with increasing amounts of FITC-labeled CD66b monoclonal antibody; the manufacturer recommended saturating concentration of this antibody is given as 2.0 µg/100 µl; correlation of sideward light scatter (*x*-axis) and CD66b staining intensity; the analysis region *R1* denotes the neutrophils, the only population with specific binding of the CD66b monoclonal antibody. **A** Healthy donor "A"; **B** healthy donor "B"; *I*, 0.8 µg/100-µl sample; II, 4.0 µg/100-µl sample; III, 8.0 µg/100-µl sample (*the numbers shown* denote the mean values of fluorescence intensity on neutrophils)

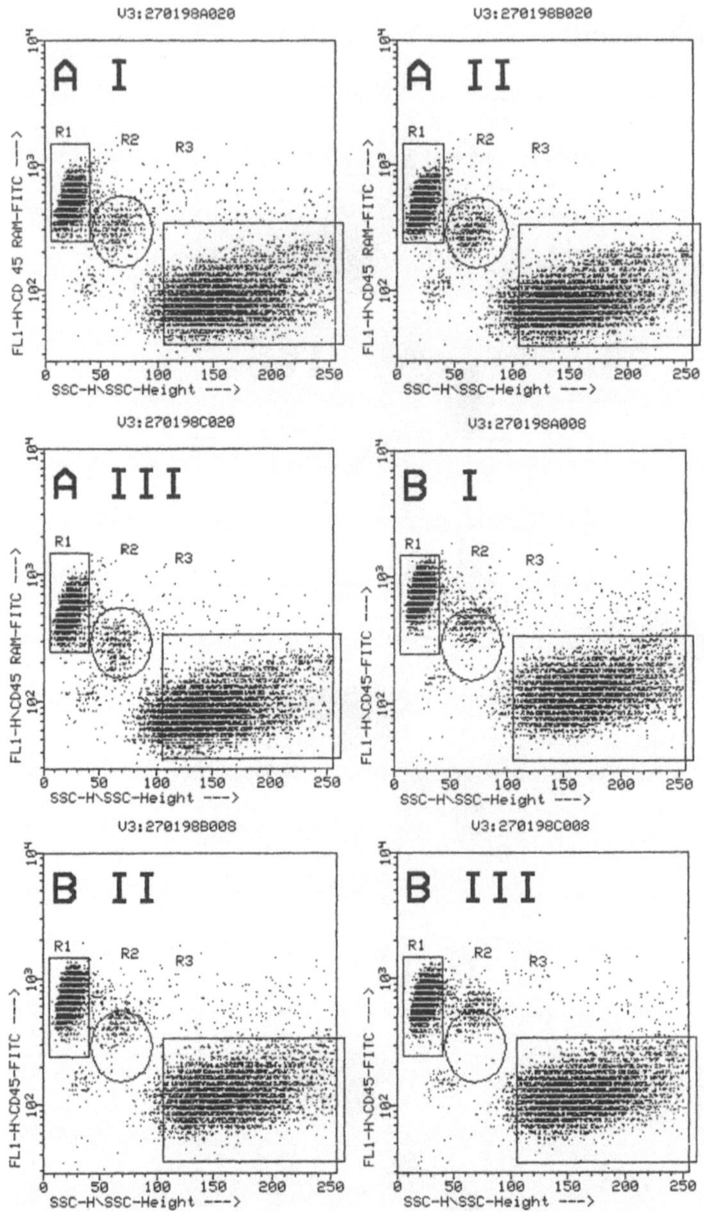

Fig. 2.15A,B. Differential effects of graded incubation times on the staining of lymphocytes, monocytes, and neutrophils with CD45 monoclonal antibody, comparing direct to indirect immunofluorescence; data from one single sample. **A** Staining by indirect immunofluorescence (CD45 monoclonal antibody+rabbit-anti-mouse-IgG-FITC). **B** Staining by direct immunofluorescence (CD45 monoclonal antibody-FITC); the analysis region *R1* denotes lymphocytes, *R2* denotes monocytes, and *R3* denotes neutrophils. *I*, staining for 30 min; *II*, staining for 45 min; *III*, staining for 60 min; whereas it is evident that, comparing **A** *I* to **A** *III*, the fluorescence intensity on monocytes drops over time in the sample stained by indirect immunofluorescence, in the sample stained by direct immunofluorescence a marked increase over time is evident on monocytes

antibody and thus to reduce expenses. This approach, however, puts one in danger in terms of not properly identifying the true binding-capacity of the cells for the respective monoclonal antibody. Figure 2.14 shows that an acceptable staining of granulocytes can be achieved with this FITC-labeled CD66b monoclonal antibody at 8 μl/100 μl blood. Figure 2.14, however, also evidences that even at 80 μl/100 μl blood there is no saturation of the CD66b antigen on neutrophils.

Again by convention, a tentative routine incubation time (blood + monoclonal antibody) is estimated to be 30 min. Although proper staining will generally occur upon this length of incubation time, prolonged incubation times reveal that while some types of cells will increasingly bind monoclonal antibody over time, other types of cells will effectively lose staining intensity, and there are differences between direct and indirect immunofluorescence (Fig. 2.15).

The most outstanding factor, however, contributing to non-standardized flow cytometric determinations resides in the subjectivity of how to position the discriminators while analyzing the list mode data. This has been clearly evidenced by us recently in the setting of determinations of CD34-expressing cells (Serke et al. 1998) . List mode data files on floppy disks have been mailed to 150 self-selected members of the two major organizations active in Europe in blood and marrow transplantation (EBMT and ISHAGE). The list mode data files contained several representative measurements of one blood sample and of one cytapheresis sample. Thus, each single participant in this survey received and analyzed identical data. The participants were asked to determine, according to the respective "in-house" protocol, the percentages of CD34-expressing cells and the subpopulation of CD34-expressing cells lacking the coexpression of the CD71 antigen. Figures 2.16 and 2.17 evidence the heterogeneity of the determinations among the 53 participants of this survey returning the filled questionnaire for analysis. It appears that the only solution to this problem is the introduction of in-built algorithm-defined software programs to analyze the list mode data without interference of the subjective operator. Realizing this potential pitfall, a number of dedicated software programs for both data acquisition and analysis have become available recently, in particular, the Simul-Set software (Becton Dickinson) for determination of the major lymphocyte subpopulations (see Sect. 2.5.1) and the Pro-Count software (Becton Dickinson) for the determination of CD34-expressing cells (see Sect. 2.5.4).

Results similar to those described above are evidenced by the data from external quality assessment surveys. In Germany, a complete set of surveys for the major diagnostic areas in flow cytometry has been established by INSTAND since 1993. In any of these surveys, two samples, differing substantially in the numbers of the cells of interest, are shipped to the participants. Ide-

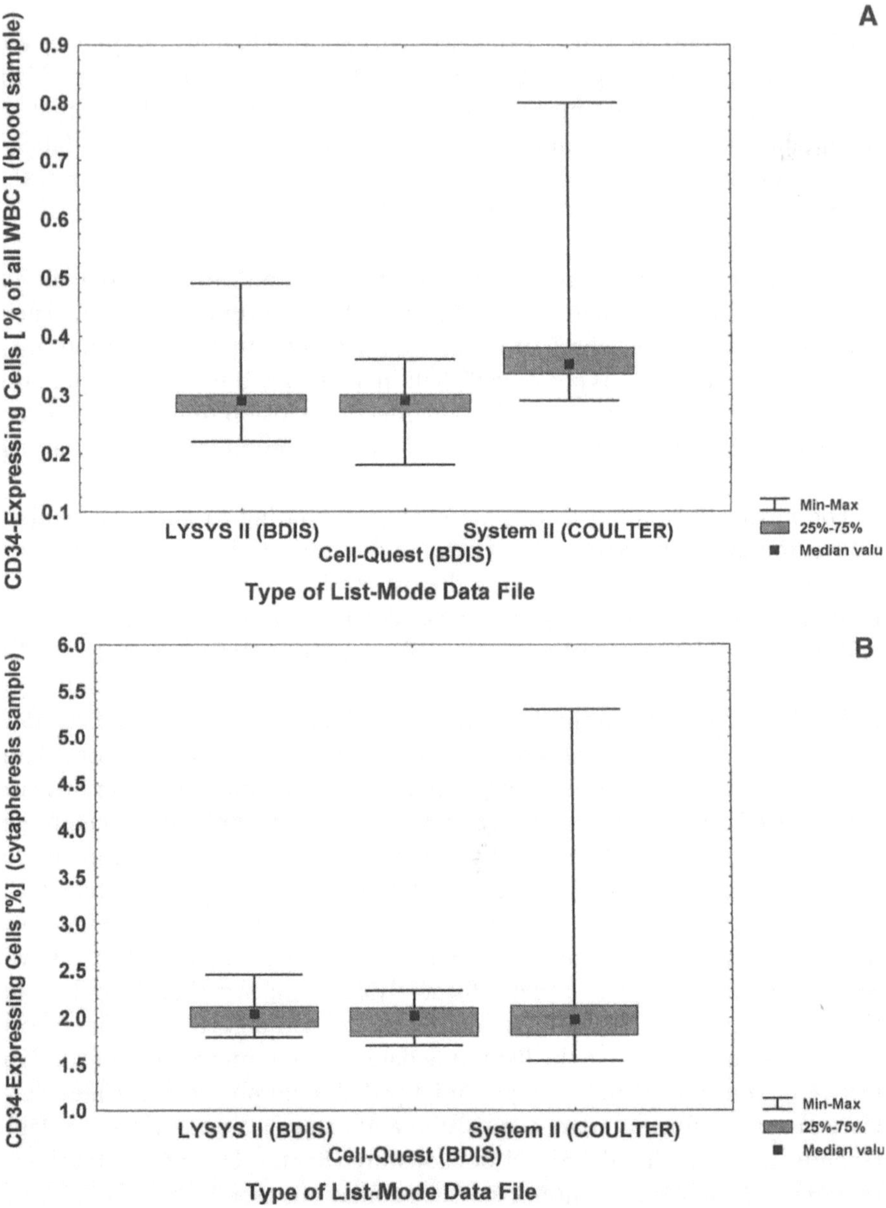

Fig. 2.16A,B. Statistical summary data from the European survey on standardization of laboratory assessment of hemopoietic stem and progenitor cells (Serke et al. 1998). Identical list-mode data shipped to the self-selected participants were analyzed by the participants; list-mode data in three different software formats (LYSYS II, Cell-Quest, SYSTEM II), but containing identical measurements, were shipped. Participants were asked to determine the percentage of the CD34-expressing cells among all leukocytes. Shown are the medians, the quartiles, and the ranges. **A** CD34-expressing cells (% of all blood cells). **B** CD34-expressing cells (% of all cytapheresis cells)

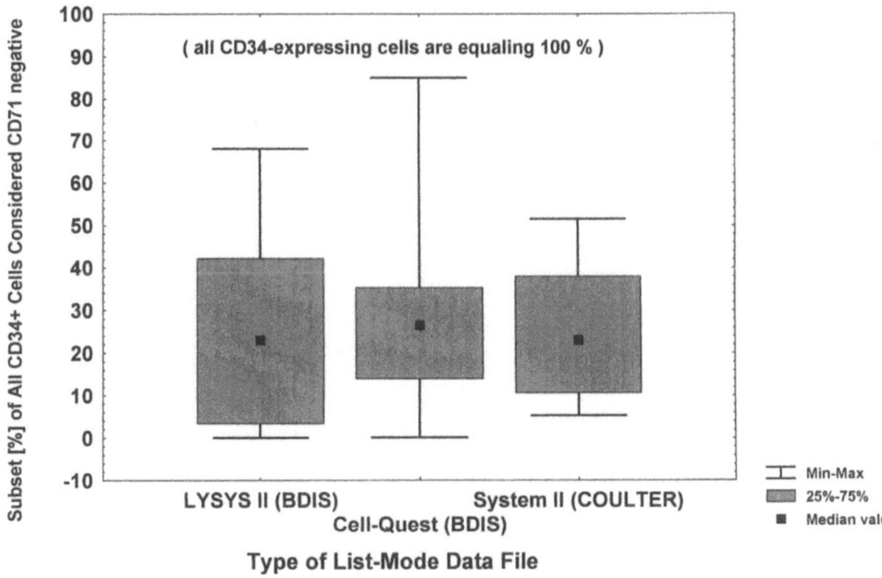

Fig. 2.17. Statistical summary data from the European survey on standardization of laboratory assessment of hemopoietic stem and progenitor cells (Serke et al. 1998); identical list-mode data shipped to the self-selected participants were analyzed by the participants; list-mode data in three different software formats (LYSYS II, Cell-Quest, SYSTEM II), but containing identical measurements, were shipped; participants were asked to determine the percentage, among all CD34-expressing cells, of the CD34-expressing cells lacking the coexpression of the CD71 antigen; the list-mode data files contained 2000 gated CD34-expressing cells, thus providing a meaningful number of CD34-expressing cells, in terms of definition of even minor subpopulations; shown are the medians, the quartiles, and the ranges

ally, the samples shipped should be identical to the diagnostic samples routinely processed. For a number of reasons, however, there are tendencies to ship stabilized samples, which, at the most, mimic clinical samples (Barnett et al. 1996). In Germany, INSTAND routinely ships samples fitting all criteria of clinical samples. The survey established most recently is that for CD34-expressing cells (Serke and Huhn 1998). The data from this survey, typically presented as Youden plots, are shown in Fig. 2.18. It is evident that there are "low counters" and "high counters" among the participants, a finding primarily described for microscopic counting of reticulocytes by Peebles et al. (1981). The substantial finding shown in Fig. 2.17, however, is that at percentages well below 0.5, and at absolute numbers of less than 20/µl, almost identical determinations of one particular cell population at various laboratories are feasible.

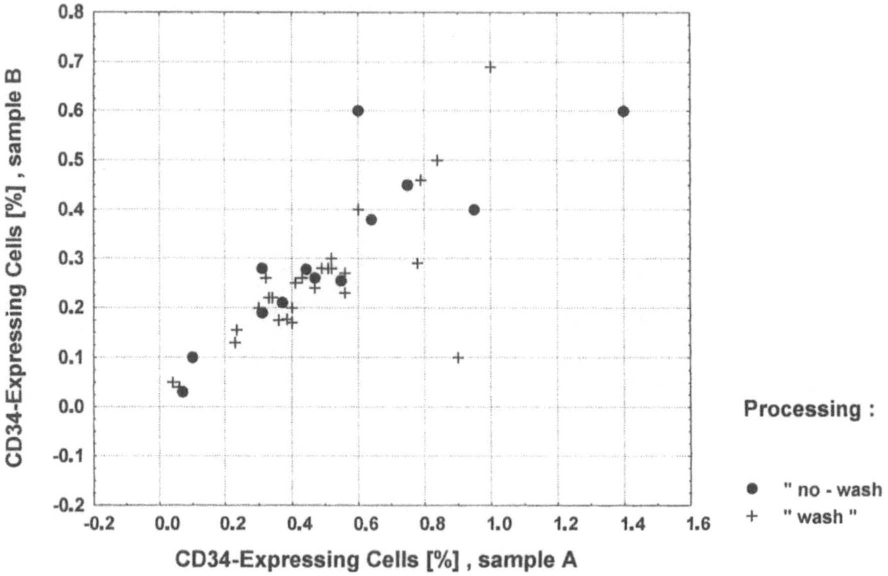

Fig. 2.18. Typical Youden plot showing the individual determinations of the participants in the April 1997 INSTAND external quality assessment survey on CD34-expressing cells; each mark denotes one individual participant; 33 participants processed the samples "wash", and 11 participants processed the sample "no-wash"; it is evident that there are "low-counting" participants and "high-counting" participants; therefore, by Pearson product-moment correlation, the *R*-values (at $P<0.01$) are: "wash", 0.68; "no-wash", 0.84

2.7 Perspectives

Although multiparameter flow cytometry is the optimal tool for a number of hematological laboratory determinations, and effectively it is the only one for some of those, this method is not an integral part of each hematological laboratory. The major obstacles to a more widespread introduction of this method are manifold. First, this technique is cost-intensive, with regard to both the flow cytometry device and the reagents. Second, the technique requires a lot of understanding of physics and cellular biology, and there is little enthusiasm among clinical hematologists to enter into these fields of "basic science". Third, the answers given by this technique, e.g. the diagnostic applications, can, seemingly, be given by alternative techniques such as immunocytochemistry. Fourth, the particular strengths of this technique are fully evidenced in applications which general laboratories are not faced with frequently. Among those applications there should be cited all the major areas of this technique as described in Sects. 2.5.1–2.5.4. It should be emphasized, however, that the laboratory hematologist not recognizing the potentials of this technique is running the risk of leaving this highly interesting area of hematological analysis to the representatives of other specialties, such as pathology and clinical chemistry, who realize the advantages and the potentials of this technique. As a consequence, this important diagnostic field will be lost as an integral part of the hematological laboratory.

References

Barclay AN, Brown MH, Law SKA, McKnight AJ, Tomlinson MG, Van Der Merwe PA (eds) (1997) The leukocyte antigen facts book. Academic Press, London

Barnett CW (1933) The unavoidable error in the differential count of the leukocytes in the blood. J Clin Invest 12:77–85

Barnett D, Granger V, Mayr P, Storie I, Wilson GA, Reilly JT (1996) Evaluation of a novel stable whole blood quality control material for lymphocyte subset analysis: results from the UK NEQAS Immune Monitoring Scheme. Cytometry 26:216–222

Bene MC, Castoldi G, Knapp W, Ludwig WD, Matutes E, Orfao A, Van't Veer MB (1995) Proposals for the immunological classification of acute leukemias. European Group for the Immunological Characterization of Leukemias (EGIL). Leukemia 9:1783–1786

Bernard A, Boumsell L, Dauset J, Milstein C, Schlossman SF (eds) (1984) Leukocyte typing. Springer Verlag, Heidelberg

Bernstein ID, Leary AG, Andrews RG, Ogawa M (1991) Blast colony-forming cells and precursors of colony-forming cells detectable in long-term marrow culture express the same phenotype (CD33- CD34+). Experimental Hematology 19:680–682

Beyer J, Schwella N, Zingsem J, Strohscheer I, Schwaner I, Oettle H, Serke S, Huhn D, Siegert W (1995) Hematopoietic rescue after high-dose chemotherapy using autologous peripheral-blood progenitor cells or bone marrow: a randomized comparison. J Clin Oncol 13:1328–1335

Bikoue A, George F, Poncelet P, Mutin M, Janossy G, Sampol J (1996) Quantitative analysis of leukocyte membrane antigen expression: normal adult values. Cytometry 26:137–147

Braylan RC, Borowitz MJ, Davis BH, Stelzer GT, Stewart CC (1997) U.S.-Canadian consensus recommendations on the immunophenotypic analysis of hematologic neoplasias by flow cytometry. Cytometry 30:213

Centers for Disease Control and Prevention (1997) 1997 Revised guidelines for performing CD4+ T-cell determinations in persons infected with human immunodeficiency virus (HIV). Morbidity and Mortality Weekly Report 46:1–29

Chance JT, Larsen SA, Pope V, Measel JW, Cox DL (1995) Instrument-dependent fluorochrome sensitivity in flow cytometric analysis. Cytometry 22:232–242

Civin CI, Strauss LC, Brovall C, Fackler MJ, Schwartz JF, Shaper JH (1984) Antigenic analysis of hematopoiesis: III. a hematopoietic progenitor cell surface antigen defined by a monoclonal antibody raised against KG-1a cells. J Immunol 133:157–161

Denny TN, Stein D, Mui T, Scolpino A, Holland B (1996): Quantitative determination of surface antibody binding capacities of immune subset present in peripheral blood of healthy adult donors. Cytometry 26:265–274

Davis BH, Foucar K, Szczarkowski W, Ball E, Witzig T, Foon KA, Wells D, Kotylo P, Johnson

R, Hanson C, Bessman D (1997) U.S.-Canadian consensus recommendations on the immunophenotypic analysis of hematologic neoplasias by flow cytometry: Medical indications. Cytometry 30:249–263

Dercksen MW, Gerritsen WR, Rodenhuis S, Dirkson MKA, Slaper-Cortenbach ICM, Schaasberg WP, Pinedo HM, Von Dem Borne AEGKr, Van Der Schoot EC (1995) Expression of adhesion molecules on CD34+ cells: CD34+ L-selectin + cells predict a rapid platelet recovery after peripheral blood stem cell transplantation. Blood 85:3313–3319

Dercksen MW, Rodenhuis S, Dirkson MKA, Schaasberg WP, Baars JW, Van Der Wall E, Slaper-Cortenbach ICM, Pinedo HM, Von Dem Borne AEGKr, Van Der Schoot EC, Gerritsen WR(1995) Subsets of CD34+ cells and rapid hematopoietic recovery after peripheral blood stem cell transplantation. J Clin Oncol 13:1922–1932

Effros RB, Allsopp R, Chiu CP, Hausner MA, Hirji K, Wang L, Harley CB, Villeponteau B, West MD, Giorgi JV (1996) Shortened telomeres in the expanded CD28-CD8+ cell subset in HIV disease implicate replicative senescence in HIV pathogenesis. AIDS 10:17–22

Groeneveld K, te Marvelde JG, Van Den Beemd MWM, Hooijkaas H, Van Dongen JJM (1996) Flow cytometric detection of intracellular antigens for immunophenotyping of normal and malignant leukocytes. Leukemia 10:1383–1389

Gutensohn K, Serke S (1996) Durchflußzytometrische Analyse CD34-experimentierender hämatopoetischer Zellen in Blut und Zytaphereseprodukten. Infusionsther Transfusionsmed 23 (Suppl 2):1–23

Krause DS, Fackler MJ, Civin CI, May WS (1996) CD34: structure, biology, and clinical utility. Blood 87:1–13

Kreissig C, Kirsch A, Serke S (1994) Characterization and measurement of CD34-expressing hematopoietic cells. J Hematotherapy 3:263–290

Macey MG, McCarthy DA, Davies C, Newland AC (1997) The Q-Prep system: effects on the apparent expression of leukocyte surface antigens. Cytometry 30:67–71

Liu Z, Hultin LE, Cumberland WG, Hultin P, Schmid I, Matud JL, Detels R, Giorgi JV (1996) Elevated relative fluorescence intensity of CD38 antigen expression on CD8+ T cells is a marker of poor prognosis in HIV infection: results of 6 years of follow-up. Cytometry 26:1–7

Mandy FF, Bergeron M, Minkus T (1997) Evolution of leukocyte immunophenotyping as influenced by the HIV/AIDS pandemic: a short history of the development of gating strategies for CD4+ T-cell enumeration. Cytometry 30:157–165

Marti G, Johnsen HE, Sutherland DR, Serke S (1998) Towards a worldwide reference method for the flow cytometric determination of CD34-expressing cells. J Hematotherapy, in press, February 1998

Metcalf D (1977) Hemopoietic colonies. Recent Results in Cancer Research 61

Ostendorf T, Nischan C, Schubert J, Grussenmeyer T, Scholz C, Zielinska-Skowronek M, Schmidt RE (1995) Heterogenous PIG-A mutations in different cell lineages in paroxysmal nocturnal hemoglobinuria. Blood 85:1640–1646

Peebles DA, Hochberg A, Clarke TD (1981) Analysis of manual reticulocyte counting. Am J Clinical Pathol 76:713–717

Porwit-MacDonald A, Janossy G, Ivory K, Swirsky D, Peters R, Wheatley K, Walker H, Turker A, Goldstone AH, Burnett A (1996) Leukemia-associated changes identified by quantitative flow cytometry. IV. CD34 overexpression in acute myelogenous leukemia M2 with t(8;21). Blood 87:1162–1169

Rothe G, Schmitz G, Adorf D, Barlage S, Gramatzki M, Hanenberg H, Höffkes HG, Janossy G, Knüchel R, Ludwig WD, Nebe T, Nerl C, Orfao A, Serke S, Sonnen R, Tichelli A, Wörmann B (1996) Consensus protocol for the flow cytometric immunophenotyping of hematopoietic malignancies. Leukemia 10:877–895

Schneider U, van Lessen A, Huhn D, Serke S (1997) Two subsets of peripheral blood plasma cells defined by differential expression of CD45 antigen. Br J Haematol 97:56–64

Schubert J, Schmidt RE (1992) Paroxysmale nächtliche Hämoglobinurie. Dtsch Med Wochenschr 117:985–989

Schwella N, Siegert W, Beyer J, Rick O, Zingsem, J, Eckstein R, Serke S, Huhn D (1995) Autografting with blood progenitor cells: predictive value of preapheresis blood cell counts on progenitor harvest and correlation of the reinfused cell dose with hematopoietic reconstitution. Ann Hematol 71:227–234

Schwella N, Beyer J, Heuft HG, Rick O, Schwaner I, Serke S, Huhn D, Siegert W (1996) Value of preapheresis cell counts on PBPC harvest and effect of reinfused cell dose on engraftment. Bone Marrow Transplant 18 (Suppl 1):8–9

Schwella N, Beyer J, Schwaner I, Heuft H-G, Rick O, Huhn D, Serke S, Siegert W (1996) Impact of preleukapheresis cell counts on collection results and correlation of progenitor-cell dose with engraftment after high-dose chemotherapy in patients with germ cell cancer. J Clin Oncol 14:1114–1121

Serke S (1988) In situ immunocytochemical staining method for haemopoietic cells grown in vitro. J Immunol Methods 115:187–193

Serke S, Huhn D (1990) Effects of various recombinant human hemopoietic growth factors (rhEpo, rhG-CSF, rhGM-CSF, rhIl-3) on the growth of peripheral blood progenitor cells (BFU-E, CFU-GM). Blut 61:25–29

Serke S, Säuberlich S, Huhn D (1991a) Multiparameter flow-cytometrical quantitation of circulating CD34^{+}-cells: correlation to the quantitation of circulating haemopoietic progenitor cells by in vitro colony-assay. Br J Haematol 77:453–459

Serke S, Säuberlich S, Huhn D (1991b) A liquid culture method for the in vitro growth of hemopoietic progenitor cells from normal human adult peripheral blood allowing for analysis by multiparameter flow cytometry. Eur J. Haematol 46:85–92

Serke S, Säuberlich S, Abe Y, Huhn D (1991) Analysis of CD34-positive hemopoietic progenitor cells from normal human adult peripheral blood: flow-cytometrical studies and in vitro colony (CFU-GM,BFU-E) assays. Ann Hematol 62:45–53

Serke S, Huhn D (1992) On the quantitative determinations of blood CD34-positive cells. Blood 80:1628–1629

Serke S, Huhn D (1993) An all leukocyte whole blood lyse method for multiparameter flow cytometry. Clin Lab Haematol 15:275–285

Serke S, Zingsem J, Zimmermann R, Huhn D, Eckstein R (1993) Optimierung der Leukozytapheresen zur Gewinnung zirkulierender hämopoetischer Stamm- und Vorläuferzellen durch Multiparameter-Durchflußzytometrie. Beitr Infusionsther 31:111–117

Serke S (1995) Detection of terminal deoxynucleotidyl transferase by permeabilization of cells using a standard red blood cell lyse reagent. Cytometry 19:189–190

Serke S, Huhn D (1996) Expression of class I, II, and III epitopes of the CD34 antigen by normal and leukemic hemopoietic cells. Cytometry 26:154–160

Serke S, Meldgard-Knudsen L, Watts M, Schneider U, Schwella N, Linch D, Johnsen HE (1996) Mobilized peripheral blood CD34-expressing cells: inverse correlation of both absolute and relative numbers to in vitro clonogenity. Br J Haematol 95:234–240

Serke S, Arseniev L, Watts M, Fritsch G, Ingles-Esteve J, Johnsen HE, Linch D, Cancelas JA, Meyer O, Kadar JG, Huhn D, Matcham J (1997) Imprecision of counting CFU-GM colonies and CD34-expressing cells. Bone Marrow Transpl 20:57–61

Serke S, Huhn D (1998) German proficiency testing survey: circulating CD34-expressing cells. J Hematotherapy, in press, January 1998

Serke S, Johnsen HE, Kvalheim G (1998) Standardizing the laboratory assessment of haemopoietic stem- and progenitor-cells: results from two European surveys. Bone Marrow Transplantation, submitted

Siegert W, Serke S (1996) Cytokine mobilized blood CD34 expressing cells are not cycling. Bone Marrow Transpl 17:467–470

Siena S, Bregni M, Brando B, Ravagnani F, Bonadonna G, Gianni AM (1989) Circulation of CD34+ hematopoietic stem cells in the peripheral blood of high-dose cyclophosphamide-treated patients: enhancement by intravenous recombinant human granulocyte-macrophage colony-stimulating factor. Blood 74:1905–1914

Stelzer GT, Marti G, Hurley A, McCoy Jr. P, Lovett EJ, Schwartz A (1997) U.S.-Canadian consensus recommendations on the immunophenotypic analysis of hematologic neoplasias by flow cytometry: standardization and validation of laboratory procedures. Cytometry 30:214–230

Stewart CC, Behm FG, Carey JL, Cornbleet J, Duque RE, Hudnall SD, Hurtubuise PE, Loken M, Tubbs RR, Wormsley S (1997) U.S.-Canadian consensus recommendations on the immunophenotypic analysis of hematologic neoplasias by flow cytometry: selection of antibody combinations. Cytometry 30:231–235

Sutherland DR, Marsh JCW, Davidson J, Baker MA, Keating A, Mellors A (1992) Differential sensitivity of CD34 epitopes to cleavage by pasteurella haemolytica glycoprotease: implications for purification of CD34-positive progenitor cells. Exp Hematol 20:590–599

Udomsakdi C, Lansdorp PM, Hogge DE, Reid DS, Eaves AC, Eaves CJ (1992) Characterization of primitive hematopoietic cells in normal human peripheral blood. Blood 80:2513–2521

3 Molecular Biology*

A. Neubauer · C. Thiede · S. Nagel

3.1 Introduction

3.1.1 General Comments

The introduction of molecular biological methods has not only changed the view of the basic scientist, but also that of the scientist involved in translational research as well as clinical medicine. This is true not only for novel diagnostic methodologies, but also for new therapeutic strategies. Molecules such as DNA and RNA can now be modified to serve as drugs, e.g. for vaccination strategies. Why molecular biology seems to have changed especially the field of hematology and oncology can only be speculated. It may be that some diseases in these subdisciplines have long served as model systems in medicine.

Molecular biology deals with methods focused on analysing and changing nucleic acids, but is also interested in investigating and modifying protein structures and functions. The molecules DNA, RNA and proteins are strictly related and depend on each other. Thus, when one wants to isolate a novel protein, in some instances it is wise to isolate the corresponding nucleic acid and then study the DNA sequence first. Knowing the DNA (or, for this matter, cDNA for copy DNA because the mRNA has been copied to DNA in order to work with it more easily) sequence then allows one to amplify, clone and manipulate the molecule.

Cancer is thought to be the result of a genetic process. These changes involve dominant proto-oncogenes such as ras, myc, or bcl-2, and recessive tumor-suppressor genes such as p53, Rb or p16/MTS-1. In addition, genes encoding for DNA repair enzymes may be mutated in cancer cells. The genetic alterations involving proto-oncogenes, tumor suppressor genes or DNA repair genes are either somatic mutations and thus occur only in the tumor cell; alternatively, germ line mutations may be detected in these genes. Most can-

*Supported by grants from the Deutsche Forschungsgemeinschaft, Wilhelm Sander Stiftung, and the German José-Carreras Foundation

cers are the result of a genetic multi-step process (Liu 1989; Fearon and Vogelstein 1990). Many different genes need to be altered in order to give rise to the growth advantage needed for malignant transformation. Rarely, a lesion in a single gene causes a malignant disease (i.e. retinoblastoma).

The lesions leading to genetic instability resulting in malignant transformation may be very different; *point mutations* causing the exchange of one single base in the DNA molecule; *genomic deletions* of genes negatively regulating cell growth or coding for DNA repair enzymes; *genomic translocations* leading to either novel fusion genes with new and tumor-specific functions (e.g. translocation t9;22 in chronic myelogenous leukemia) or resulting in an over-expressed normal gene product (e.g. translocation t14;18 in follicular lymphomas). The reason for acquiring somatic mutations is not clearly understood yet. Why is one single cell able to accumulate many different genetic lesions? Recent studies point to the oxygen supply as an important factor in sustaining normal growth control in tissues (Graeber et al. 1996; Polyak et al. 1997); in addition, different growth rates may result in different mutation rates in a similar genetic background (Richards et al. 1997). Concerning genomic translocations, there have been recent reports that, for example, the bcr-abl translocation (t9;22) may be the result of a wrong "crossing-over", since in human hematopoietic cells, normal chromosome 9q and 22q are structurally close to each other. A DNA break in both chromosomes may then lead to a mistake in linking both DNA strands, while the cells try to fix the DNA breaks (Kozubek et al. 1997).

Figure 3.1 shows the interaction of DNA, RNA, and protein. In mammals this is thought to be a one way route (i.e. DNA→RNA→protein). The process of synthesizing RNA out of DNA is called *transcription*, that of protein out of RNA *translation*. The primary transcript is subject to splicing, which is not known in bacteria. Splicing shortens the RNA significantly and enables the RNA to cut out sequences which may not be translated into protein (i.e. intronic sequences).

Molecular techniques target all stages described above: investigation on the genomic level and detection of gene expression using either RNA or protein as molecules. With regard to the genomic level, the chromosomes can be examined using standard cytogenetic techniques. In recent years, a technique called fluorescence in situ hybridization (FISH) has been introduced into hematologic laboratories because of its ease and beauty. Cytogenetics and fluorescence in situ hybridization are described somewhere else in this book (chapter by Prof. Dr. Fonatsch). Genomic level also means *genomic DNA*. Since DNA is a rather large molecule, it is difficult to prepare DNA in vitro without shearing the high molecular weight DNA. For isolating large intact DNA [fragments above 50–100 kilobases (kb) in size], different protocols have to be used compared to the standard DNA isolation procedure. The large DNA fragments are needed, e.g. in pulsed-field gelelectrophoresis. DNA suit-

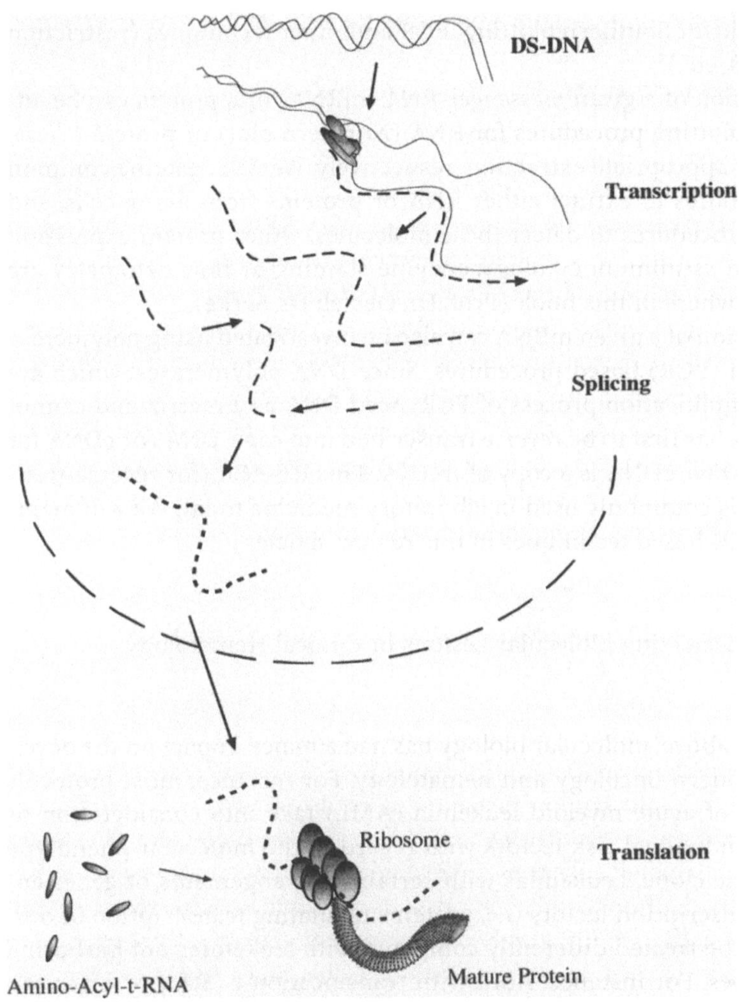

Fig. 3.1. Displays the organization of a single cell. DNA is the genetic material which, given appropriate transcription factors, gives rise to a transcribed RNA. This transcribed RNA is then spliced (i.e. shortened, intronic sequences are cut out) and translocated into the cytoplasm. Here, the transcript is translated at the ribosome into a protein, which may then be subject to chemical (e.g. glycosylation) or physical changes. After the mature protein has been synthesized and modified, the protein encounters its function (e.g. hemoglobin in red cells, rhodopsin in retinal cells, myoglobin in myocytes)

able for pulsed-field gelelectrophoresis may be isolated using agarose beads. However, there are too few applications in diagnostic hematology and oncology to discuss the isolation in detail. Instead, we will describe regular DNA extraction protocols yielding a fragment size of approximately 25–30 kb. This

DNA is suitable for Southern blotting, PCR and other techniques (restriction endonucleases, etc.).

The expression of a given *messenger-RNA* (mRNA) or a *protein* can be analyzed using blotting procedures for RNA (Northern blot) or protein (Western blot) after appropriate extraction, respectively. We will describe common routine procedures to extract either RNA or proteins from living cells, and the blotting procedures to detect these molecules. Other protein expression measures such as immunocytology, enzyme staining or flow cytometry are discussed elsewhere in this book (Prof. Dr. Oertel; Dr. Serke).

The expression of a given mRNA can also be investigated using polymerase chain reaction (PCR) based procedures. Since DNA polymerases, which are used in the amplification process of PCR, need DNA as a matrix and cannot use RNA, RNA has first to be *reverse* transcribed into *copy*-DNA (or cDNA for that matter). Thus, cDNA is a copy of mRNA. This RT-PCR (for reverse-transcribed PCR) is commonly used in laboratory medicine today. We will mainly focus on PCR-based techniques in this review article.

3.1.2 Usefulness of Detecting Molecular Lesions in Clinical Hematology and Oncology

As mentioned above, molecular biology has had a major impact on the development of modern oncology and hematology. For instance, most protocols for treatment of acute myeloid leukemia (AML) take into consideration or even stratify individual risk factors with regard to the molecular phenotype of the leukemic clone. Leukemias with certain rearrangements of genes encoding for transcription factors (i.e. proteins regulating transcription of other genes) will be treated differently compared with leukemias not harboring these genotypes. For instance, AML with translocation t (8;21) or inversion inv (16) may be best treated in the post-induction therapy and thus probably cured with one or more courses of high-dose cytosine arabinoside, whereas leukemias with complex genomic changes, deletions of chromosomes 5 and 7 or rearrangements of chromosome 11q23 harbor a poor prognosis and thus are best referred to allogeneic bone marrow transplantation in first remission (reviewed in Look 1997).

Another example is the presence (or absence, for that matter) of the Philadelphia chromosome encoding the bcr-abl-fusion gene in acute lymphoblastic leukemias (ALL) in adults, which can be detected in approx. 30% of de novo ALL cases. Patients with this phenotype have a very poor prognosis, as opposed to patients without this lesion (reviewed in Look 1997).

In oncology, different treatment modalities may be chosen because of the molecular genotype of a patient´s sample; for instance, deletion of the p53 gene, the most frequently mutated/deleted gene in human cancer, harbors poor prognosis in many cancers, such as breast or colon cancer, and leukemias (Chen et al. 1991; Runnebaum et al. 1991; Hamilton 1992; Thompson et al. 1992; Bergh et al. 1995; Döhner et al. 1995). In addition, it has been shown that gene amplification/overexpression of the receptor tyrosine kinase gene c-erbB2 in principal worsens the prognosis of individuals with breast and ovary cancer; however, in breast cancer, treatment with dose intensification of anthracyclins is of benefit especially in this subgroup (Thor et al. 1989; Muss et al. 1994).

Molecular oncology may thus not only be important for risk stratification, but also for planning the optimal therapy. In addition, gene therapy may be coming to the clinic soon. First trials have shown that there may be promising results, for example, with strategies expressing wild-type P53 in chemotherapy-resistant lung cancers (Roth et al. 1996).

3.2 Methods

3.2.1 Separation of Blood or Bone Marrow Cells for Further Molecular Studies

3.2.1.1 *Principle of Method*

Cells which are in suspension are easily prepared for the extraction of nucleic acids and proteins. If the cells of interest are mixed with other cells (e.g. leukocytes of peripheral blood), separation may be performed using either Ficoll-gradient separation or simple buffy-coat preparations.

3.2.1.2 *Detailed Description of Method*

We prefer blood and bone marrow anticoagulated with 20 U/ml heparin. The heparin should be free of any preservatives. EDTA may also be used. Since EDTA is not appropriate for FISH analysis (see extra chapter), heparin is the drug of choice. The blood sample should be submitted to the molecular laboratory using the fastest way possible. We do not recommend cooling or sending the sample on ice. During extreme climate (outside temperature above 30°C or below −10°C), samples may be altered such that DNA and especially RNA may not be extracted any more.

After arrival in the laboratory, the blood/bone marrow sample is transferred into a new plastic tube labeled with the identification code. After appropriate mixing, blood samples are diluted with one fifth volume with a 5% dextrane solution, mixed and incubated at room temperature for 40 min. Nucleated cells are then separated and washed once in cold PBS. Bone marrow samples are not put on dextran and transferred to the next step immediately, which is lysis of red cells. This is accomplished by mixing the cell pellet obtained from washing or the bone marrow sample with any red cell lysis solution. After incubation, cells are centrifuged and the pellet is washed with cold PBS twice. An alternative for the above protocol is separation with a Ficoll gradient (d=1.077). In either case, cells can be processed further after separation.

3.2.2 Separation of Solid Tissue for Further Molecular Studies

3.2.2.1 *Principle of Method*

Isolation of nucleic acids/protein from cells deriving out of solid tissues have to be performed differently. We prefer to extract RNA, DNA and protein from cells snap frozen in liquid nitrogen.

3.2.2.2 *Detailed Method*

Small tissue samples are frozen down in appropriate tubes without the addition of buffer or sodium chloride. For extraction of nucleic acids/proteins, the tissue is not thawed but put onto a Petri dish precooled with liquid nitrogen. The tissue is then minced and directly put into the extraction buffer (see below). When RNA is extracted, it is important to make sure that the correct cell number is used.

By following this protocol, degradation of nucleic acids/proteins is mainly avoided.

3.2.3 Extraction of High-Molecular Weight DNA from Living Cells

3.2.3.1 *Principle of Method*

DNA is a rather stable molecule. It is, however, a large molecule, and thus extraction of high-molecular weight DNA needs special precautions. Nucleated cells are put into single cell suspension. Cells are lysed and the DNA is extracted using standard phenol-chloroform procedures and ethanol precipitation. Alternatively, columns may be used instead, according to the manufacturer. The optimal procedure has to be defined by each laboratory.

3.2.3.2
Detailed Method

After incubating the cells in appropriate buffer solutions, approx. 10E6 to 5×10E6 cells are incubated in 4 ml STE (1× STE, pH 8.0=150 mM NaCl; 1 mmM Tris, 1 mM EdTA). After mixing, 100 μl of a 20 mg/ml proteinase K solution are added and cells are mixed; 2.5 ml of a 10% SDS solution are added in order to lyse cellular membranes. The solution is mixed by inverting the reaction tube very carefully. Caution: too vigorous shaking may result in degradation of high molecular weight DNA. The solutions is incubated at 55°C overnight. One volume of high quality buffer saturated phenol is added and the tube put onto a shaker for 15 min. The tube is centrifuged at 12,000 *g* for 10 min and the aqueous phase is put into a new tube. It is important to avoid contamination with the protein or the organic phase. The phenol step has to be repeated once. After that, chloroform is added at equal volume. The tube is put onto a shaker for 15 min and centrifuged at 12,000 *g* for 10 min. Again, the aqueous phase is extracted and put into a fresh tube; 0.1 volume of a 3 M sodium acetate solution, and 2 volumes ice-cold ethanol (best quality) are added. Immediately, spinning-out of high-molecular weight DNA is performed using, e.g. a glass pipette. The DNA is then washed twice with 70% ethanol and dried for 12 h. Thereafter, it is transferred either into aqua destillata or 1× TE (TE, pH 8.0=10 mM Tris, 1 mM EDTA).

3.2.4
Southern Blotting: Quantitative Southern Blotting

Two discoveries were important for developing Southern blotting: cutting high-molecular weight DNA with appropriate DNA restriction enzymes; and blotting techniques. Southern blots (Maniatis et al. 1982) require the presence or absence of a given DNA in a sample, or its different or similar restriction pattern in the genomic DNA.

The most important principle for this technique is that of hybridization. Hybridization refers to pairing of complementary nucleic acids. Due to the basic rule of Crick-Watson base pairing, specific bases will bind to other bases: Adenine binds thymine (in DNA) or uracil (in RNA), guanine binds to cytosine, respectively. Thus, when knowing a single DNA strand, one can automatically deduce its complementary strand:

...A T G C A A T T C G C G...

results in pairing with

...T A C G T T A A G C G C....

The binding of complementary DNA or RNA is called hybridization. Hybridization is the important principle by which certain DNA sequences can be detected by specific, complementary DNA probes. In addition, hybridization takes place during the annealing of DNA primer molecules to cDNA or genomic DNA in the process of the exponential polymerase chain reaction. Schematically, a typical Southern blot consists of the following different steps:

1. Extraction of high-molecular weight DNA from cells isolated from different tissues.
2. Cutting the DNA with appropriate restriction enzymes, which cut the DNA at specific DNA sites.
3. Running the cut sample on a 0.8% agarose gel to separate the DNA molecules by size.
4. Blotting the separated DNA onto a filter paper.
5. Probing the paper with an, e.g. radioactively labeled probe containing the sequence of the gene of interest or parts of it, and washing off the unhybridized probe.
6. Exposing the paper to an X-ray sensitive film and developing this film.

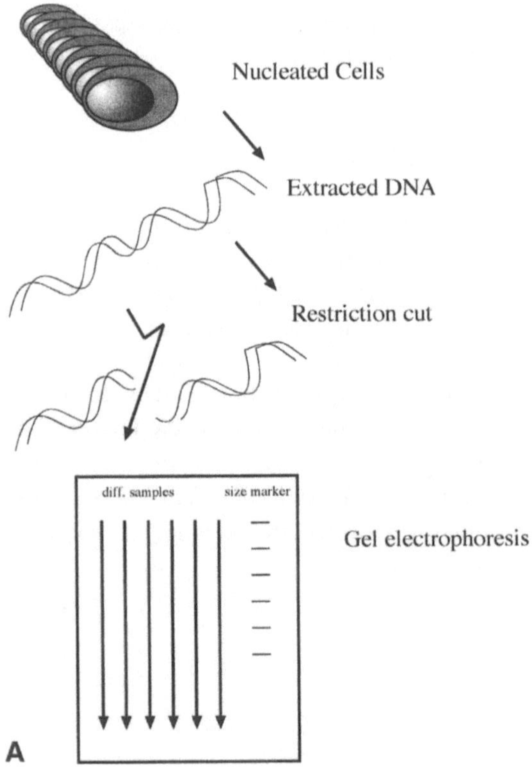

Fig. 3.2A,B. Southern blot. **A** displays the basic principle behind the technique and **B** a typical blot probed for the calcitonin gene (copyright Stockton Press: see Ritter et al. 1995). In this particular sample, high-molecular weight DNA was extracted from different leukemia cell lines, cut with restriction enzymes Msp I (*lanes 2, 4, 6, and 8*) and Hpa II (*lanes 1, 3, 5, and 7*), and probed with a calcitonin-gene probe kindly provided by Dr. S. Baylin

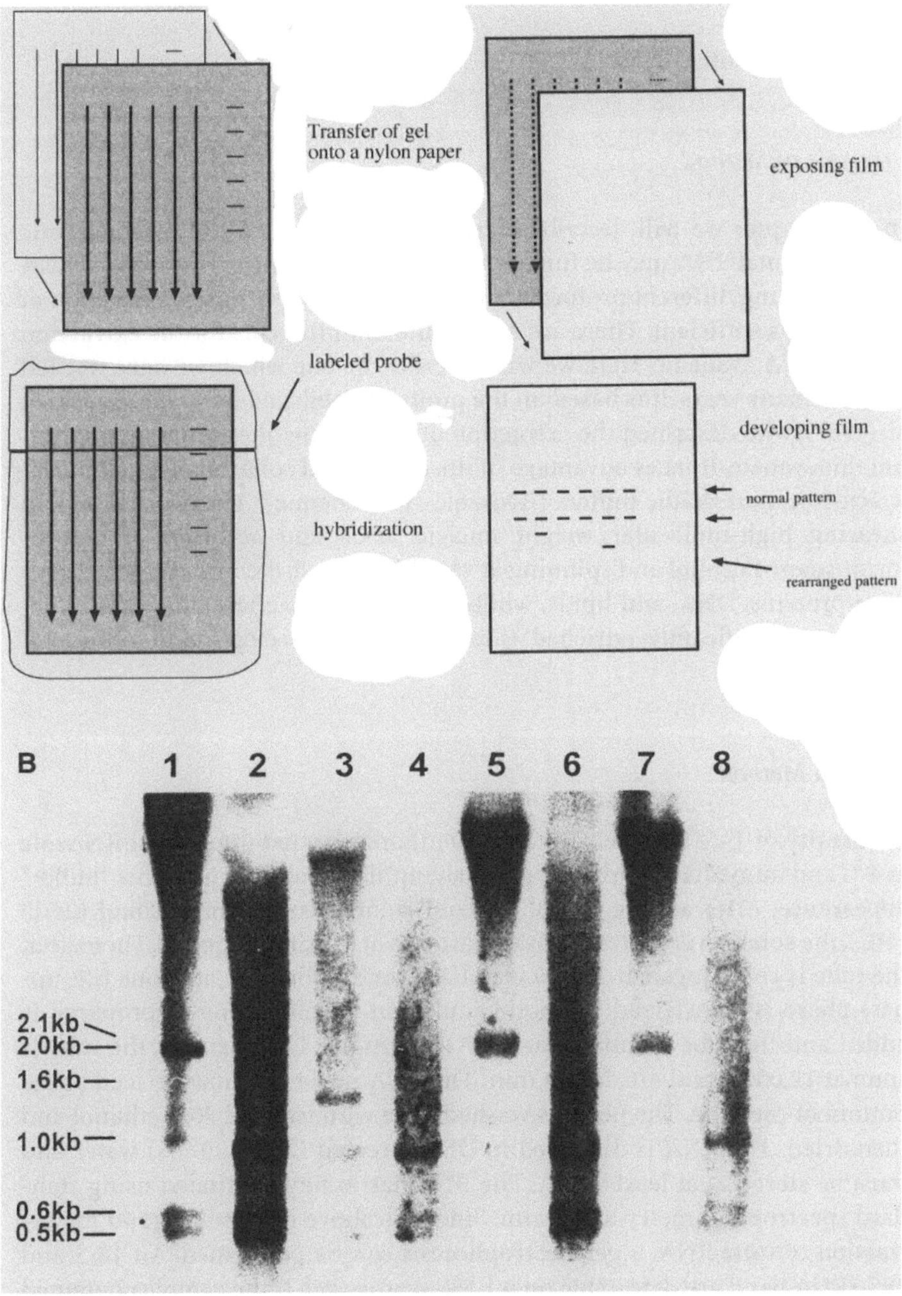

Figure 3.2 displays the principle of a Southern blot (A) and a typical example (B) as a cartoon. For a more detailed description of the method of Southern blotting, see Maniatis (Maniatis et al. 1982; Ausubl 1997).

3.2.5
Extraction of Total RNA

3.2.5.1
Principle of Method

In this chapter we will describe extraction of total RNA out of eukaryotic cells. This total RNA may be further processed to obtain, e.g. messenger RNA (mRNA) using different protocols. However, for most purposes, extraction of total RNA is sufficient. There are many different protocols for the extraction of total RNA available. Here we will describe the one which we have worked with for many years. It is based on the protocol published by Chomczynski et al. (1987), who described the extraction of RNA using phenol and guanidinium thiocyanate. It takes advantage of the differential solution of small nucleic acids in more acidic buffers (RNAzole, AGS Chemie). After vortexing and shearing high-molecular weight nucleic acids and addition of chloroform/isoamylalcohol and spinning at very high speed, the organic phase contains proteins, DNA, and lipids, while in the aqueous phase, the RNA molecules are significantly enriched (i.e. transport, messenger, and ribosomal RNAs).

3.2.5.2
Detailed Method

A quantity of 1–5ˇ10E6 cells (in, e.g. 50 µl) are pipetted into 900 µl RNAzole at 4°C and immediately mixed vigorously, until the solution has got a "milky" appearance. After adding 100 µl ice-cold chloroform/isoamylalcohol (25:1) (4°C), the solution is vortexed for at least 30 s at maximum power. Thereafter, the tube is centrifuged at 12,000 *g* and 4°C for 20 min. The aqueous (i.e. upper) phase is transferred to another tube, an equal volume isopropanol is added and the tube incubated at –20°C overnight. The next day, the tube is spun at 12,000 *g* and 4°C for 20 min. The RNA pellet can now be seen at the bottom of the tube. The pellet is washed once with ice-cold 70% ethanol and then dried. The RNA is dissolved in DEPC-treated (DEPC: 0.1%) water and must be stored at at least –80°C. The RNA has to be quantitated using standard spectrophotometry at 260 nm. Since the above protocol is good for extraction of total RNA, a gel electrophoresis can be performed. An 18 S and 28S-rRNA band are detectable on a 1.5% agarose gel. If the sample contained degraded RNA (often a problem with clinical samples shipped a long way!), a smear of low-molecular weight nucleic acids may be seen, instead of the 18S and 28S rRNA. Frequently, a dilution of the primary material may yield in better and non-degraded RNA. The RNA may now be modified, e.g. using a column or special beads, to enrich mRNA species.

3.2.6
Northern Blotting

3.2.6.1
Principle of Method

Total or mRNA can be used for Northern blotting. Since RNA molecules are much smaller compared to genomic DNA, the samples are electrophoresed directly on a gel. The gel is prepared using formalin to denature RNA and prevent formation of secondary structures (Ausubl 1997). After electrophoresis, the RNA is transferred onto a filter paper and afterwards probed using a directly labeled probe.

3.2.6.2
Detailed Method

Since Northern blotting is currently not routinely performed in hematology and RT-PCR is replacing this laborsome technique, for a detailed description of Northern blotting we refer to standard descriptions (Maniatis et al. 1982; Ausubl 1997).

3.2.7
DNA Polymerase Chain Reaction (PCR)

3.2.7.1
Principle of Method

PCR remains the most frequently used molecular technique throughout laboratories all over the world. PCR is a technique of in vitro amplification of DNA in a test-tube. For example, within 3 h, one DNA copy may be amplified to approx. 5˘10E6 copies. Because of this sensitivity, PCR harbors the danger of contamination. Precautions to avoid contamination have been reported (McPherson et al. 1991). They include that pre-PCR work has to be separated physically from post-PCR procedures (e.g. different building).

The scheme of PCR is displayed in Fig. 3.3. It shows the potential exponential amplification of DNA. In theory, the amplification process should follow a 2 *E n* equation, where *n* is the amount of PCR cycles. This is, however, only true in the first PCR cycles. After a certain amount of cycles, the amplification process switches from an exponential to a linear scale. This implies the biggest advantage of PCR: its invention enabled researchers to use it as an easy technique to amplify a target DNA sequence. In other words, PCR is a novel cloning technique. PCR may not only be used for research purposes, but also

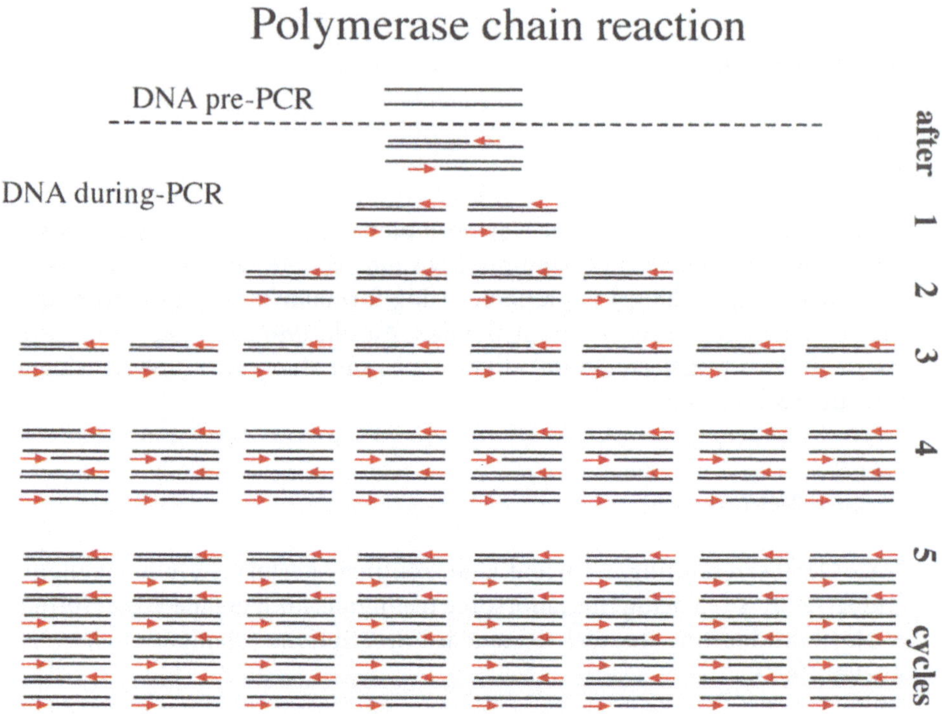

Fig. 3.3. Polymerase chain reaction (PCR). PCR is an in vitro method to clone or amplify genetic material. As source nucleic acid, either genomic DNA or cDNA may be used. The DNA is pipetted together with different PCR reagents and put into a machine cycling through different steps of temperature. One can see that the DNA is amplified by 2 *E n*, where *n* is the amount of PCR cycles. The primers (or PCR-start molecules) are *depicted in red*. Details of PCR are described in the text

for diagnosis in human medicine. There, a target molecule may be derived from human DNA sequences (e.g. presence of certain germ line or somatic mutations), bacterial or viral sequences (detection of *Mycobacterium tuberculosis*; *Helicobacter pylori* or cytomegalovirus).

PCR is an enzymatic reaction taking advantage of heat-stable DNA polymerases derived from *Thermophilus aquatus*. Besides DNA polymerase, small DNA molecules, PCR primers, are used to start (or: prime) the amplification process. The primers are flanking the DNA sequence to be amplified, one primer (the "sense"- or 5′-primer) represents the sense orientation, the remaining (the "anti-sense"- or 3′-primer) the antisense orientation (the other strand). Figure 3.3 denotes the primers in red. These primers are synthesized in machines and commercially available upon the customer′s request. It is important to avoid primer structures which may cause DNA loops or 3′-

prime overhangs. Computer programs (e.g. MacMolly or Laser-Gene) can help to find the optimal DNA sequence of both primers of a given DNA sequence. In addition to enzyme and primers, deoxynucleotides (tri-phosphates or dNTPs) are needed to complete the new DNA strand. All these reagents are put into a PCR buffer containing Mg, potassium, and gelatin. At the end, the target DNA is pipetted into the probe. Then, the sample is transferred to a thermal cycler, a machine which changes its temperatures through different steps (i.e. different temperatures) and cycles (i.e. repeating the incubations several times). These steps are: DNA denaturation at high temperature (94°C), then primer annealing (=hybridization) to the target sequence (depending on their base composition, between 50 and 72°C), and elongation (or polymerization) by the DNA polymerase at 72°C. These incubation steps are automatically performed by the thermal cycler, which repeats these steps between 20 and 35 times (= cycles).

Although easy to perform, it is important to understand the pitfalls of PCR. Since one molecule may be amplified to more than 10ˇ10 E6 within 1 or 2 h, contamination is a serious problem. In most instances, contamination stems from a post-PCR sample. In rare cases, contamination may also be derived from the technician setting up PCR (e.g. amplification of male DNA sequences in pregnant women should always be performed under extreme precautions when a male technician is setting up PCR). For instance, if one tries to detect viral sequences in a given sample, and a truly *negative* sample is contaminated with viral sequences generated in a previous PCR of a different sample, this sample will certainly turn positive. Thus, when setting up a PCR laboratory, the most important step is to take any precaution to avoid PCR contamination. We recommend strictly separating the pre- and post-PCR laboratories. The best advice is to separate these two laboratories in different buildings. Equipment formerly used in a post-PCR room should never be transferred to a pre-PCR situation. Another disadvantage of PCR is its comparable high error rate with regard to the induction of DNA mutations. This is especially important when searching for DNA mutations and in attempts to clone PCR-generated DNA fragments. The reason for this high artificially induced mutation rate is that the mostly used enzyme, *Taq*-DNA polymerase, lacks proofreading activity. Other enzymes are now commercially available which overcome this problem. Another problem frequently encountered in PCR is lack of specific gene amplification. This may be caused by different reasons, for instance: primers, dNTP concentrations, buffer composition, etc.

3.2.7.2
Detailed Description of Method

PCR comes in very different modalities. As source nucleic acid, either genomic DNA or copy-DNA (derived from RNA) may be used. However, the very principle of PCR is always the same (see above).

While the reaction mixture of PCR is pipetted together, it is important to work at low temperature (4°C) to avoid wrong start and mispriming of the PCR. A typical set-up for a PCR starting from genomic DNA is described in Table 3.1. The DNA may be either pipetted before or as the very last reagent. Typically, we use approx. 50 ng genomic DNA, and 1/10 of a cDNA reaction (containing approx. 100 ng reverse-transcribed RNA) for a PCR.

The conditions have to be optimized for each target sequence to be amplified. If PCR amplification is either of poor yield or gives unspecific results, concentrations of primers, dNTPs and Mg may be subject to change. In addition, a different primer sequence may be worth testing.

In order to guarantee full denaturation of genomic DNA, we first denature at 94°C for 3 min, then anneal at 50 to 72°C for 30 s, then do the elongation at 72°C between 30 and 120 s. The respective protocol heavily depends on the sequence to be amplified. After the end of the amplification process, the success of it is checked using a regular agarose-gel stained with ethidium bromide, a molecule which gives a red color upon intercalation with double-stranded DNA when viewed under UV light.

Table 3.1. PCR conditions used in a typical PCR

Reagent	Storage	Concentration in PCR
PCR primer	–20°C	0.25 μM/l
Taq polymerase	–20°C	0.5–1 U
dNTPs	–20°C	200 μM/l each
Mg	–20°C	1.5 mM
KCl	–20°C	50 mmol/l
Tris HCl pH 8.3	–20°C	10 mmol/l
Gelatin	–20°C	0.001% (w/v)

3.2.7.3
Reverse-Transcriptase PCR (RT-PCR)

3.2.7.3.1
Principle of Method

RT-PCR is performed to detect *expressed* (or better: *transcribed* genes) genes. One can take advantage of this fact to look for gene expression of normal gene sequences or specific fusion genes, e.g. in the case of translocated genes (bcr-abl in chronic myelogeneous leukemia). RT-PCR has, because of its sensitivity and ease, replaced Northern blotting in most instances, when one is looking for the level of expression of specific mRNA molecules. For RT-PCR, even heavily degraded RNA may be used. Thus, it is ideally suited for clinical purposes, since the shipping of clinical samples is frequently associated with degradation of RNA molecules.

RNA is extracted from living cells as described above. In a second step, it is reverse-transcribed into copy-DNA (or cDNA), since the polymerases used in PCR may not utilize RNA. This cDNA is then PCR-amplified and the amplification process controlled as decribed above in the case of DNA PCR.

3.2.7.3.2
Detailed Description of Method

Caution. All pipetting steps are to be performed on ice. 1 µg total RNA is dissolved in 8 µl water. As an alternative, 20 ng mRNA may be used instead of 1 µg total RNA. To this solution, 5 µl dNTPs (2.5 mM each), 2 µl 10˘ PCR buffer (see above), 2 µl 0.1 M DTT (Sigma); and 1 µl 100 µM random hexamers (Pharmacia) are added. The solution (20 µl) is put on 90°C for 5 min, then transferred onto ice for 5 min; 1 µl RNAse-inhibitor (Promega) and 0.7 µl reverse transcriptase (we recommend Superscript, Gibco BRL) are added, the mixture is vortexed, shortly spun down and then incubated for 10 min at room temperature, 40 min at 42°C. After this, the tube is put on a thermal block preheated at 90°C for 5 min to inactivate the enzyme. This solution can now be stored at –20°C for some time.

For PCR, approx. 0.5–2 µl of the mixture is removed and used as described above instead of the genomic DNA (see Sect. 3.2.7.2). One has to be aware that cDNA is a single stranded DNA molecule; thus, it is not as stable as genomic DNA; secondly, the amplification process may not be as efficient as when one starts from genomic DNA.

3.2.7.3.3 Quantitative RT-PCR for bcr-abl

3.2.7.3.3.1 General Description

In general, PCR is not a quantitative method. Since the amplification process dramatically depends upon many different parameters (primary and secondary structure of DNA and primers; buffer and dNTP concentrations, enzyme used, etc.), it is not possible to use this process to quantitate the amount of DNA in the sample without changing the setup of the PCR protocol. Of special interest is to quantitate the amount of RNA to measure the expression of certain genes. For this purpose, different methods have been published. Nearly all are based on the usage of so-called "competitors", i.e. molecules with identical primer binding sites but a somewhat different sequence compared to the target sequence (either differing from the target molecule by length or by sequence), which are pipetted in known concentrations into the reaction mixture before PCR is started. Using these competitors as internal standard, one can then quantitate the amount of target molecules from the ratio competitor/target molecule. One of these quantitative approaches is described in this chapter. It is used to measure the amount of bcr-abl molecules in chronic myelogeneous leukemia (CML) (Fig. 3.4).

3.2.7.3.3.2 Detailed Description

The technique takes advantage of the co-amplification of two competitors [one targeting bcr-abl, the other a so-called reference gene, in this case porphobilinogen-deaminase (pbdg)]. A reference gene amplification and co-amplification of its competitor is included because of the variability of the RNA quality of clinical samples. A plasmid construct is used as a common competitor for both genes, thus avoiding pipetting errors (i.e. both competitors are always put into the reaction at identical concentrations). Then, different concentrations of the respective competitor are set-up in order to analyze a given sample. The procedure may also be used in a nested fashion in order to increase sensitivity. A detailed description is given in Nagel et al. (1996).

After PCR has been completed, four different bands may be detected on the agarose gel: one for each competitor, and one for each target gene (bcr-abl and pbdg). These differ in size, so that they can easily be distinguished (see Fig. 3.4). The intensities of each individual band are quantitated using a standard gel scanner and give a good measure for the level of expression. The amount of cDNA molecules in the sample of question is equivalent to the amount of competitor molecules where both bands give identical densitometry results (Fig. 3.4).

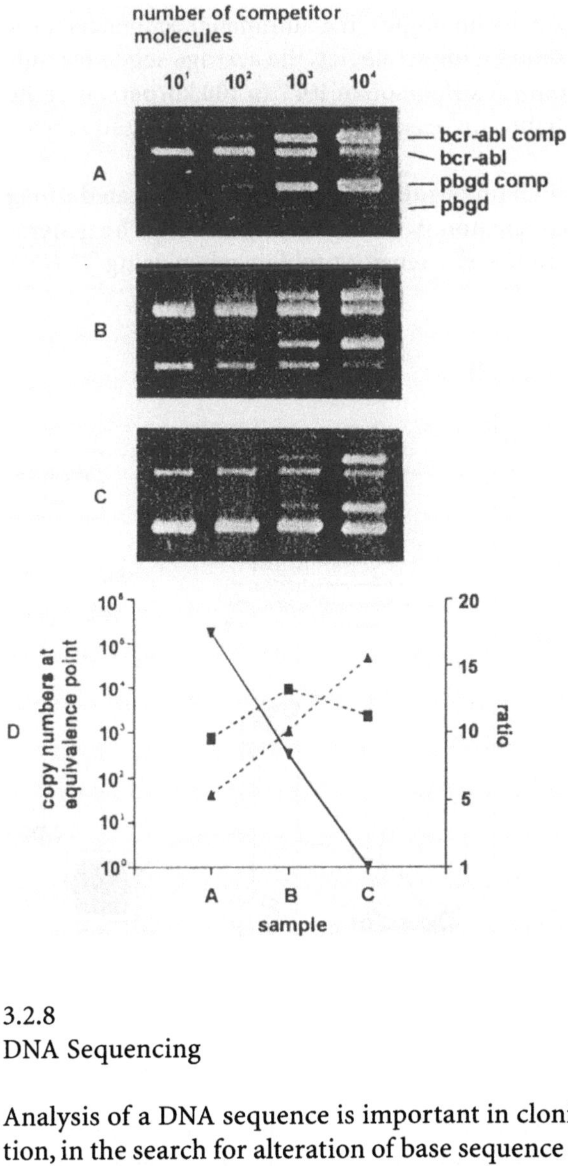

Fig. 3.4. Quantitative RT-PCR for the amount of bcr-abl transcripts in different samples. A novel technique was used to quantitate bcr-abl-transcript number. (Copyright Oxford University Press: see Nagel et al. 1996)

3.2.8 DNA Sequencing

Analysis of a DNA sequence is important in cloning new genes; and, in addition, in the search for alteration of base sequence of critical genes. Changes of base compositions (i.e. mutations) are a common mechanism in the development of human malignancies as well as several hereditary diseases (see "Introduction"). Thus, sequence analysis is an important method in modern molecular medicine.

The most frequently used methods for DNA sequence analysis are the procedures published by Maxam and Gilbert and by Sanger in 1977 (Maxam and Gilbert 1977; Sanger et al. 1977). In the majority of the laboratories, the dideoxy chain termination method published by Sanger is used. However, due to the development of new technologies like automated sequencers, robotic workstations and new sequencing strategies, the average sequence output per year has increased from 1.5 kb/person in 1977 to 100 kb/person in the early 1990 s, and has been further increased by high throughput sequencers (Chen 1994).

The principle of the Sanger chain termination method is illustrated in Fig 3.5. The setup of the sequence reaction is very similar to a PCR. The generation of the necessary single strands was a major problem when using T7 DNA

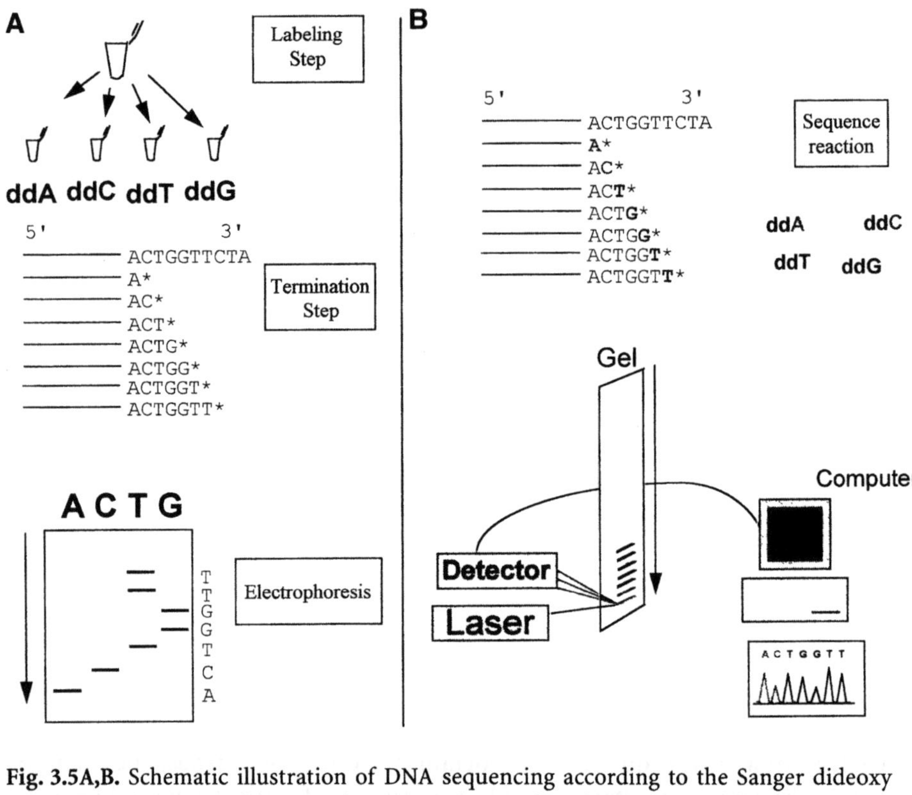

Fig. 3.5A,B. Schematic illustration of DNA sequencing according to the Sanger dideoxy method. **A** This figure illustrates the principal procedure for the Sanger dideoxy method for chain termination sequencing. In a first step, the DNA strand is labeled using a S^{35} or P^{32}. In second step, these prelabeled molecules are than aliquoted in four vials containing the appropriate didyeoxy nucleotides. After chain termination, samples are than loaded on separate lanes on high resolution PAA gels. The sequence can be read from bottom to top. **B** This scheme illustrates sequencing reaction using the dye termination chemistry. The Sanger chain termination reaction is carried out in the presence of dye labeled dideoxy molecules. Upon incorporation of the dye-dideoxy molecule, the strand is labeled. The reaction is than loaded in one lane. Fluorescent labels are activated using a laser beam and the resulting fluorescence is detected in a photomultiplier

polymerase several years ago and required the use of M13 phages, asymmetrical PCR or solid phase approaches. With the widespread use of Taq cycle sequencing, this is no longer a problem. Using an appropriate primer molecule, DNA strands are synthesized in the presence of radiolabeled nucleoside triphosphates (S^{35} or P^{32}). These prelabeled strands are then elongated in the presence of four different dideoxy molecules, which – when incorporated – induce the termination of the strand, since they lack the 5′-deoxy moiety necessary for elongation. This step is carried out in four different reaction vessels in the classical radioactive procedure and in all dye primer approaches. If separated on high resolution polyacrylamide gels (PAA) in four different lanes, a band indicates that a strand had been terminated at this particular base position (Fig. 3.5A).

The chemical basis of modern fluorescence based strategies is similar to the classical procedure; however, labeling is achieved by the attachment of fluorescent dyes to the primer molecule used for sequencing. This still requires four different reaction tubes. A major improvement was achieved by the invention of the dye terminator chemistry. In this approach, the terminator molecules themselves are labeled by four different fluorescent dyes, which enables labeling and termination to be carried out in the same reaction tube (Fig. 3.5B). These samples are loaded on an automated sequencing device. The fluorescent dye is activated using a laser device and the emitted fluorescence is then detected. Processing of the raw data and sequence analysis is then performed on a personal computer. Using this technology on the ABI 377XL, 64 samples can be analyzed in parallel. Read length, i.e. the number of bases which can be read with at least 98% accuracy, is about 650 bases. Best results according to read length and accuracy are obtained using the dye primer chemistry. However, major drawbacks are the limited flexibility and the time needed. Cycle sequencing using the Taq dye terminator approach has been improved substantially recently by the invention of a modified Taq enzyme. These polymerases carry point mutations, which increase their acceptance for the dye dideoxy-nucleotides and the development of novel dye molecules with increased sensitivity. Thus major drawbacks of these technique, like high variability in peak height and sequence gaps, have now been overcome and make this very easy and rapid procedure the method of choice for most sequencing applications.

3.2.8.1
Future Perspectives of DNA Sequencing

Recently, micro-chip based strategies for the screening of known DNA fragments for the presence of mutations (Lipschutz et al. 1995; Kozal et al. 1996) have been invented. This techniques takes advantage of light activated syn-

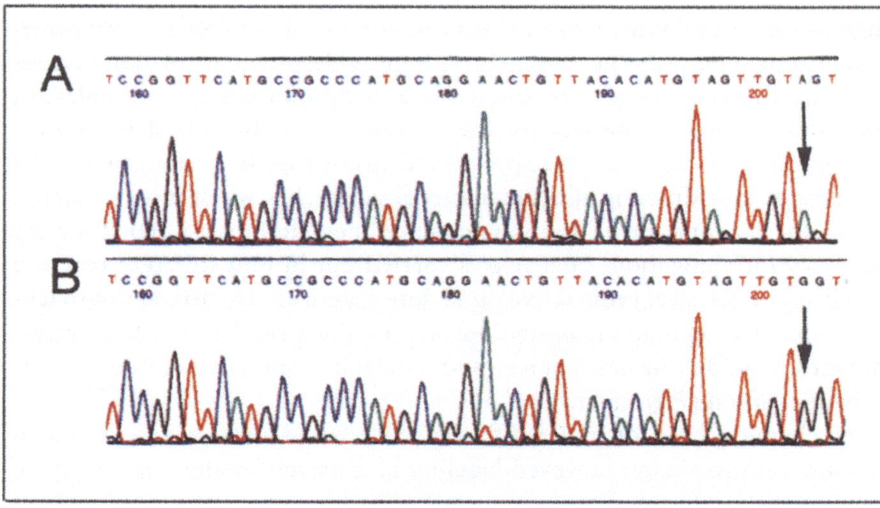

Fig. 3.6A,B. DNA sequencing reaction of a representative portion of the p53-tumor-suppressor gene in two different samples using an automated DNA sequencing machine. The reaction was performed as described in Fig. 3.5. The pictures show a sequencing reaction of the antisense strand of DNA around codon 234 of the p53 gene. Thus, the gel has to be read in antisense orientation *from the right to the left. The arrow* depicts the first base of codon 234, which in its wildtype form is: T A C (encoding tyrosine). In **A** the wildtype sequence is displayed. Since the gel has to be read *from right to left*, and is the antisense, A T G has to be translated to: T A C. In contrast, in **B**, sequence of the B-cell line Raji is shown, which reads G T G, or C A C, encoding histidine. Thus, a T to C mutation can be observed in this B-cell line (*arrow*)

thesis of large panels of 16mer DNA probes on micro chips (up to 20,000/cm^2) covering the whole sequence of a DNA fragment. These arrays enable the screening for every polymorphism in a given sequence. Since this techniques offers the opportunity for automated processing and computer based analysis, high throughput screening of individuals for certain mutations, for example, mutations of the p53 gene, seems possible in near future (Fig. 3.6).

3.2.9
Extraction of Proteins from Living Cells

3.2.9.1
General Description

In contrast to all the other methods mentioned above dealing directly with the genomic message, working with proteins means getting information filtered by the cellular expression machinery, because expression of a distinct protein is often not correlated to raised levels of its specific mRNA molecule.

Because cellular proteins vary in their stability and can easily degrade, resulting in poor detection, one must handle them with the same precautions compared to RNA.

This chapter describes a basic protocol which should be suitable for western blot analysis of most cellular proteins. There also is a variety of other lysis protocols, not mentioned here, which are used when only proteins of a distinct cellular fraction are to be examined. In general, composition and concentration of certain detergents is varied resulting in more or less complete lysis of membranes and organelles.

3.2.9.2
Detailed Description

(The detailed protocol is performed similar to that of Santa Cruz Biotechnology Inc., Research Applications.) Approximately 10E5 to 5×10E6 cells in suspension are collected from cell culture or isolated peripheral blood lymphocytes (PBL) prepared according to the method described in Sect. 3.2.1.2, pelleted by low speed centrifugation (250 *g*) for 5 min and washed twice with PBS at room temperature, carefully removing the supernatant after each centrifugation step. Cell pellets prepared this way can be frozen at –70°C for delayed further processing.

Caution. Beyond this step the complete procedure is carried out on ice taking care not to raise the temperature above 4°C. Then 120–300 µl cold RIPA-lysis buffer (1× PBS, 1% NP40, 0.5 sodium deoxycholate and 0.1% SDS) which has been supplemented immediately before use with 10 µl of a protease inhibiting mix (prepare stock solutions, mix and freeze in aliquots containing 50 µg/ml aprotinin (in 0.01 M HEPES, pH 8.0), 50 µg/ml pepstatin (in ethanol), 50 µg/ml leupeptin (in water) and 20 µl of 100 mM PMSF (in propanol) is added to the cell pellet. Cells are further disrupted and homogenized through repeated aspiration with a 21 gauge needle. The lysate is then centrifuged at 15,000×g for 20 min at 4°C. Alternatively the crude cell lysate can be homogenized by centrifugation through QIA suredders (QIAGEN luc., Hilden, Germany) at 15,000×g for 2 min at 4°C. The supernatant fluid being the total cell lysate is then dispensed into aliquots and can now be stored at –70°C for further use. Protein concentration of the total protein lysate is measured using the BCA (BCA Protein Assay Reagent Kit, PIERCE, Rockford, USA) method following manufacturer´s recommendations.

When dealing with long cellular proteins like the p210 $^{Bcr\text{-}Abl}$ oncoprotein and samples of known protein content are used, a short lysis protocol in electrophoresis sample buffer (according to Santa Cruz, containing 1 ml glycerol, 0.5 ml α-mercaptoethanol, 3 ml 10% SDS, 1.25 ml 1.0 M Tris-HCl pH 6.7, 1–2 mg bromphenol blue, store frozen in small aliquots) and direct submission to polyacrylamide gel electrophoresis (PAGE) has proven to be useful in our lab, because degradation by proteinases is a matter of time and manipulating steps and can such be minimized. Using this strategy photometric analysis of protein content by the BCA method is not possible!

3.2.10
Western Blotting (p210 *bcr-abl*)

3.2.10.1
General Description

Determination of the oncoprotein p210 Bcr-Abl is thought to be a predictive disease marker in Philadelphia chromosome positive leukemic cells. Therefore Bcr-Abl Western blotting and PCR techniques are both used for quantitation of this marker. Usually detected Bcr-Abl levels are then compared to wildtype Abl tyrosine kinase or a convenient reference gene to allow for standardization of results.

We use an Abl tyrosine kinase specific antibody that will also detect the p210 Bcr-Abl oncoprotein.

3.2.10.2
Detailed Description

Prior to polyacrylamide gel electrophoresis (SDS-PAGE) total protein lysate equalling 40-60 µg protein are now mixed with an equal volume of electrophoresis sample buffer or, with the short lysis protocol, directly used and boiled for 3 min on a heating block. Samples are then immediately loaded onto a precast discontinuous SDS-PA gel consisting of a 7,5% separating (lower) and a 3% stacking (upper) gel and run under the following conditions: 60 V for 15 min and 150 V for about 1 h on a BioRad Mini Protean II electrophoresis chamber.

After electrophoresis the gel is equilibrized in blotting buffer (Trizma-Base 3,03 g/l, Glycine 8,55 g/l, 10% Ethanol or Methanol) during assembly of the tank blotting unit. Blotting is performed at 200 mA for approximately 1.5 h on a nitrocellulose membrane. Blotting efficiency can be controlled by staining with Ponceau red.

Non-specific binding of antibodies is blocked by soaking membranes in TBST (TBS with 0,05% Tween 20) with 5% low-fat milk powder for at least 15 min at room temperature. We usually do this overnight at 4°C on a rocking platform.

Membranes are now incubated in primary antibody at 0.5 μg/ml in TBST with 2% milk powder for 45–60 min at room temperature and subsequently washed three times in TBST. We have tested several different Abl antibodies; of all Abl tyrosine kinase specific antibodies available, we have had the best results with the mouse-derived clone 8E9 from Pharmingen (San Diego, USA).

Secondary antibody incubation is carried out for 30–45 min using a horseradish peroxidase conjugated anti-mouse antibody diluted 1:2000 in TBST with 2% milk powder. This is again followed by a three times wash in TBST for 5 min each and one time for 5 min with TBS.

To visualize the formed protein-antibody complexes, membranes are processed using the enhanced chemiluminescence (ECL) method.

3.2.10.3
Application of Molecular Techniques

The techniques described in this chapter can be applied in any disease in hematology/oncology which is caused by genetic alterations. As mentioned above, mutations in cells may be the result of a hereditary process (i.e. the germ line is mutated), or a somatic mutation (only the cells of the tissue in question are affected).

Molecular diagnostic steps in human cancer as a genetic disease are subject to all the mentioned techniques. Depending on the lesion in question, one will either be interested in the genomic characterization of the alteration (e.g. genomic rearrangement in the bcr-abl genes; mutations in the ras protooncogene), or the expression of a given gene (bcr-abl-fusion gene; HER2/neu gene, etc.). In addition, in many areas detection of point mutations leading to altered protein functions is important.

3.2.10.3.1
Application of Molecular Techniques to Detect Neoplasia

Since cancer is, in most cases, the result of a genetic multistep process, the detection of one single aberration (be it a single point mutation, a translocation, or a gene deletion) is not sufficient to diagnose "cancer" in most instances. There may be some exceptions to this rule, for example, the detection of p53 mutations in bronchial epithelial cells or urine, which is a very strong predictor for the presence of a malignant disorder. In contrast, the detection of ras mutations in the stool or in the pancreatic juice is in no way sufficient to state that a patient suffers from a malignant disease. In addition, even the long-thought "leukemia/lymphoma-specific" fusion genes may be detected in blood or bone marrow from healthy, normal blood donors albeit at very low levels. Thus, one has to be very careful using molecular medicine to diagnose "cancer".

However, molecular techniques may be used to discover the genetic background of a given disease and thus highlight the biology behind a malfunctioning tissue. This, on the other hand, may lead to a specific way to treat this disorder [e.g. all-trans-retinoic acid in acute promyelocytic leukemia (AML-M3)]. In addition, detection of genetic lesions may also help the clinician to categorize a disorder as a specific disease (e.g. the presence of the bcr-abl fusion gene in the peripheral blood cells derived from a patient suffering from leukocytosis strongly suggests the diagnosis of chronic myelogeneous leukemia). And lastly, hematologists and oncologists have learned in recent years that molecular biology may yield in more risk-adapted anti-cancer treatment strategies; e.g. patients suffering from acute myeloid leukemia with expression of the fusion genes AML1-ETO or CBFβ-MYH11 may best be treated by high-dose cytosine arabinoside and may not be need allogeneic stem cell transplantation in first remission, in contrast to any other patients with AML. We, and others, have recently shown that PCR may be a more sensitive method to detect inversion inv (16) in de novo AML samples compared to classical cytogenetics (Fischer et al. 1996; Ritter et al. 1997). This may have important consequences for the diagnostic steps in AML, since inv (16) may be one of the cytogenetic markers with the impact of a better prognosis.

Chronic myelogeneous leukemia has been classically defined by means of cytomorphology, histology, and the presence of the Philadelphia chromosome. The introduction of molecular biology into clinical medicine has changed many aspects in the diagnosis, and treatment, of CML. Today the presence of the fusion transcript bcr-abl, which is the hallmark of the Philadelphia chromosome, in a peripheral blood sample is a fast and easy means to detect early CML without the need of a bone marrow puncture. This may be important in the differential diagnosis of a patient suffering from mild leukocytosis. However, to corroborate the diagnosis, cytogenetic analysis is still needed; in addition, further chromosomal aberrations, such as trisomy 8, isochromosome 17q, or other lesions, may only be detected using classical cytogenetical analysis. Another advantage of cytogenetics, quantification, has recently been challenged by methods such as quantitative PCR approaches. In these techniques, a competitor is co-amplified together with the target gene, in order to give a means to quantitate the exact amount of bcr-abl moieties (see above) (Hochhaus et al. 1996; Nagel et al. 1996).

One problem associated with RT-PCR diagnosis of CML is that RNA is needed for the analysis. Often, the blood sample arrives in the laboratory after a long journey, and RNA may be degraded, especially in times of very cold or hot weather. Therefore, it is crucial to run "reference" genes as controls to check for intact RNA quality (see Fig. 3.4). In our lab, we monitor the RNA quality on a 1.8% agarose gel, and samples with heavily degraded RNA are not subjected to RT-PCR. In addition, RT-PCR out of samples derived from single colonies is especially tricky and should only be performed using extensive controls. When one performs all necessary controls, however, this technique may enable detailed analysis of expression pattern of the fusion gene bcr-abl, and, together with a FISH analysis, characterize early and very early hematopoietic progenitor cells in patients with CML as "malignant" or "nonmalignant".

RT-PCR, and especially quantitative RT-PCR for bcr-abl, is very well suited to detect malignant cells after allogeneic bone-marrow transplantation (BMT). For this purpose, a nested protocol has to be employed. Patients suffering from a relapse after BMT may be treated with donor lymphocytes in order to induce a graft versus leukemia reaction. This seems to be more efficacious in a situation where minimal amounts of leukemia cells are present in the host (Van Rhee et al. 1994). Thus, monitoring of the leukemia load with a sensitive method such as PCR is very attractive. Once RT-PCR turns positive, or the quantitative method indicates a rising leukemia load, donor cells may be given. This is now clinical routine practice in many institutions. We always recommend to repeat RT-PCR, especially when a PCR turns positive, after a long period of negative PCR. PCR, especially in its nested form, is a technique with the problem of false-positivity. We refer to the chapters above for this special problem. Performing PCR in a diagnostic laboratory requires certain precautions as detailed above.

A serious problem with the ultra-sensitive RT-PCR is that some authors have detected bcr-abl fusion transcripts in normal adult persons not suffering from CML at all (Biernaux et al. 1995). These authors used an extreme variant of nested PCR with a sensitivity of approx. 10 E -8 (!). However, this level of sensitivity is not common in RT-PCR laboratories. Thus, it may actually not be responsible for "false positivity". On the other hand, it is interesting to speculate why up to 40% of adult normal persons should carry fusion transcripts for an activated oncogene. More investigations are necessary to clarify this issue.

3.2.10.3.2
Application of Molecular Techniques to Detect Monoclonal B-Cell Proliferation

Since most lymphomas in Western countries are derived from B cells, we will discuss detection of monoclonal B-cell proliferation here in more detail. B cells are characterized by its ability to recombine, or rearrange, the genes coding for the immunoglobulin molecules. This enables a B cell to produce a single type of antibody with a given specificity. The B cell rearranges its immunoglobulin genes following a certain feature detailed. Out of a polyclonal background, monoclonality may be detected by conventional Southern blotting, or by PCR amplification of genomic DNA with PCR primers specific for certain areas of the immunoglobulin genes (typically consensus primers for frame work region and joining region). Whereas Southern blotting is laboursome and requires radioactivity, it has a big advantage over PCR: it is not dependent on primers which may fail amplification because of a wrong primer sequence. However, since Southern blotting requires masses of DNA compared with PCR, in most instances in the routine laboratory situation, PCR will be used to detect a monoclonal B-cell proliferation. Protocols are given in the literature (Rudolph et al. 1997). The two disadvantages of this procedure must, however, never be forgotten: (a) a negative PCR does not exclude monoclonal B-cell proliferation (i.e. follicular center lymphomas or marginal zone B-cell lymphomas of MALT-type are PCR-positive in 70%–80%, whereas CLL is positive in over 90%). This depends on the differentiation of the monoclonal B cell: whether the follicular center had been entered or not (with the consequence of mutations in the immunoglobulin gene). (b) The second problem with detection of monoclonal B cells: does monoclonality mean malignancy? This, for sure, is an open question and will certainly be an interesting issue for many researchers: for instance, monoclonal B cells within a gastric mucosa sample certainly do not mean that a lymphoma is present (see: Savio et al. 1996; Rudolph et al. 1997). Gastritis with dense lymphoid infiltrates due to infection with *Helicobacter pylori* may, in some cases, also lead to infiltration with monoclonal B cells.

3.2.10.3.3
Application of Molecular Techniques to Detect Hereditary Disorders

In recent years it has been established that cancer is the result of a genetic multi-step process involving dominant acting proto-oncogenes and recessive tumor-suppressor genes. In addition, involvement of genes coding for DNA repair enzymes seems to be a key step in the genetics of many, especially solid tumors. These cancer genes can be mutated in somatic cells (i.e. the tumor cells), or mutations within these genes may be inherited in the germ-line leading to a higher susceptibility to acquire cancer during the entire life-span. Hereditary cancers with mutations in critical genes involving the germ-line are, however, rare compared to sporadic cancers where the same genes may be targeted by somatic mutations. In some instances mutations in genes leading to hereditary cancer may only very rarely be observed in sporadic tumors, e.g. breast cancer gene BRCA-2. In other malignant diseases, the genes targeted by hereditary states are frequently also mutated in "sporadic" (i.e. non-hereditary) cancers.

Today, hereditary cancer syndromes are important in the clinical practice not only for the individual suffering from this particular type of cancer, but also for the whole family of this individual. Screening of families is therefore not only a biochemical problem, but also an ethical issue, since the consequences of a "positive" (i.e. mutated) germ-line for the well-being of an individual not suffering from any disease has not very well studied yet. Probably the most frequent inherited cancer syndromes are the HNPCC states (for: human non-polyposis colorectal cancer syndrome, Lynch syndrome). These syndromes are caused by germ-line mutations in critical DNA repair genes, and were detected by the biological read-out of these enzymes: lesions causing DNA mismatch-repair deficiency. Three genes involved have been isolated and characterized (hMSH2; hMLH1, hPMS2). The human genes are relatives of bacterial genes encoding mismatch-repair enzymes. The mutations leading to these cancer syndromes may thus either be detected by screening the sequence of the respective genes, or by analyzing repeated DNA sequences anywhere in the genome, where, once a mutation has occurred in the repair genes, replacement errors can be detected leading to the presence of more than the expected bands.

Besides HNPCC, other cancer syndromes are not as frequent: FAP (familiar adenomatosis coli with mutations of the APC gene on chromosome 5q; this syndrome is characterized by the occurrence of hundreds to thousands of polyps in the colon, leading to cancer early in life of affected individuals); Li-Fraumeni syndrome (caused by germ-line mutations of the "genome watcher" p53, leading to colon, breast, throat cancer and leukemia and lymphoma). Recently, mutations in the breast cancer causing genes BRCA1 and BRCA2 have been described in families with high-risk for breast cancer. Mutations in either gene will lead to different patterns in affected families. Both genes may encode for transcription factors playing a critical role in the development of breast epithelial cells (Monteiro et al. 1996). Again, mutations in families may be detected by sequencing the critical portions of both genes.

Current calculations assume that approx. 10%–15% of all cancers seen in Western countries are caused by hereditary mutations. The remainder are thought to be the result of somatic mutations. Recently, another very interesting aspect has come to attention; i.e. immunogenicity of tumor cells. For instance, leukemia cells may be subject to killing by autologous cytotoxic T cells. The T cells must be primed to kill leukemia cells by specific immune mechanisms. For a T-cell clone to proliferate, presentation of a leukemia-specific peptide within the HLA molecule is a prerequisite. Thus, specific peptides may be, depending on the HLA background of the host, more or less immunogenic. For example, presentation of the CML-causing peptide Bcr-Abl can only take place in the background of HLA-A3 and HLA-B7, respectively. As a consequence, human beings with HLA-A3 may be somehow "protected" in acquiring CML. And indeed, recently, it has been demonstrated that people with HLA-A3 have a highly significant lower risk of suffering from CML compared to other HLA subtypes (Posthuma et al. 1997) Thus, besides hereditary cancers caused by mutations in cancer genes (with dominant or recessive traits), the incidence of certain cancer types may also be influenced by immune mechanisms leading to a somewhat higher or lower, for that matter, incidence of specific types of cancers.

3.2.10.3.4
Application of Molecular Techniques to Detect Infectious Diseases

Infections are a leading cause of human mortality. Obviously, the level of immunocompetence is of extreme importance for the susceptibility to acquire a given infection. Classical techniques to diagnose infectious diseases are either direct (i.e. cultural), or indirect (i.e. serum antibodies) measures. In recent years, new ways to detect infectious states have challenged these classical methods: Since most infectious diseases are caused by nucleic-acid-carrying organisms, the direct and sensitive detection of a given nucleic acid in a clinical sample is an attractive method. In most instances, PCR has been used to search for foreign DNA/RNA in human samples. However, since the detection of a certain nucleic acid within a given organism does not tell anything about the relevance of this finding, one has to be careful with the interpretation of "positive" PCR findings. Since most infectious diseases in hematology/oncology are to be found in the background of immunocompromised patients (either inborn, acquired or induced by physicians (e.g. chemotherapy)), diseases occurring in these patients will be discussed in this chapter.

PCR may be used to amplify foreign DNA or RNA in human specimens. In immunocompromised patients, certain opportunistic infections are especially abundant: cytomegalovirus (CMV) infections, aspergillus infections, or infections with *Pneumocystis carinii*. For all of these pathogens, PCR technques have been described for early and sensitive diagnoses (Cathomas et al. 1993). The pitfalls are obviously that PCR in most of these assays is not quantitated, and that one cannot state if a positive PCR test indeed means an infected individual. However, for CMV, it has been well established that early intervention after conversion of the PCR status (i.e. negative PCR to positive PCR) leads to lower mortality of the infection. Thus, for CMV, early diagnosis is crucial.

Many PCR assays have been described for other pathogens, e.g. *Mycobacterium tuberculosis*, or viral infections. In the clinic, PCR has been mostly used to detect early hepatitis C-RNA in the blood of suspected patients. Here, different assays have been performed. For a detailed analysis, the reader is referred to the original literature.

References

Ausubl FM (ed) (1997) Current protocols in molecular biology, vol 1–3. Wiley and Sons, New York

Bergh J, Norberg T, Sjögren S, Lindgren A, Holmberg L (1995) Complete sequencing of the p53 gene provides prognostic information in breast cancer patients, particulary in relation to adjuvant systemic therapy and radiotherapy. Nature Med 1:1029–1034

Biernaux C, Loos M, Sels A, Huez G, Stryckmans P (1995) Detection of major bcr-abl rearrangement at very low level in blood cells of some healthy individuals. Blood 86:3118–3122

Cathomas G, Morris P, Pekle K, Cunningham I, Emanuel D (1993) Rapid diagnosis of cytomegalovirus pneumonia in marrow transplant recipients by bronchoalveolar lavage using the polymerase chain reaction, virus culture, and the direct immunostaining of alveolar cells. Blood 81:1909–1914

Chen EY (1994) The efficiency of automated DNA sequencing. Academic Press, London

Chen LC, Neubauer A, Kurisu W, Waldman F, Ljung BM, Goodson W, Goldman E, Moore D, Balazs M, Liu E, Mayall B, Smith HS (1991) Loss of heterozygosity on the short arm of chromosome 17 is associated with high proliferative capacity and DNA aneuploidy in primary human breast cancer. Proc Natl Acad Sci U S A 88:3847–3851

Döhner H, Fischer K, Bentz M, Hansen K, Benner A, Cabot G, Diehl D, Schlenk R, Coy J, Stilgenbauer S, Volkmann M, Galle PR, Poustka A, Hunstein W, Lichter P (1995) p53 gene deletion predicts for a poor survival and non-response to therapy with purine analogs in chronic B-cell leukemia. Blood 85:1580–1589

Fearon ER, Vogelstein B (1990) A genetic model for colorectal tumorigenesis. Cell 61:759–767

Fischer K, Scholl C, Salat J, Fröhling S, Schlenk R, Bentz M, Stilgenbauer S, Lichter P, Döhner H (1996) Design and validation of DNA probe sets for a comprehensive interphase cytogenetic analysis of acute myeloid leukemia. Blood 88:3962–3971

Graeber TG, Osmanian C, Jacks T, Hausman DE, Koch CJ, Lowe SW, Glaccia AJ (1996) Hypoxia-mediated selection of cells with diminished apoptotic potential in solid tumors. Nature 379:88–91

Hamilton SR (1992) Molecular genetic alterations as potential prognostic indicators in colorectal carcinoma. Cancer 69(6 Suppl):1589–1591

Hochhaus A, Lin F, Reiter A, Skladny H, Mason PJ, Van Rhee F, Shepherd PC, Allan NC, Hehlmann R, Goldman JM, Cross NCP (1996) Quantification of residual disease in chronic myelogeneous leukemia patients on interferon-a therapy by competitive polymerase chain reaction. Blood 87:1549–1555

Kozal MJ, Shah N, Shen N, Yang R, Fucini R, Merigan TC, Richman DD, Morris D, Hubbell E, Chee M, Gingeras TR (1996) Extensive polymorphisms observed in HIV-1 clade B protease gene using high-density oligonucleotide arrays. Nature Med 2:753–759

Kozubek S, Lukasova E, Ryznar L, Liskova A, Govorun RD, Krasavin EA, Horneck G (1997) Distribution of ABL and BCR genes in cell nuclei of normal and irradiated lymphocytes. Blood 89:4537–4545

Lipschutz RJ, Morris D, Chee M, Hubbell E, Kozal MJ, Shah N, Shen N, Yang R, Fodor SPA (1995) Using oligonucleotide probe arrays to access gene diversity. Biotechniques 19:442–447

Liu E (1989) Oncogenes in human leukemias and lymphomas. In: Benz C, Liu E (eds) Oncogenes, cancer treatment and research edn. Kluwer Academic Publisher, Boston

Look AT (1997) Oncogenic transcription factors in the human acute leukemias. Science 278:1059–1064

Maniatis T, Frisch EF, Sambrook J (eds) (1982) Molecular cloning: A laboratory manual, 2nd edn. Cold Spring Harbor Laboratory, Cold Spring Harbor

Maxam AM, Gilbert W (1977) A new method for sequencing DNA. Proc Natl Acad Sci U S A 74:560–564

McPherson MJ, Quirke P, Taylor GR (eds) (1991) PCR: A practical approach, 1st edn. IRL Press, Oxford

Monteiro ANA, August A, Hanafusa H (1996) Evidence for a transcriptional activation function of BRCA1-terminal region. Proc Natl Acad Sci U S A 93:13595–13599

Muss HB, Thor AD, Berry DA, Kute T, Liu ET, Koerner F, Cirrcione CT, Budman DR, Wood WC, Barcos M, Henderson IC (1994) c-erbB2 Expression and response to adjuvant therapy in women with node-positive early breast cancer. New Engl J Med 330:1260–1266

Nagel S, Schmidt M, Thiede C, Huhn D, Neubauer A (1996) Quantification of Bcr-Abl transcripts in human leukemias by competitive and differential PCR. Nucl Acids Res 24:4102–4103

Polyak K, Xia Y, Zweier JL, Kinzler KW, Vogelstein B (1997) A model for p53-induced apoptosis. Nature 389:300–305

Posthuma EFM, Falkenburg JHF, Apperley JF, Jeannet M, Schipper RF, Schreuder GMT, D´Amaro J, Biezen JH, Hermans J, Willemze R, Niederwieser D (1997) HLA-A3 and HLA-B8 may protect against acquiring chronic myeloid leukemia (abstract). Blood 90 Suppl 1:250a, #1102

Richards B, Zhang H, Phear G, Meuth M (1997) Conditional mutator phenotypes in hMSH2-deficient tumor cell lines. Science 277:1523–1526

Ritter M et al (1995) Detection of DNA methylation in the calcitonin gene in human leukemias using differential polymerase chain reaction. Leukemia 9:915–922

Ritter M, Thiede C, Schäkel U, Schmidt M, Alpen B, Pascheberg U, Mohr B, Ehninger G, Neubauer A (1997) Underestimation of inversion (16) in acute myeloid leukemia using standard cytogenetics as compared with polymerase chain reaction: Results of a prospective investigation. Br J Haematol 98:969–972

Roth JA, Nguyen D, Lawrence DD, et al. (1996) Retrovirus-mediated wild-type p53 gene transfer to tumors of patients with lung cancer. Nature Med 2:985–991

Rudolph B, Bayerdörffer E, Ritter M, Müller S, Thiede C, Neubauer B, Lehn N, Seifert E, Otto P, Hatz R, Stolte M, Neubauer A (1997) Is the polymerase chain reaction or cure of Helicoabcter infection of help in the differential diagnosis of early gastric MALT lymphoma? J Clin Oncol 15:1104–1109

Runnebaum IB, Nagarajan M, Bowman M, Soto D, Sukumar S (1991) Mutations in p53 as potential molecular markers for human breast cancer. Proc Natl Acad Sci USA 88:10657–10661

Sanger F, Nicklen S, Coulson R (1977) DNA-sequencing with chain-terminating inhibitors. Proc Natl Acad Sci U S A 74:5463–5467

Savio A, Franzin G, Wotherspoon AC, Zamboni G, Negrini R, Buffoli F, Diss TG, Pan L, Isaacson PG (1996) Diagnosis and posttreatment follow-up of Helicobacter pylori positive gastric lymphoma of mucosa-associated lymphoid tissue: Histology, polymerase chain reaction, or both? Blood 87:1255–1260

Thompson AM, Anderson TJ, Condie A, Prosser J, Chetty U, Carter DC, Evans HJ, Steel CM (1992) p53 allele losses, mutations and expression in breast cancer and their relationship to clinico-pathological parameters. Int J Cancer 50:528–532

Thor AD, Schwartz LH, Koerner FC, Edgerton SM, Skates SJ, Yin S, McKenzie SJ, Panicali DL, Marks PJ, Fingert HJ, Wood WC (1989) Analysis of c-erbB2 expression in breast carcinomas with clinical follow-up. Cancer Res 49:7147–7152

Van Rhee F, Cullis J, Spencer A, Cross NCP, Chase A, Garicochea B, Bungey J, Barrett J, Goldman JM (1994) Relapse of chronic myeloid leukemia after allogeneic bone marrow transplant: The case for giving donor leukocyte transfusion before the onset of hematologic relapse. Blood 83:3377–3383

4 Classical and Molecular Cytogenetics

C. Fonatsch · B. Streubel

4.1 Introduction

Cytogenetic analysis provides information of diagnostic and prognostic importance for malignant diseases, after all for hematological malignancies. Furthermore, it may contribute to the elucidation of the course of disease before, during and after different therapeutic measures. The main goal of the tumor cytogeneticist is the discovery of primary non-random chromosome abnormalities specific to a certain tumor type and playing a role in tumor development. In addition, he has to study the so-called secondary chromosome abnormalities, since in most cases they herald a disease aggravation, e.g. the transition from pre-leukemia into overt leukemia or from a low-grade lymphoma into a high-grade lymphoma.

Moreover, the identification of recurrent chromosomal breakpoints in leukemias, lymphomas and a number of solid tumors have expedited the cloning of genes whose aberration-induced deregulation causes malignant transformation.

Karyotype analyses rest mostly on classical chromosome banding techniques that have the distinct advantage that the entire genome can be analyzed in a single experiment. Using a Giemsa banding technique, one can achieve a typical visual resolution of a single band in the range from 5 to 10 million base pairs. Poorly spread or contracted metaphase chromosomes and highly rearranged karyotypes with numerous marker chromosomes, common in tumor cell preparations, however, are often difficult to interpret unambiguously. Furthermore, chromosome preparations are labor-intensive and time-consuming and the interpretation of cytogenetic findings requires extensive experience.

Fluorescence in situ hybridization (FISH) overcomes some of these limitations. Based on results of classical cytogenetic investigations FISH analysis helps to identify marker chromosomes and to determine the origin of complex rearranged chromosomes. In some cases FISH increases the resolution power, shortens the reporting time and bypasses the culturing process to accommodate less viable specimens. Commercial availability of many different types of FISH probes has accelerated their rapid acceptance by clinical laboratories. In this connection it has to be remarked that FISH analysis is associated with high expenses.

4.2
Principle of the Method

4.2.1
Classical Cytogenetics

A prerequisite for chromosome analysis are dividing (mitotic) cells. Bone marrow and/or peripheral blood are the tissues of choice for the cytogenetic study of most hematological disorders. Malignant lymphomas are best investigated from lymph node biopsies, and solid tumors are studied cytogenetically from tumor tissue, mostly after short-term or long-term cultivation.

If dividing cells are suspected in the tissue to be examined, a *direct preparation* after short incubation is recommended, in order to study the chromosome constitution as present in vivo. In direct preparations of mitotic cells two goals have to be aspired: First, cells in the stage of metaphase, as many as possible, should be available for chromosome preparation – this is attained by incubation in culture medium containing the spindle poison colcemid. Secondly, overlaying of chromosomes must be avoided by treatment of cells by a hypotonic solution. Cultivation with synchronic action of colcemid and hypotonic solution lasts for half an hour until 2 h maximally and is performed in an incubator at 37°C.

The cell cultivation over a period of 24–72 h (*short-term culture*) can yield a higher amount of analyzable metaphases than the direct preparation, since cells pass through divisions in vitro. Moreover, in certain malignancies (e.g. acute promyelocytic leukemia) direct preparations may lead to false negative results, because only metaphases with a normal karyotype have been found.

Since extensive cytogenetical and molecular genetic studies are limited by the restricted amount of material obtainable by short-term cultures, it is tried to establish *long-term cultures* from bone marrow or blood samples, lymph nodes, spleen, ascites, pleural effusion and of solid tumor tissue. Thus, the number of malignant cells desired for investigation can be enriched. However, in many cases, the establishment of permanently growing cell lines is not successful. Another disadvantage of long-term cell cultures consists in the occurrence of karyotype deviations in vitro which may lead to incorrect cytogenetical as well as molecular genetic findings. Moreover, as a result of genetical in vitro aberrations, other features and functions of cells can be altered, as for example morphology, immunophenotype or the expression of cytokines, etc.

After the preparation and fixation of the cells and dropping on ice cold slides, chromosome staining procedures are applied. For each chromosome a specific pattern is obtained by using different chromosome banding techniques. These banding patterns allow the assignment of homologous chromosomes, the identification of supernumerary or of missing chromosomes as well as of structural aberrations. The fluorescence banding technique using quinacrine derivatives (quinacrine mustard, quinacrine dihydrochloride) is based on the intercalation of the acridine nucleus into the DNA molecule and on ionic binding of the side chain to the phosphate groups of DNA. AT-rich DNA is stained more intensively than GC-rich regions by quinacrine stains. For achievement of Giemsa banding patterns pre-treatment of chromosomes by trypsin or by 2× saline sodium citrate (2×SSC) is required. The mechanism of Giemsa banding is not yet fully understood; the different distribution of chromosome proteins and of DNA along the chromosomes presumably induces the expression of dark and light G-bands. Other chromosome banding techniques are used to produce a reverse banding pattern (R-bands) or telomeric staining (T-bands) or centromeric staining (C-bands). Moreover, nucleolus organizer regions (NORs) located in the short arms of acrocentric chromosomes are stainable by silver nitrate ($AgNO_3$).

The purpose of the analysis of stained chromosome preparations is the examination of the number as well as of the structure of chromosomes in order to detect karyotype deviations. Furthermore, it has to be tested whether a so-called *mosaic* status is present, this is the combination of cells with a normal and with an abnormal karyotype or with several abnormal karyotypes within one tissue. Various chromosome banding techniques are used to identify the involvement of specific chromosomes and chromosome bands in abnormalities.

A verification or falsification of aberrations detected by chromosome banding analysis and in many cases additional information concerning karyotype abnormalities are achieved by fluorescence in situ hybridization.

4.2.2 Molecular Cytogenetics

Cell cultivation and chromosome preparation are performed as described in Sect. 4.2.1. In the fluorescence in situ hybridization (FISH) procedure differentially labeled DNA probes, specific for distinct chromosomal regions or whole chromosomes, are hybridized to prepared specimens and commonly visualized with fluorochrome-conjugated reagents. The two DNA strands of a double stranded DNA probe and of target DNA must be separated before hybridization (DNA denaturation). After placing single strands of probe DNA on a slide containing denatured chromosomes, DNA strands with complementary base sequences can be allowed to hybridize (DNA renaturation or annealing). Complementary probe DNA strands can reanneal to form homoduplexes, as can complementary target DNA strands. However it is the annealing of probe DNA strands to complementary chromosomal target DNA strands to form labeled heteroduplexes that defines the usefulness of a FISH.

Most genomic DNA probes of higher eukaryotes contain ubiquitously occurring interspersed repetitive sequences (IRS). The IRSs result in various background stainings of the chromosomes. Protocols, termed "chromosomal in situ suppression" (CISS) hybridization, have been developed that suppress the signals from the IRSs within probe sets by a hybridization reaction with competitor DNA and include an additional preannealing step after the probe denaturation.

Following hybridization, excess probe which did not associate with the metaphase chromosomes and interphases is removed from the slide by washing. The annealed probe which is labeled by the incorporation of modified nucleotides obtaining bindings to reporter molecules (e.g., biotin or digoxigenin) is incubated in a solution containing fluorochrome-conjugated reporter-binding molecules (avidin or streptavidin for the reporter molecule biotin, anti-digoxigenin for the reporter molecule digoxigenin). One biotin- and one digoxigenin-labeled probe can be simultaneously detected on the same slide by incubating the hybridized preparation with different fluorochromes (mostly fluorescein and rhodamine or Texas red) for each of the two reporter-binding molecules. Finally, chromosomal DNA is counterstained with 4′,6-diamidino-2-phenylindole (DAPI) for the identification of the chromosomes. The hybridized slide is examined with a fluorescence microscope with epi-illumination and a filter set appropriate for the fluorochromes used.

In order to take advantage of the FISH technique as a powerful assistance and completion to classical cytogenetics it is important to consider the potential use and the limitations of the different FISH probes for the detection of rearrangements.

4.2.2.1
Whole Chromosome Painting Probes (WCPP)

Each WCPP is composed of a mixture of many probes, complementary in sequence to a specific site along the length of a single chromosome. If many of those sequence-specific probes are mixed together in a single hybridization reaction, the whole chromosome of interest lights up and therefore appears "painted". WCPPs are especially useful in the accurate identification of small markers and complex rearranged chromosomes. A limitation for this class of probes is that it may not completely cover the whole chromosome, especially in cryptic regions. Furthermore, WCPPs are not useful for structural changes within the same chromosome, like inversions and small deletions. Moreover, the chromosomal origin but not the specific region of small inserted segments can be identified with WCPPs.

FISH is usually limited to the simultaneous hybridization of only two differentially labeled DNA probes to prepared specimens and is therefore mainly utilized to confirm the presence of previously characterized or suspected aberrations. The difficulty of choosing the right chromosome-painting probe is attempted to be eliminated by the development of multicolor-labeling probes. In the future, two recently developed sophisticated systems [M-FISH (Speicher et al. 1996), SKY (Schröck et al. 1996)] will probably allow the simultaneous detection of all human chromosomes in one reaction.

4.2.2.2
Centromeric Probes

Centromeric probes contain repetitive DNA sequences found in the centromeric or pericentromeric regions of human chromosomes. These probes can be utilized for both metaphase chromosome and interphase nuclei hybridization. Centromeric probes are powerful and rapid diagnostic tools for the identification of numerical chromosomal abnormalities. The drawback here is that a structurally imbalanced chromosome cannot be distinguished from a normal one. For example, a deleted chromosome 5 with an intact centromere region generates the same signal as a completely normal one. Because of this limitation, centromeric probes are best used for rapid preliminary diagnoses of numerical abnormalities which are subsequently confirmed by further cytogenetic studies. Other applications include the rapid assessment of the outcome of a sex-mismatched bone marrow transplant, the determination of the percentage of abnormal cells in patients with mosaic numerical abnormality and the identification of dicentric chromosomes. This class of probes is also useful for detecting numerical chromosome abnormalities in interphase nuclei from neoplastic specimens, where the process of culturing may present a problem.

4.2.2.3
Unique Sequence DNA Probes (USP)

The USP class of FISH probes contains locus-specific DNA segments and is suitable for hybridizing both metaphase and interphase nuclei. Since each USP is region/gene-specific and mainly composed of unique sequences, it is perfect for detecting microdeletions, microduplications and cryptic translocations of a specific chromosome region which are undetectable by classical cytogenetic techniques. USPs are also useful for the identification and follow-up investigations of known recurring translocations found in certain types of leukemia patients, such as the translocation t(15;17)(q22;q21) in patients with ANLL M3. Apart from commercially available unique sequence DNA probes, FISH hybridization can be applied to genomic DNA fragments from all sources, cloned in plasmid, phage, cosmid, or YAC (yeast artificial chromosome) vectors.

4.2.2.4
Telomeric Probes

The telomeres are the terminal cap segments of each chromosome. They are vital for survival because intact telomeres are important for the replication and stability of chromosomes. Telomeres are speculated to be involved in breakage and healing events that can result in terminal deletions, gene amplifications, and cryptic translocations. Moreover, the human telomere bands are known to contain the highest gene concentration in the whole genome. The importance of FISH with unique telomere probes for each arm of all chromosomes for the identification of cryptic rearrangements in routine protocols of clinical laboratories must be verified.

4.3
Fields of Application

The main question with which tumor cytogeneticists are confronted reads as follows: Which role do chromosome abnormalities play in cancer origin and progression? The development of methods of chromosome preparation, including in situ hybridization techniques, and the combination of cytogenetic with molecular genetic findings helped greatly in clearing up the correlation of karyotype deviation and tumor development in some cases. For example, chromosome deletions may lead to loss of tumor suppressor genes (e.g. *RB* gene loss by chromosome 13 deletion in retinoblastoma). The translocation of chromosomal segments can cause the formation of new hybrid genes (e.g. *ABL-BCR* fusion gene as a consequence of the Philadelphia translocation in chronic myeloid leukemia, acute lymphoblastic leukemia and acute myeloid leukemia) or causes the activation of oncogenes by juxtaposition of promoter or enhancer sequences (e.g. activation of c-*MYC* oncogene by juxtaposition with immunoglobulin gene sequences in Burkitt´s lymphoma). The amplification of genes, e.g. oncogenes, may lead to cytogenetically identifiable structures, designated as homogeneously staining regions (HSR) or double minutes (dmin) (e.g. N-*MYC* amplification in neuroblastoma).

Beneath the dealing with scientific questions classical and molecular tumor cytogenetics are concerned with the correlation of chromosome findings with clinical data. In this field cytogenetics have gained great importance. Cytogenetics are helpful in diagnosis, staging and prognosis as well as in therapy planning of different malignant diseases, after all in hematological neoplasias. The sequential analysis of karyotype deviations during the clinical course may contribute to the clarification of biological mechanisms underlying tumor development and expansion. The combination of cytogenetic results with clinical, but also with immunological and molecular genetic, data allows conclusions concerning relationships of malignancies, furthermore leading to the identification of the cell type affected by the neoplasia and of the molecular genetic events occurring in this cell.

4.4 Types of Material and Material Gain

4.4.1 Leukemias and Lymphomas

In hematoproliferative disorders bone marrow, peripheral blood, lymph node and spleen tissue, more rarely ascitic and pleural effusions, are used for cytogenetic examinations. These tissue types are affected by malignant transformation; they are characterized by abnormal proliferation and/or cell differentiation.

The success of a cytogenetic analysis mostly depends on the quality of material to be investigated. Therefore, neither the first drops nor the last morsels of a bone marrow aspirate should be used for cytogenetic diagnosis; but cell-rich material which comes in plenty in the middle part of the bone marrow punction is most suitable. The tissue drawing must be performed under sterile conditions, since the chromosome analysis is in most cases preceded by cell cultivation, which is only possible with sterile material. The syringe used for bone marrow or blood withdrawal must be heparinized (10 IE heparin/ml tissue) to avoid clumping of blood components. Heparin is added also to lymph node and spleen tissue after surgical removal.

The shorter the time interval between removal of tissue samples and preparation in the cytogenetic laboratory, the greater the chances for a successful chromosome analysis with a correct result. The time span should not exceed 24 h. In many cases conveyance by mail is unavoidable; then express mail is needed and the material must be packaged well and protected from leaking out. After arrival the tissue specimen is lead to different methods of culturing and preparation, depending on the amount of material.

4.4.2 Solid Tumors

Chromosomes from human solid tumors are often difficult to prepare depending on the type and stage of tumors. The tissue sample is obtained by fine needle aspiration or, more often, by surgical removal. Operation specimens should be immersed in culture medium or in sterile balanced salt solution, as isotonic sodium chloride. Tissue retains viability for 2–3 days; after overnight storage tumor cells have no impaired growth capacity in comparison to freshly obtained cells.

A major problem, for example in intestinal tumors, may be contamination with micro-organisms. To avoid infection of cultures exposure to anti-microbial agents is recommended. The samples can be treated in a balanced salt solution containing benzylpenicillin and streptomycin (200 IU/ml and 400 μg/ml) or neomycin sulfate (50 μg/ml) against bacteria, and amphotericin B (2.5 μg/ml) against yeasts and moulds for 30–60 min.

Most solid tumor samples are "contaminated" by stromal fibroblasts which after a few days in culture overgrow the tumor cells. Therefore, before disaggregation of the biopsy the removal or at least the reduction of the fibroblasts is required for a successful culture of solid tumor parenchyma cells.

Also fat, clotted blood, and necrotic tissue should be removed from the tumor tissue, because growing of tumor cells may be disturbed by these components.

The tumor tissue first is minced as finely as possible with scissors or scalpels and then cultures are started in different ways with or without foregoing enzymatic disaggregation (by incubation in medium containing collagenase for 15–30 min).

4.5 Methods

4.5.1 Direct Tissue Preparation

4.5.1.1 *Material and Reagents*

- Sterile bone marrow (BM) or peripheral blood (PB) mixed with anti-coagulants (vetrene, liquemine, heparin)
- Culture medium for BM and PB: 9 ml hypotonic solution (potassium chloride 0.075 M) and 1 ml trypsin (0.25%) plus 0.1 μg colcemid/ml medium
- Fixative: methanol: glacial acetic acid, 3:1

4.5.1.2 *Procedure*

Before culture start tubes have to be marked (patient number, medium description, date, etc.). Cultivation for 0.5–1 h at 37°C follows.

- Culture tubes (plastic ware 12 ml) are used as centrifuge tubes too; they are spun at 700–800 rpm for 10 min (step 1)
- The supernatant is discarded with a pipette; the sediment is gently moved (step 2)
- Under permanent gentle agitation of the sediment, ice-cold fixative is added drop by drop by pipette (step 3)
- Cell suspension is centrifuged at 1000 rpm for 10 min (step 4)
- The supernatant is removed again and the pellet is shaken up (step 5)
- Fresh fixative is added and then cell suspension is stored within the refrigerator at 4°C or at room temperature for 30 min (step 6).

A further centrifugation step and renewal of the fixative follow. Steps 4 and 5 are repeated one to three times, until the cell suspension after red and brown color has reached white and clear consistency. After a last centrifugation, removal of the fixative and adding a few drops of fresh fixative, the cell suspension is dropped on ice cold wet slides. Cooling of slides in a distilled water containing vessel at 4°C leads to spreading of metaphase chromosomes. About three drops of the cell suspension are distributed on each slide. This leads in most cases to the cell density desired, which is examined via a phase contrast microscope.

4.5.2
Short-Term Cultivation of Different Tissues and Cytogenetic Preparation

4.5.2.1
Material and Reagents

- Sterile bone marrow, peripheral blood, mechanically and/or enzymatically minced and disaggregated lymph node, spleen, or solid tumor tissue mixed with coagulation inhibitors (see Sect. 4.5.1, but not EDTA)
- Depending on cell density:
  1–10 drops in 2.5 ml culture medium
  2–10 drops in 5 ml culture medium
- Culture media:
  RPMI 1640, McCoy´s 5 A, Ham´s F10
  Mixed with fetal calf serum (final concentration: 10%–20%), bicarbonate as a buffer (final concentration: 1%), antibiotica-antimycotica mixture (final concentration: 1%)

- Mitogen: phytohemagglutinin (PHA, 25 µg/ml medium)
- Spindle poison: colcemid (final concentration: 0.02–0.1 µg colcemid/ml medium)
- Hypotonic solution: potassium chloride 0.075 M
- Fixative: methanol: glacial acetic acid, 3:1

4.5.2.2
Procedure

Before culture start tubes have to be marked (patient number, medium designation, culture time, date).

- Dependent on the amount of material available, several parallel cultures using different nutrient media in 12 ml sterile plastic tubes are set up from bone marrow, blood, lymph node, spleen and solid tumor tissue and incubated for 24 h, 48 h and 72 h at 37°C (step 1)
- Colcemid in final concentrations of 0.02 and 0.1 µg/ml medium is added 2 h or 30 min, respectively, before harvesting (step 2).
- Culture tubes function as centrifuge tubes; they are spun at 1000 rpm for 10 min (step 3).
- Supernatant is discarded and cells are treated with hypotonic solution (potassium chloride 0.075 M) at room temperature for 20 min (step 4).
- Then cell suspension is centrifuged at 700–800 rpm for 8–10 min; supernatant is removed and the cell pellet is gently agitated (step 5).
- Ice-cold fixative is added to the cell pellet drop by drop (step 6).

Further steps are analogous to the steps described in Sect. 4.5.1 beginning with step 4.

To present the constitutional karyotype, 72 h blood cultures containing PHA (25 µg PHA/ml medium) are used.

4.5.3
Long-Term Cultivation

Materials and reagents as described in Sect. 4.5.2 are used.

4.5.3.1
Procedure

- Lymph node, spleen or solid tumor tissue is minced by use of fine surgical scissors or a scalpel in a culture medium containing petri dish in order to produce a dense cell suspension. The cell suspension is mixed with culture medium RPMI 1640 (0.5–1 ml suspension and 4–8 ml medium) and transferred in sterile plastic culture flasks (50 ml). Cell density is examined under a microscope. Flasks containing solid tumor cells are stored horizontally; flasks containing hematopoietic malignant cells are stored vertically in an incubator at 37°C and under 5% CO_2.

- After 2–3 days one-third to half of the culture medium is changed dependent on microscopically examined cell growth and replaced by fresh medium.
- Cell proliferation is inspected twice per week; at sufficient cell growth splitting of cells, i.e. distribution of cells into two flasks, is performed. In case of poor cell proliferation only half of the medium is changed and replaced by fresh medium.
- Last medium exchange is performed 24 h before cytogenetic preparation. One-half or 2 h before cell harvesting colcemid in final concentrations of 0.3–0.75 μg/ml medium is added to the suspension culture in order to arrest mitosis in the stage of metaphase.
- Cell suspension is transferred from culture flasks into centrifuge tubes and is then spun, treated by hypotonic solution and fixed in methanol-acetic acid, as described in Sects. 4.5.1 and 4.5.2.

Afterwards, the cells are dropped on ice-cold slides and the cell density is checked using phase contrast optics.

4.5.4
Chromosome Banding Methods

4.5.4.1
Giemsa Banding Using 2xSSC Pretreatment (GAG)

4.5.4.1.1
Reagents

- Giemsa stock solution (azureB-eosin-methylene blue)
- Phosphate buffer (modified Sörensen buffer, pH 6.8): 5.7 g sodium phosphate dibasic (Na_2HPO_4) and 2.45 g potassium phosphate monobasic (KH_2PO_4) dissolved in 5000 ml distilled water.
- Giemsa staining solution: 10 ml Giemsa stock solution is mixed with 90 ml phosphate buffer
- 2×SSC: 5.54 g sodium chloride (NaCl) and 8.82 g trisodium citrate, 2 hydrate – dissolved in 1000 ml distilled water
- Eukitt for mounting the slides

4.5.4.1.2
Procedure

After drying the slides for 1–4 days they are stained by the Giemsa banding technique described by Sumner et al. (1971) and modified by Fonatsch et al. (1980). In brief, the slides are incubated in staining vessels of plastic containing 2× saline sodium citrate (2×SSC) solution at 59°–61°C for 17–21 h. Then they are stained in phosphate buffered Giemsa solution for 1–3 min, rinsed in distilled water and the stain intensity is microscopically examined. If the staining is adequate, the slides are air dried and mounted using Eukitt.

4.5.4.2
Fluorescence Banding Using Quinacrine Mustard (QFQ)

4.5.4.2.1
Reagents

- Quinacrine mustard, 5 mg dissolved in 100 ml distilled water
- Phosphate buffer (modified Sörensen´s buffer, see Sect. 4.5.4.1)

4.5.4.2.2
Procedure

The slides are stained in quinacrine mustard solution for 20–30 min in the dark. Then they are rinsed in running tap water to remove excess quinacrine for 10 min, afterwards with distilled water and finally mounted in phosphate buffer. The slides are examined under a fluorescence microscope using a wavelength of 450–500 nm. In contrast to Giemsa banding preparations, which are long-lasting, fluorescence preparations fade and are of limited usability.

4.5.4.3
C-Banding Using Barium Hydroxide [Ba(OH)$_2$ Pretreatment] (CBG)

4.5.4.3.1
Reagents

- Phosphate buffered Giemsa solution (see Sect. 4.5.4.1)
- $Ba(OH)_2$, 5% (5 g/100 ml distilled water)
- HCl solution, 0.2 N (10 ml 2 N HCl, standardized, in 100 ml distilled water)
- 2×SSC (see Sect. 4.5.4.1)

4.5.4.3.2
Procedure

The $Ba(OH)_2$ solution (5%) is pre-warmed at 60°C in a glass vessel in the incubator for 2 h. The slides are treated for 1 h with 0.2 N HCl at room temperature, then rinsed with distilled water and incubated within the barium hydroxide solution at 60°C for 30–60 s. Then the slides are rinsed thoroughly in several changes of distilled water and incubated in 2×SSC solution at 60°C for 60 min.

Then staining with Giemsa in phosphate buffer for 15 s until 2 min follows: Whereas specific banding patterns along the whole chromosome are produced by Giemsa or fluorescence banding techniques, C-banding allows the presentation of heterochromatic blocks at centromeres of all chromosomes and of the distal part of the long arm of the Y chromosome.

4.5.4.4
Silver Staining of Active Nucleolus Organizer Regions on Acrocentric Chromosomes (AgNOR Staining)

4.5.4.4.1
Reagents

- $AgNO_3$, 50% (5 g/10 ml distilled water)
- Phosphate buffered Giemsa solution (see Sect. 4.5.4.1)

4.5.4.4.2
Procedure

Fresh unstained chromosome preparations are overlaid with 50% silver nitrate solution, covered with a cover glass and transferred in a humid chamber to prevent drying, for example, a high-grade steel box with wet filter paper. The humid chamber is incubated at 37°C for about 17 h. Then the staining is examined by microscope; when the chromosomes are stained to the required intensity, the cover glass is removed, the slide is rinsed thoroughly in distilled water. Eventually staining is repeated or – if it is sufficient – the slide is stained with Giemsa solution for 5 s. When staining was successful, the nucleolus organizer regions especially localized in the satellite stalks of short arms of acrocentric chromosome pairs 13–15, 21 and 22 are visible as dark brown structures.

Besides the chromosome staining methods described, R-banding and T-banding techniques have to be mentioned. By these methods banding patterns reverse to the G- or fluorescence banding patterns are achieved. T-banding makes visible, after all, the telomeres.

In addition to the chromosome banding techniques fluorescence in situ hybridization with DNA probes specific to centromeres (α-satellite probes), whole chromosome painting probes and smaller DNA probes (YACs, cosmids, BACs = bacterial artificial chromosomes setc.) containing whole genes or segments of genes is used (see below, Sect. 4.5.7).

4.5.5
Analysis of Chromosome Preparations

4.5.5.1
Instruments and Accessories

- Photomicroscope, with epifluorescence equipment
- Slide projector
- Films of different sensitivity

4.5.5.2
Procedure

Chromosome analysis is performed either via a microscope at 1000 times magnification or after microphotography of metaphases by examination of the film via a slide projector. Nowadays computer-aided chromosome analysis systems are in use that are timesaving, but produce chromosome pictures of minor quality. If available, at least 20 banded metaphases per tissue type are analyzed concerning the number and the banding pattern of chromosomes. The description of bands follows the International System for Human Cytogenetic Nomenclature (ISCN 1991, 1995). Two and more karyograms are made from each patient. For that all chromosomes of a metaphase are cut out from a photographic picture and ordered systematically according to their size, the location of the centromere and banding pattern along each arm.

4.5.6
Nomenclature of the Banded Mitotic Chromosomes

International standing committees of cytogeneticists have established the nomenclature of human chromosomes and chromosomal changes in several conferences since 1960. The most recent and authoritative document in which all recommendations are considered and previous ISCN documents are included is An International System for Human Cytogenetic Nomenclature (1995).

Karyotype means the chromosome complement specific to a cell but also to an individual, defined by the number and configuration of chromosomes. The systematic order of chromosomes of a cell according to their size, location of the centromere and banding pattern is called a karyogram. Normal diploid human cells contain 46 chromosomes, 22 pairs of autosomes and one pair of gonosomes (sex chromosomes).

Chromosome banding techniques allow the identification of each chromosome, leading to the designation of autosome pairs with 1–22 and of gonosomes with X and Y. In describing a karyotype the total number of chromosomes is firstly recorded followed by a comma and then the sex chromosome constitution. 46,XY, for example, means a normal male and 46,XX a normal female karyotype. If chromosome anomalies are present, they are recorded after the gonosomes, separated by a comma.

The short arm of each chromosome is designated as p (from French "petit"), the long arm as q. The chromosome is divided into the short and the long arm by the centromere, also called primary constriction. Secondary constrictions are constrictions outside the centromere. According to the location of the centromere metacentric, submetacentric and acrocentric chromosomes are distinguished. The centromere is situated in the middle of metacentric chromosomes, in submetacentric chromosomes the short arm is markedly shorter than the long arm and in acrocentric chromosomes the short arm is very short compared to the long arm; the centromere seems to be telomeric. In mitosis the chromatids (half chromosomes) are separated longitudinally and every chromatid moves into a daughter cell. During the synthesis phase following the mitosis each chromatid is duplicated and the chromosome, consisting of two chromatids, is formed.

The various chromosome banding techniques allow the longitudinal differentiation of individual chromosomes by producing a specific continuous series of bands, the chromosome-specific banding pattern. Thus, the assignment of homologous chromosomes to pairs, the identification of additional or missing chromosomes and of structural abnormalities become feasible.

Each chromosome arm consists of one or several regions. A region is defined as any area of a chromosome lying between two adjacent landmarks. Landmarks are for example morphologic chromosomal characteristics such as the ends (telomeres) of chromosome arms or the centromeres (Fig. 4.1). A region comprises different chromosome bands which may be subdivided into subbands. A band is defined as part of the chromosome clearly distinguishable from its adjacent segment by its differential staining property.

Regions and bands of a chromosome arm are numbered from the centromere outward. The regions adjacent to the centromere are labeled 1 in the short arm as well as in the long arm; adjacent distally are situated regions 2 and so on (Fig. 4.1). For the description of a specific band the chromosome number (1–22, X, Y), the arm designation (p or q), and the region number and band number within the region are necessary. 22q11 means therefore band 1 in the region 1 in the long arm of chromosome 22.

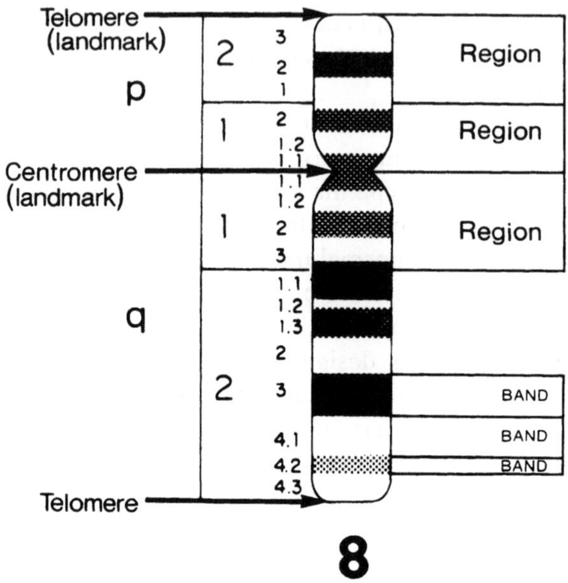

Fig. 4.1. Idiogram of a G-banded chromosome 8 showing short arm p and long arm q, centromere and telomere (landmarks), regions and bands

4.5.7
Fluorescence In Situ Hybridization (FISH)

4.5.7.1
FISH with Whole Chromosome, Centromere, and Telomere Probes

4.5.7.1.1
Reagents

- 20×SSC solution: NaCl – 350.7 g, tri-Na-citrate-dihydrate – 176.4 g in 2 l distilled water
- Ethanol
- Formamide
- 10×PBS solution: NaCl – 80 g, KCl – 2 g, $Na_2HPO_4 \cdot 7H_2O$ – 21.6 g (or $Na_2HPO_4 \cdot 2H_2O$ – 14.24 g), KH_2PO_4 – 2 g in 1 l distilled water.
- 10×PBD solution: 500 ml 10×PBS +2.5 ml Triton X 100
- Vectashield (VECTOR Cat.: H-1000)
- DAPI solution: 1 ml 1×PBS +5 μl DAPI stock solution

4.5.7.1.2
Procedure

Slide Pretreatment. Allow the slides containing metaphase chromosomes to air dry for 1 day. In case of archival preparations pretreat the slides before

FISH by soaking them in xylene for approximately 7 days until the coverslips detach spontaneously (El-Rifai and Knuutila 1996). Incubate the slides in 2×SSC solution at 37°C for 30 min. Dehydrate slides in 70%, 80%, 95% ethanol at room temperature for each 1 min. Allow the slides to air dry for 30 min.

Slide Denaturation (Denaturation of Chromosomal Target DNA). Incubate the slides in a Coplin jar with a 70°C 70% formamide/2×SSC denaturation solution for 3 min. Check the temperature of the denaturation solution inside the Coplin jar to be sure that it is 70°C. The quality of the formamide in the denaturation solution is critical. Do not leave the denaturation solution in the water bath longer than 30 min because the pH will drop. Fresh denaturation solution should generally be used for each experiment. Dehydrate the slides in −20°C cold 70%, 80% and 95% ethanol for 2 min each. Allow the slides to air dry for 30 min.

Probe Preparation. It is recommended to follow the manufacturer´s instructions. Here, a standard procedure for biotin and/or digoxigenin labeled whole chromosome probes containing blocking DNA for suppression of repetitive DNA sequences is presented.

Prewarm the probes at 37°C for 5 min, vortex and centrifuge briefly. For one color FISH take at least 10 μl of probe per 24×24 mm area; for dual color FISH aliquot 6–9 μl of two different labeled probes into one tube and mix well. Denature the probes at 72°C for 5 min and incubate them at 37°C for 1 h. Suppression of repetitive sequences is achieved by preannealing with Cot-1 DNA (see Sect. 4.2.2).

Hybridization (of Probe DNA to Chromosomal Target DNA). Put the slides with the denatured metaphase chromosomes on a 37°C slide warmer for 5 min. Centrifuge the probes briefly and apply the hybridization volume to the prewarmed slide. Cover the area with a 24×24 mm coverslip. Remove any large air bubbles with gentle pressure, seal with Fixogum and incubate overnight (16 h) in a moist chamber at 37°C.

The slide should not get dry at any time after the hybridization procedure!

Post-Hybridization Wash (Removal of Excess Probe DNA). Remove slides from the moist chamber. Peel off Fixogum, remove the coverslips carefully and transfer the slides to 2×SSC at room temperature. Wash hybridized slides 5 min in a 72°C post-hybridization wash solution (painting probes should be treated with 1×SSC, α-satellite probes with 0.25×SSC, telomere probes with 2×SSC). Transfer the slides in 1×PBD, wash solution at room temperature for 2 min.

You can vary the temperature and the salt concentration of the post-hybridization wash solution. Lower salt concentration and higher temperature result in a higher stringency, but this can lead to loss of signal. Higher salt concentration and lower temperature (lower stringency) result in non-specific binding of the probe to other sequences. If you want to combine different kinds of probes on one slide, you should use the post-hybridization wash solution with the lower stringency.

Detection of the Hydridized Probe. Remove the slides from the 1×PBD wash solution and drain excess wash solution from the slides. Apply 70 µl of the detection reagent (e.g. the fluorochrome Texas red combined with the reporter-binding molecule anti-digoxigenin and the fluorochrome FITC combined with the reporter-binding molecule avidin) to each slide and cover the slides with 24×60-mm coverslips. Incubate the slides in a moist chamber at 37°C for 30 min. Remove the coverslips carefully and wash the slides 3×2 min in 1×PBD wash solutions at room temperature.

Counterstain (for the Identification of the Chromosomes). Place slides in 1×PBS and treat slides separately now. Blot excess fluid from the edge of the slide and apply 120 µl of the DAPI solution. Cover with a 24×60-mm coverslip and place in a dark box for 3 min. Wash in 1×PBS for 5 s without agitation. Apply one drop of Vectashield antifade, cover with a 24×60-mm coverslip, place in a drying block and press gently to remove any excess fluid. (Do not move the coverslip!)

Store the slides at 4°C in a dark box until evaluating with the fluorescence microscope. For long term storage seal the edges of the coverslip with Fixogum and store in the dark at –20°C.

4.5.7.2
FISH with Small DNA Probes (such as YACs, Cosmids, and BACs)

4.5.7.2.1
Reagents

- 2×SSC (see Sect. 4.5.7.1)
- Ethanol
- Formamide
- 3 M sodium acetate
- Hybridization cocktail (20% dextran sulfate, 2×SSC)
- Cot-1 DNA
- 1×PBD (see Sect. 4.5.7.1)
- 1×PBS (see Sect. 4.5.7.1)

- 4×SSC: 200 ml 20×SSC, 1 ml Triton X-100 at 1 l distilled water
- BSA
- Vectashield (VECTOR Cat.: H-1000)
- Fluorescein-avidin DCS (Vector Laboratories)
- Biotinylated anti-avidin D antibody (Vector Laboratories)
- DAPI solution (see Sect. 4.5.7.1)

4.5.7.2.2
Procedure

For slide pretreatment see procedure in Sect. 4.5.7.1. For slide denaturation (denaturation of chromosomal target DNA) see procedure in Sect. 4.5.7.1.

4.5.7.2.3
Probe Preparation

Probes are generally labeled by nick translation, but other methods such as random oligonucleotide-primed labeling are also effective (Telenius et al. 1992). Biotin-labeled and digoxigenin-labeled deoxynucleotides are most frequently used for labeling. Probes should contain fragments of 100–500 bp with the majority at 250–300 bp. Larger fragments produce significant background with little or no detectable hybridization signal.

Pipette 100 ng of labeled probe in a vial. For suppression of repetitive sequences add 10 µg human Cot-1 DNA to the labeled DNA probe to be hybridized. Adjust the volume with ddH_2O to at least 10 µl, add 1/30 vol 3 M sodium acetate, vortex, add 2 vol cold 100% ethanol, vortex, and incubate at –20°C for at least 30 min. Spin in a table-top centrifuge for 10 min at high speed, discard the supernatant, add 100 µl 70% ethanol, spin as before, discard the supernatant, and dry the pellet in a vacuum concentrator.

Dissolve the pellet first in 5 µl deionized formamide, add 5 µl hybridization cocktail and mix well. For denaturation incubate probe for 5 min at 95°C. Transfer the tube quickly to 37°C to allow preannealing for 15 min. (The preannealing time can be considerably increased.)

4.5.7.2.4
Hybridization (of Probe DNA to Chromosomal Target DNA)

See procedure in Sect. 4.5.7.1.

Post-hybridization wash (removal of excess probe DNA). During the last 30 min of the hybridization, warm two Coplin jars with 50% formamide/2×SSC wash solution and two Coplin jars with 2×SSC wash solution in a 42°C water bath. Remove the slides from the moist chamber. Peel off the Fixogum, remove the coverslips carefully and transfer the slides to a coplin jar with 2×SSC solution at room temperature for 5 min. Wash the hybridized slides 2×5 min in the prewarmed 50% formamide/2×SSC wash solutions and 2×5 min in the prewarmed 2×SSC wash solutions. Transfer the slides in a Coplin jar with 1×PBD wash solution for 2 min.

4.5.7.2.5
Detection of the Hybridized Probe

See procedure in Sect. 4.5.7.1. For counterstain (for the identification of the chromosomes), see Sect. 4.5.7.1. Amplification of hybridization signals is carried out (if necessary). Signals of both biotin- and digoxigenin-labeled probes can be amplified if necessary. Because the signal-to-noise ratio decreases with successive amplifications, amplification is recommended only when the probe yields weak fluorescence with very little background. Amplification can be performed at any point after the post-hybridization washes, including after viewing, and it may be repeated. Here the amplification procedure of a biotin-labeled probe starts directly after the post-hybridization wash step. The procedure should be performed with minimum exposure to ambient light.

Wash the hybrdized slides in a 0.1% Triton X-100/4×SSC solution at 42°C for 5 min.

Drain excess wash solution from the slides and add 100 µl of a 2–5 µg/ml fluorescein-avidin DCS (Vector Laboratories) in a 4×SSC/1% (w/v) BSA (fraction V) solution to each slide. Incubate the slides in a moist chamber at 37°C for 30 min.

Wash the slides for 2×5 min in 0.1% Triton X-100/4×SSC solution at 42°C.

Drain excess wash solution from the slides and add 100 µl of a 1–3 µg/ml biotinylated anti-avidin D antibody (Vector Laboratories) in a 4×SSC/1% (w/v) BSA (fraction V) to each slide. Incubate the slides in a moist chamber at 37°C for 30 min.

Wash the slides 2×5 min in a 0.1% Triton X-100/4×SSC solution at 42°C. Drain excess wash solution from the slides and add 100 µl of a 2–5 µg/ml fluorescein-avidin DCS (Vector Laboratories) in a 4×SSC/1% (w/v) BSA (fraction V) solution to each slide. Incubate the slides in a moist chamber at 37°C for 30 min.

Wash the slides 2×5 min in a 0.1% Triton X-100/4×SSC solution at 42°C. Continue now with the counterstain procedure.

4.6 Results – Numerical and Structural Chromosome Abnormalities in Different Malignant Diseases

4.6.1 Numerical Chromosome Abnormalities (Genome Aberrations)

Numerical chromosome abnormalities are caused by non-disjunction of single chromosomes or of a whole chromosome set. Gain or loss of a sole or a few chromosomes leads to an aneuploid karyotype; e.g. the gain of a chromosome 8 leads to trisomy 8, the threefold presence of a chromosome 8 within a cell; or loss of a chromosome 7 leads to monosomy 7, the presence of a single chromosome 7 within a cell (Fig. 4.2). The karyotype designation 47,XX,+8 means that in a female cell a chromosome 8 is supernumerary; the karyotype 45,XY,-7 indicates a male cell with loss of a chromosome 7.

Karyotypes containing more than 46 chromosomes are referred to as hyperdiploid, karyotypes with less than 46 chromosomes are designated as hypodiploid, both are nearly diploid. If a chromosome set does contain 46 chro-

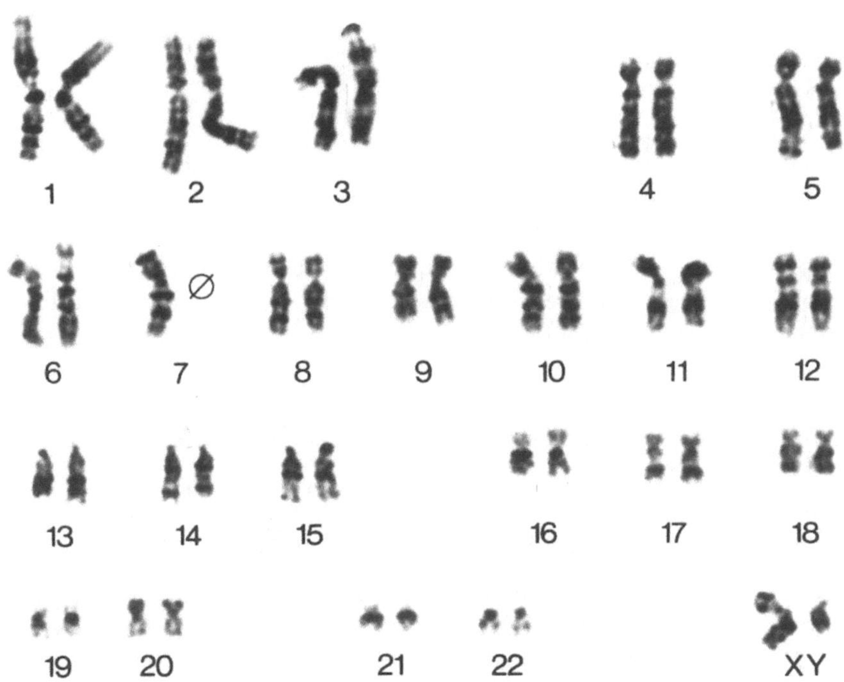

Fig. 4.2. G-banded karyogram of a bone marrow cell of a patient with myelodysplastic syndrome and monosomy 7

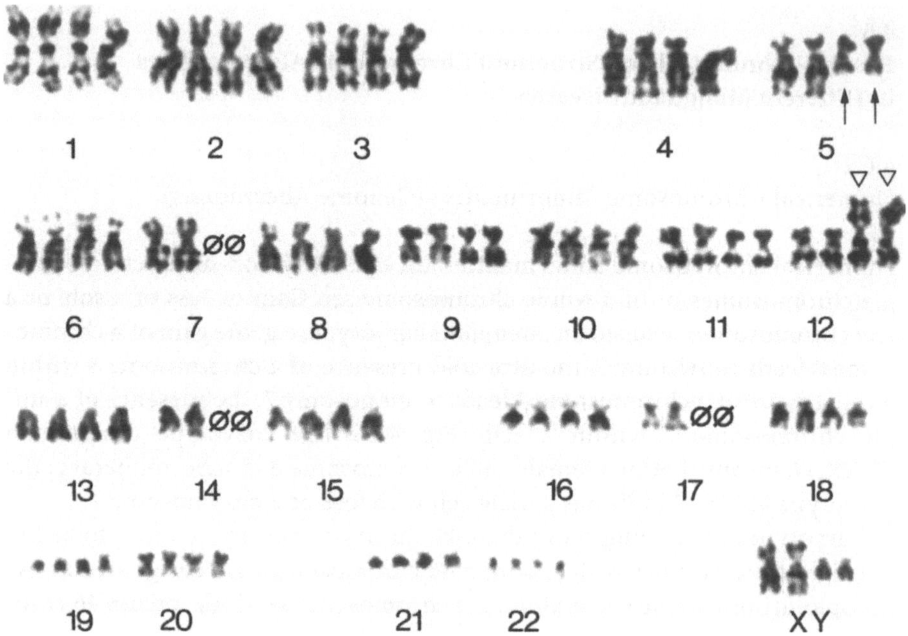

Fig. 4.3. G-banded karyogram of a bone marrow cell of a patient with myelodysplatic syndrome and a near-tetraploid karyotype, missing chromosomes 7, 14, and 17, and structural aberrations in chromosomes 5 and 12 (arrows)

mosomes, but has structural abnormalities or numerical abnormalities, which lead to the chromosome number 46, the karyotype is called pseudodiploid.

Polyploidies are multiplications of the haploid chromosome set, for example triploidy (threefold presence of the haploid set), tetraploidy (fourfold) (Fig. 4.3), pentasomy (fivefold), and so on.

4.6.2
Structural Chromosome Abnormalities (Chromosome Aberrations)

Structural chromosome abnormalities are based on breaks, with one exception. The following anomalies are restricted to a single chromosome:

1. Deletions are due to an interstitial or a terminal loss of a part of the chromosome. A deletion in the short arm of chromosome 12 is designated as del(12)(p11.2p13), if a chromosome segment between subband p11.2 and band p13 is lost or as del(12)(p11.2), if the whole short arm from subband p11.2 is missing (Fig. 4.4a,b).

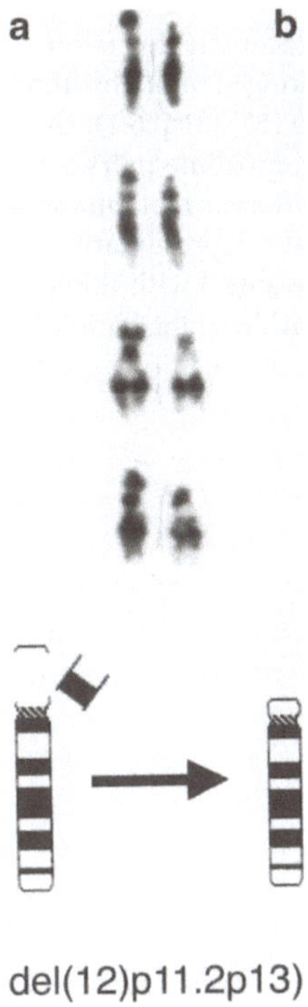

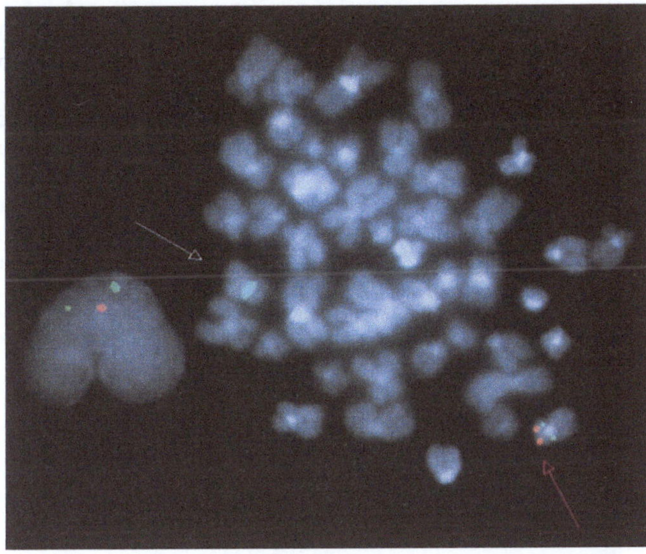

Fig. 4.4. a Deletion in the short arm of chromosome 12 – del(12)(p11.2p13): G-banded chromosome pairs 12 from 4 different metaphases and schematic representation; the chromosome at the right-hand of each pair shows the deletion. **b** FISH with a centromeric probe for chromosome 12 (green) and a YAC probe containing the ETV6 gene (red), showing a red YAC signal on the normal chromosome 12 (red arrow) and loss of the ETV6 region on the chromosome with del(12)(p11.2p12) (white arrow)

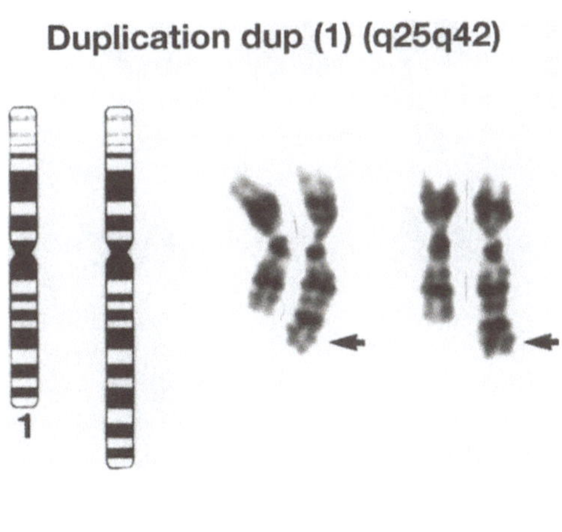

Fig. 4.5. Duplication within the long arm of chromosome 1– dup (1)(q25q42): G-banded chromosome pairs 1 from two different metaphases and schematic representation; the chromosome 1 bearing the duplication is on the right-hand of each pair

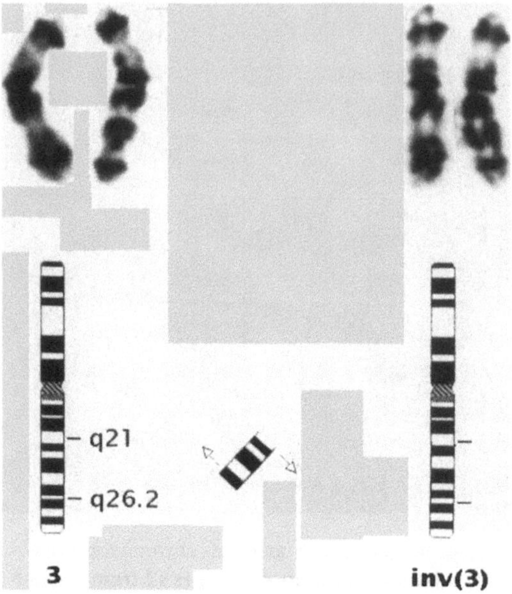

Fig. 4.6. Paracentric inversion within the long arm of chromosome 3 – inv(3)(q21q26.2): G-banded chromosome pairs 3 from two different metaphases and schematic representation; the chromosome 3 with the inversion is on the right-hand of each pair

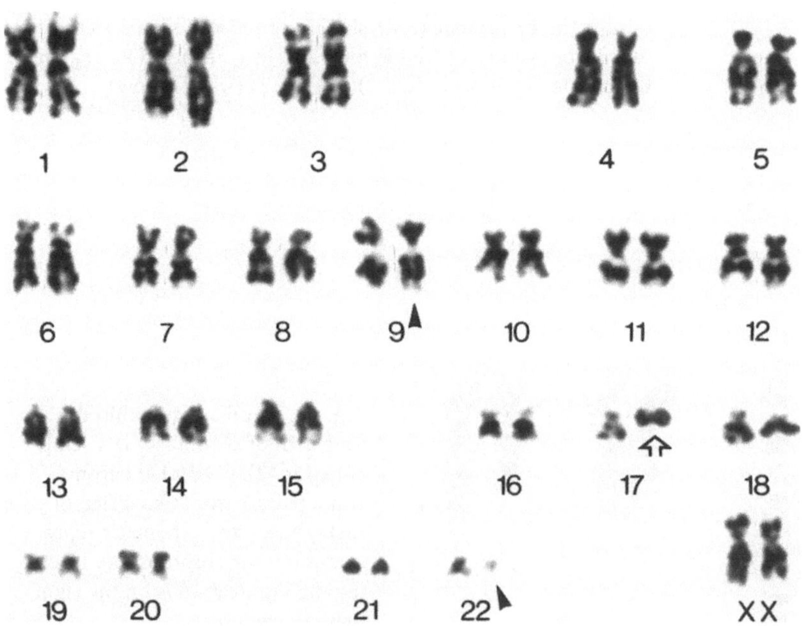

Fig. 4.7. G-banded karyogram from a bone marrow cell of a patient with chronic myeloid leukemia and the standard Philadelphia translocation t(9;22)(q34;q11) (arrowheads) and a ring chromosome 17 – r(17)(p13q25) (open arrow)

2. Duplication means that a chromosome segment is present twofold within a chromosome; dup(1)(q25q42) signifies a duplication of bands 25–42 within the long arm of chromosome 1 (Fig. 4.5).
3. An inversion occurs after two breaks, by turning of the chromosome segment through 180° and insertion back in the original chromosome. If the breakpoints are in different chromosome arms, the inversion is described as pericentric, if they are both in the same arm, then it is described as paracentric. The designation inv(3)(q21q26) for example means that a paracentric inversion within the long arm of chromosome 3 is present (Fig. 4.6).
4. A ring chromosome is formed, if a break occurs on both arms of a chromosome and the break sites fuse together under loss of the chromosome seg-

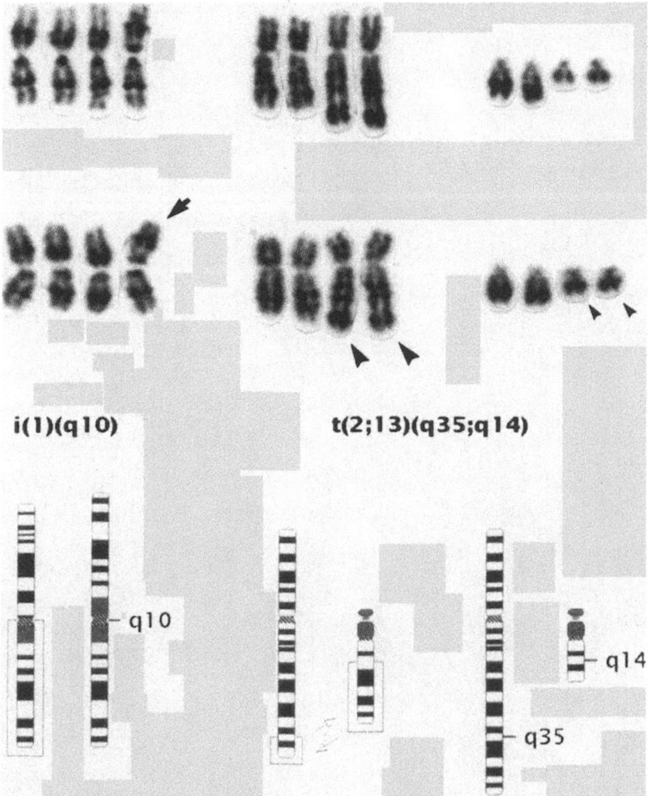

Fig. 4.8a. Partial karyotypes and schematic representation of a near tetraploid alveolar rhabdomyosarcoma (ARMS) with an isochromosome of the long arms of chromosome 1 – i(1)(q10) (arrow) – and a translocation between the long arms of chromosomes 2 and 13 – t(2;13)(q35;q14) (arrowheads).

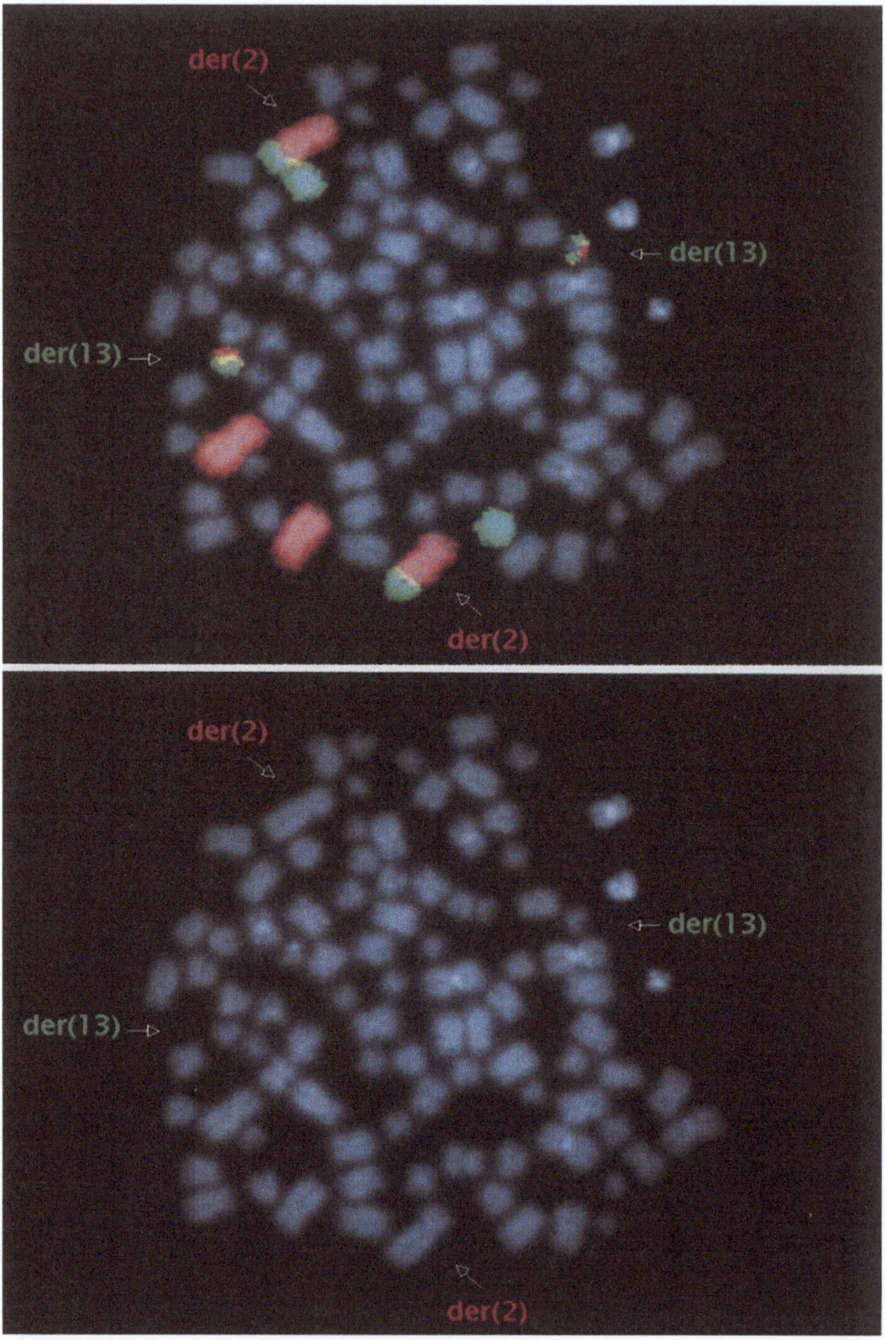

Fig. 4.8b. FISH with painting probes for chromosomes 2 (red) and 13 (green) of an ARMS cell (upper part); same metaphase after DAPI staining only (lower part)

ments distally of the breakpoints: r(17)(p13q25) indicates that breakage in the short arm of chromosome 17 within band 13 and in the long arm within band 25 led to ring-formation (Fig. 4.7).

Two and more chromosomes are involved in translocations and dicentrics:

5. Reciprocal translocations are produced by interchange of parts of two chromosomes; t(2;13)(q35;q14) – a translocation specific to the alveolar rhabdomyosarcoma – means that segments of the long arms of each of the two chromosomes are reciprocally exchanged (Fig. 4.8a,b). Insertion represents a specific type of translocation, the intercalary rearrangement of a chromosomal segment, often recognizable only by FISH.
6. If two centromere bearing segments fuse together, a dicentric chromosome will arise characterized by two centromeres. The description is dic(7;9)(q10;q10), if the long arms of chromosomes 7 and 9 are joined under preservation of both centromeres (Fig. 4.9).
7. Whereas all chromosome abnormalities described under points 1–6 are due to chromosome breakage events, so-called isochromosomes result from the abnormal division of the centromere. If the separation of chromatids during mitosis does not proceed longitudinally but transversally at or near the centromere, both the short and the long arm of the chromosome behave as chromatids and go into different daughter cells. Replication during synthesis phase leads to chromosomes consisting of two identical chromosome arms, an isochromosome of the long arms and an isochromosome of the short arms. As an example an isochromosome of the long arms of chromosome 1 is shown – i(1)(q10) (Fig. 4.8a).

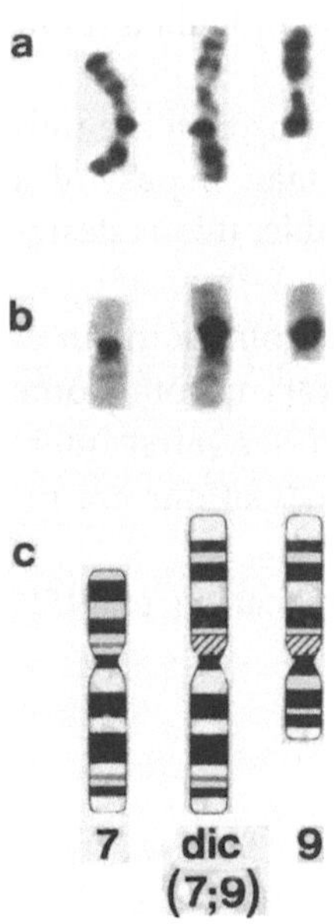

Fig. 4.9a–c. Dicentric chromosome consisting of the long arms of chromosomes 7 and 9 – dic(7;9)(q10;q10). **a** G-banded normal chromosome 7 (left) and 9 (right) and dicentric (middle). **b** C-banding. **c** Schematic representation

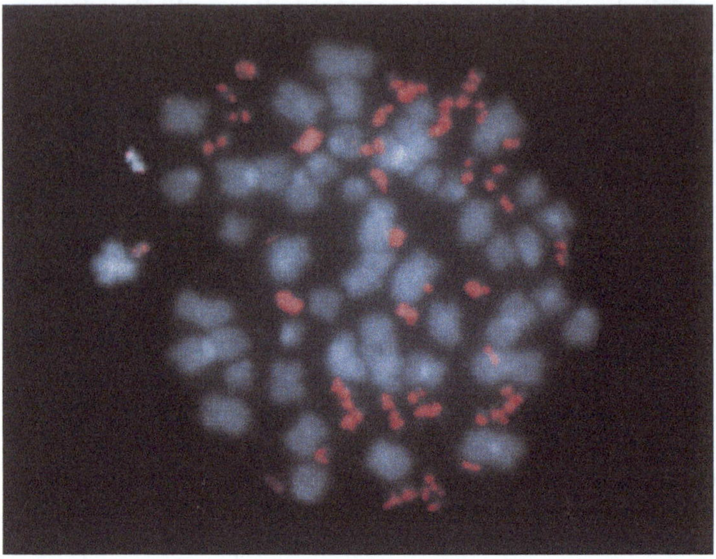

Fig. 4.10. DNA probe containing the c-MYC gene (red signal) hybridizes to double minutes in a bone marrow cell of a patient with AML and trisomy 4

The amplification of genes, most of them encoding oncogenes or enzymes which inhibit cytostatic drugs, leads to cytogenetic phenomena called double minutes (dmin) (Fig. 4.10) and homogeneously staining regions (HSR). dmin and HSR mainly occur in solid tumors and only in rare cases of leukemias or lymphomas.

Structurally altered chromosomes whose origin and composition are unidentifiable are called marker chromosomes, abbreviated mar. If part of a marker chromosome, after all the centromere, is recognizable, this is designated as a derivative chromosome, der.

As a clonal abnormality is defined loss of an identical chromosome in at least 3 metaphases or presence of an identical supernumerary chromosome or of an identical structural aberration in at least 2 metaphases (First International Workshop 1978). Non-clonal sporadic karyotype deviations are recorded, too.

For a detailed karyotype description, including the application of FISH techniques, the new ISCN (1995) is recommended.

References

El-Rifai W, Knuutila S (1996) Fluorescent in situ hybridization on archival G-banded slides. Cytogenet Cell Genet 73:322–324

First International Workshop on Chromosomes in Leukaemia 1977 (1978) Chromosomes in acute non-lymphocytic leukaemia. Br J Haematol 39:311–316

Fonatsch C, Schaadt M, Kirchner H, Diehl V (1980) A possible correlation between the degree of karyotype aberrations and the rate of sister chromatid exchanges in lymphoma lines. Int J Cancer 26:749–756

ISCN 1991 Guidelines for Cancer Cytogenetics, Supplement to an International System for Human Cytogenetic Nomenclature (1991) Mitelman F (ed) S. Karger, Basel

ISCN 1995 An International System for Human Cytogenetic Nomenclature (1995) Mitelman F (ed) S. Karger, Basel

Schröck E, du Manoir S, Veldman T, Schoell B, Wienberg J, Ferguson-Smith MA, Ning Y, Ledbetter DH, Bar Am I, Soenksen D, Garini Y, Ried T (1996) Multicolor spectral karyotyping of human chromosomes. Science 273:494–497

Speicher MR, Gwyn Ballard S, Ward DC (1996) Karyotyping human chromosomes by combinatorial multi-fluor FISH. Nature Genetics 12:368–375

Sumner AT, Evans HJ, Buckland RA (1971) New technique for distinguishing between human chromosomes. Nature 232:31–32

Telenius H, Carter NP, Bebb CE, Nordenskjöld M, Ponder BA, Tunnacliffe A (1992) Degenerate oligonucleotide-primed PCR: General amplification of target DNA by a single degenerate primer. Genomics 13:718–725

References

[illegible]

5 New HLA Typing Methods

R. Blasczyk

5.1 Introduction

5.1.1 History of HLA

The human major histocompatibility complex (MHC) was discovered during studies initiated by J. Dausset, R. Payne and J. J. van Rood describing a genetically inherited system of alloantigens [1–3]. Initially histocompatibility research generated little interest among biologists, primarily because of the artificial nature of the underlying phenomenon, that is, rejection of organ transplants. Later, however, the MHC attracted a great deal of attention, and this as a result of immunological research, which demonstrated that histocompatibility molecules restrict the specificity of the antigen receptor expressed on the surface of T lymphocytes, and thus play a major role in the regulation of the immune response [4].

During the early 1960s multi-transfused patients and parous women were shown to have often circulating antibodies towards the alloantigens or HLA antigens now known to be products of the human MHC genes. 'HLA', as a term, originated in discussions among pioneers in the field and is probably a shortening of '*H*uman *L*eukocyte antigens series *A*', meaning the first histocompatibility locus. More often and appropriate, though strictly speaking incorrect, HLA is used to mean *human leukocyte antigens.*

Following the detection of the first leukocyte alloantigen in 1954 [1] which was called Mac (now HLA-A2), the sophisticated analysis of leuko-agglutination reaction patterns demonstrated shortly thereafter the existence of a second gene for leukocyte antigens which was named FOUR and shown to have two alleles – 4a (now Bw4) and 4b (now Bw6) [5]. In 1964 a related system of three alleles, named LA, was discovered [6] and later shown to be identical with the gene encoding the Mac antigen. Segregation analysis by family studies proved that the two polymorphic systems LA and FOUR were closely linked [7]. They later became known as HLA-A and HLA-B, respectively. First serological evidence for the existence of a third antigen system, named AJ and renamed later HLA-C, was obtained in 1970 [8] and definitively confirmed 1973 [9]. A second class of antigens was discovered with the help of the mixed lymphocyte culture (MLC) technique [10–12] showing that MLC reactivity could be induced in HLA-A and B identical unrelated individuals [13] and vice versa that MLC identity could be found in HLA different unrelated pairs [14]. Segregation analysis by family studies proved the existence of a MLC locus closely linked to the classical HLA genes [15]. This locus became known as HLA-D. With the help of homozygous typing cells used in the MLC several alleles of this locus were defined [16]. Later, sera were found which allowed the identification of MLC determinants on B lymphocytes and monocytes [17]. These antigens were designated HLA-D related or HLA-DR. Further analysis of more sera succeeded in the discovery of the MB gene (now HLA-DQ) [18]. The existence of a third HLA class II locus – named SB (now HLA-DP) – was demonstrated by the use of a secondary MLC, the primed lymphocyte test (PLT) [19, 20].

The impressive knowledge of the human MHC and its antigenic products has been gathered in only 30 years. A series of collaborative international histocompatibility workshops and conferences (IHWC) has brought together scientists at regular intervals to discuss results of testing of shared reagents. The IHWCs have also been an opportunity for the introduction of new techniques and for the testing of a common set of reagents on many different human populations throughout the world. Following each IHWC, a WHO Nomenclature Committee has met to update the universally accepted vocabulary of HLA. The WHO Nomenclature reports are published in relevant scientific journals and serve as the standard for all workers in the field [21]. The WHO nomenclature Committee designates recognized HLA alleles and specificities according to standard genetic practice [22].

Many individuals have contributed to current knowledge of histocompatibility, and Benacerraff, Dausset, and Snell were awarded the Nobel Prize in 1980 for their work on the role of the MHC in the immune response, the discovery of human MHC antigens, and in mouse immunogenetics, respectively. Zinkernagel and Doherty have been awarded the Nobel Prize in Physiology and Medicine 1996 for the discovery of how the immune system recognizes virus-infected cells. They found that lymphocytes must recognize both the virus and the major histocompatibility antigens in order to kill the virus-infected cells. This principle of simultaneous recognition of both, self and foreign molecules, called MHC restriction, has since then constituted a foundation for the further understanding of the specificity of the cellular immune system.

5.1.2
Genomic Organization of the HLA Complex

Histocompatibility genes are found in a closely linked complex in all well-studied endothermic vertebrates, and similar histocompatibility systems, or elements of them, are found in some exothermic (cold-blooded) vertebrates, as well [23]. The human MHC spans a region of approximately 4000 kb on the short arm of chromosome 6 (6p21.3) comprising a series of about 200 tightly linked pseudogenes, expressed genes and genes of unknown function [24, 25].

The MHC is split into three subregions based on similar structure and function of the coded proteins (Fig. 5.1). The class I region at the telomeric end of the MHC spans about 1800 kb and contains the genes coding for the classical transplantation antigens HLA-A, B and C, other nonclassical class I-related genes (e.g. HLA-E, F, G), pseudogenes (e.g. HLA-H, J, K, L, X) and gene fragments. The class II region is located most centromeric and comprises about 800 kb. This subregion contains the class II loci HLA-DRA, DRB, DQA, DQB, DPA, DPB, DNA, DMA, DOB, several pseudogenes and genes involved in antigen presentation LMP1, LMP2, TAP1, and TAP2. The genes and gene products coded for in the region between HLA-DRB and HLA-B were grouped in class III. This central region spans about 1100 kb and contains about 35 genes of different roles, most of them not related to immune functions. Examples for genes of the class III region are the genes encoding for the serum complement components C4B, C4A, Bf, and C2, the heat shock protein genes (HSP-70) and the tumor necrosis factor genes TNF-A and TNF-B.

The gene density varies considerably in the different regions. The class II region contains one gene in every 40 kb of DNA, while the class III region contains one gene in every 15 kb of DNA. The class I region is the least characterized, but recent data indicate that the gene density is similar to the class III region. The most updated map of the human MHC region on chromosome 6 is available via the World Wide Web pages of The Sanger Centre (The Sanger Centre, Hinxton, Cambridge, CB10 1SA, UK, http://www.sanger.ac.uk/chr6/).

The complex of alleles of closely linked loci found on a single chromosome is defined as a haplotype [7]. HLA haplotypes are formed by class I, class II and class III alleles. Two haplotypes in one individual constitute the HLA genotype. Haplotypes are genetically transmitted as codominant traits in a Mendelian fashion. Both, the maternal and the paternal copies, encode proteins that are expressed together on each single cell. Some alleles from different loci do occur together more often than expected by chance from the allele frequencies. This phenomenon of linkage disequilibrium arises because of conserved HLA haplotypes. Haplotype frequency also depends on the eth-

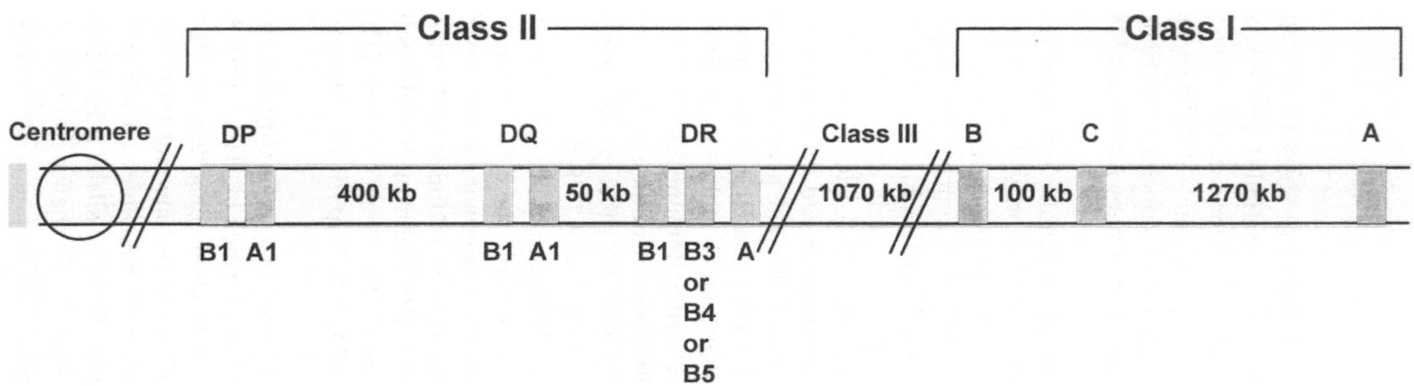

Fig. 5.1. Map of the human MHC containing the expressed HLA class I and class II genes. The DR region varies between haplotypes (see Fig. 5.2). The class I pseudogenes are clustering around HLA-A. HLA-K, -H, – G and -F are located in this order telomeric from HLA-A. HLA-J, -L, -E and -X are located in this order centromeric from HLA-A

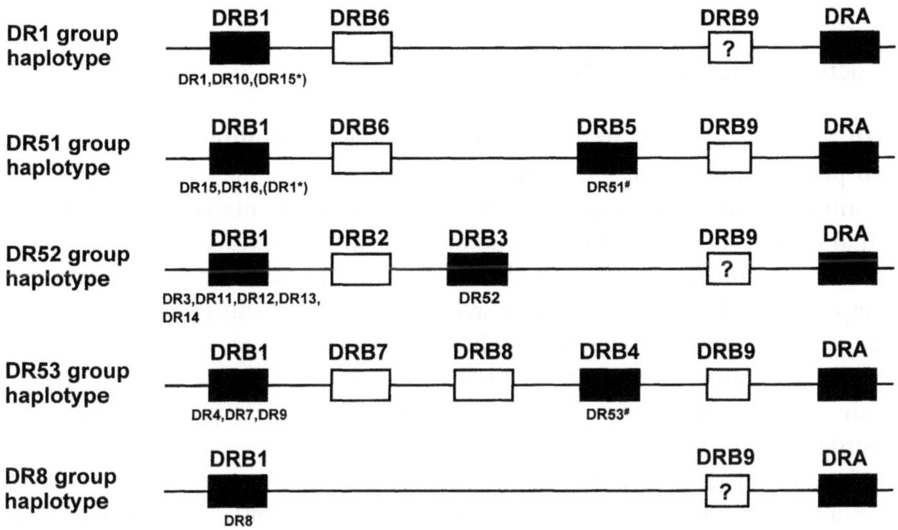

Fig. 5.2. DRB gene organization with different composition of the haplotypes depending on the allele present on the DRB1 gene. *The open boxes* indicate loci believed to be pseudogenes. *Rare haplotypes; #DR51 and DR53 are not expressed on certain haplotypes (DRB5*0108 N; DRB4*0103102 N)? The presence of DRB9 in these haplotypes needs to be confirmed

nic background of the population and differs considerably between the races [26].

The genes of the class III region encoding for the serum complement components C4B, C4 A, Bf, and C2 are also polymorphic and give rise to the complement haplotypes called the complotype. Extended haplotypes were defined by studying the distribution of complotypes in relation to HLA-B and HLA-DR showing a significant three-point linkage disequilibrium between these regions [27].

The number and size of genes can differ considerably between haplotypes giving rise for haplotype polymorphisms. Differences in DNA content between haplotypes have been observed in the class II subregion between DRA and DQA1 (Fig. 5.2). Depending on the individual allele present on the DRB1 gene, the composition of the haplotypes can vary characteristically [28]. In the class III region, the number of C4 and the flanking CYP21 genes is known to vary due to deletions and duplications, and the number of genes present can vary from 1 to 4 [29]. Size variation of the C4 genes is due to a varying length of intron 9 from 0.35–6.5 kb [30]. Differences in DNA content have also been observed in the class I region. Individuals expressing certain HLA-A alleles possess haplotype differences of up to 90 kb between HLA-E and HLA-A [31]. In addition, certain haplotypes possess a 50 kb deletion that falls between the HLA-A and HLA-G genes and includes the HLA-H gene [32].

5.1.3 Structure of HLA Class I Molecules and Genes

MHC class I molecules are non-covalently linked heterodimers composed of two polypeptide chains [33]. The 45 kDa heavy or alpha chain is encoded within the MHC and spans the membrane bilayer, orientated with its N-terminal major portion on the outside of the cell. The extracellular portion of the heavy chain has been divided into three domains called α1, α2, and α3, composed of 90, 92, and 92 amino acids, respectively, and encoded by separate exons. Following the α3 domain is a membrane spanning-region of 25 amino acids and a cytoplasmatic tail of 30 amino acids [34, 35]. The light chain is a non-MHC encoded (chromosome 15) 12 kDa protein called β2-microglobulin (β2 m) [36–38].

The tertiary structure of HLA class I molecules has been revealed by X-ray crystallography first of HLA-A2 in 1987 and subsequently in HLA-A68, B27, B35 and B53 [39–44]. A class I molecule is composed of two sets of structurally homologous domains, one set being the membrane-proximal conserved α3 and β2m domains, and the other being the membrane-distal diverse α1 and α2 domains. The α3 and β2m domains are folded into β-sandwich structures resembling Ig constant regions. The α1 and α2 domains sit on the top of these Ig-like domains forming a platform consisting of β-pleated sheets

A

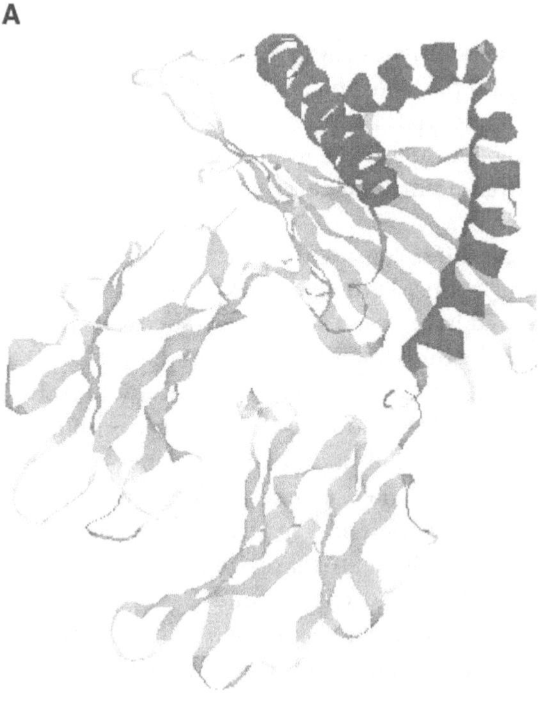

Fig. 5.3A. Side view of the HLA class I molecule (HLA-A2) showing the C-backbone as ribbons. The groove which accommodates a peptide of usually nine amino acids is formed by β-pleated sheets and two α-helices of the α1 and α2 domain. This peptide presenting membrane-distal part of the molecule is stabilized by β2-microglobulin, supporting the α1 and α2 domain against the membrane-proximal α3 domain.

B

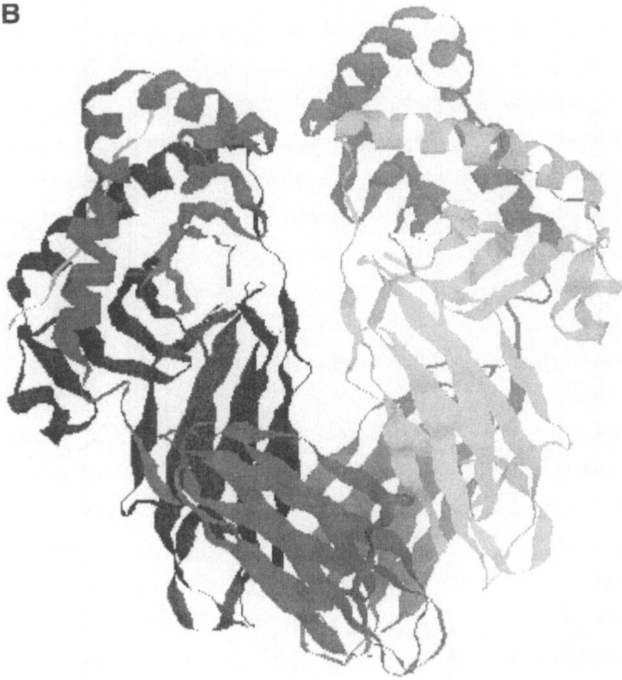

Fig. 5.3B. Side view of the MHC class II dimer of the class II αβ heterodimers seen in the crystal forms of HLA-DR1. The structure of the heterodimer (the α chains are *colored light*, the β chains *dark*) is similar to the class I molecule. The peptide binding cleft accommodates peptides of 15–24 residues which are in contrast to class I molecules allowed to overhang the ends of the groove. If the HLA class II dimer of dimers is a crystallization artifact, an intrinsic property of DR1 or a physiological phenomenon is still unclear. The figures were made with the program rasmol 2.6 [191]

topped by two long α-helices that lie diagonally across the sheet. The two α-helices form a deep cleft between them that functions as the binding site for antigenic peptides with a length of 8–10 amino acids. The extracellular portion of the molecule is about 70 Å high, and cross-sectional dimensions are about 50 Å and 40 Å (Fig. 5.3A).

The β2m domain interacts extensively with all three α-domains stabilizing the three-dimensional structure of HLA class I molecules. The heavy chain loses its structure when separated from β2m, and β2m is required for biosynthesis and cell surface expression of HLA class I heavy chains. The loss of β2m synthesis is associated with a complete loss of HLA class I cell surface expression [45, 46].

The structure of the HLA class I genes has first been elucidated in a HLA-A3 and Cw3 allele in 1984 [47, 48]. HLA class I genes carry the principal features of eukaryote genes. The coding sequences are interrupted by non-cod-

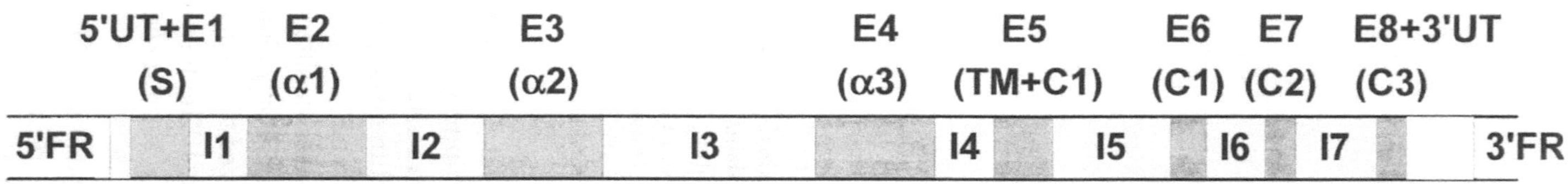

Non-coding regions	Size (bp)	Transcribed region (mRNA)	Size (bp)	Amino acid position
Promoter	200	5' UT	23	
Intron 1	130	Exon 1	73	-24 - -1
Intron 2	241	Exon 2	270	1 - 90
Intron 3	601	Exon 3	276	91 - 182
Intron 4	97	Exon 4	276	183 - 274
Intron 5	438	Exon 5	117	275 - 313
Intron 6	140	Exon 6	33	314 - 324
Intron 7	169	Exon 7	48	325 - 340
		Exon 8	5	341
		3' UT	405	
Total size	2.0 kb		1.5 kb	341 AA

Total size of the gene	3.5 kb	
Total size of the polypeptide		341 AA

Fig. 5.4. Structure of HLA class I genes. The polymorphism is nearly exclusively restricted to the 2nd and 3rd exon. α1-α3, α1-α3 domains; *C*, cytoplasmatic part; *FR*, flanking region; *UT*, untranslated region; *E*, exon; *I*, intron; *S*, signal peptide; *TM*, transmembrane part

ing sequences which make up more than two-thirds of these genes. The mature mRNA has a length of about 1.1 kb from the ATG start codon to the TGA stop codon. The corresponding genes span 3.3 kb from the cap-site to the AATAAA box in the 3′ untranslated region. Together with regulatory promoter elements in the 5′ flanking region of at least 0.2 kb, HLA class I genes are about 3.5 kb in size. Their intron/exon organization, reflecting the structure of the class I heavy chain, includes 8 exons and 7 introns (Fig. 5.4). Exon 1 encodes for the signal peptide, the exons 2 and 3 encode for the polymorphic α1 and α2 domains, exon 4 for the conserved α3 domain, exon 5 for the transmembrane part and the first 5 amino acids of the cytoplasmatic tail, and exons 6 and 7 for the remaining cytoplasmatic region. In HLA-A and C, exon 8 carries the 2nd and 3rd nucleotide of the carboxy-terminal amino acid, the TGA stop codon and the 3′ untranslated region. In HLA-B, exon 8 bears exclusively the 3′ untranslated region.

The size of the introns varies from 97 bp in intron 4 to about 600 bp in intron 3. This 3rd intron separates the gene physically in a 5′ part carrying the variable 2nd and 3rd exons and a 3′ part carrying the conserved exons 4–8. The HLA class I introns are type I introns having their splicing sites behind the first nucleotide of the first codon of the following exon. The 5′ flanking region carries several regulatory elements about 100 bp upstream of the ATG start codon which have been summarized as "class I regulatory complex" (Fig. 5.5) [49]. This complex exhibits significant sequence variations between the different HLA class I genes as well as between the alleles of a single locus [50, 51].

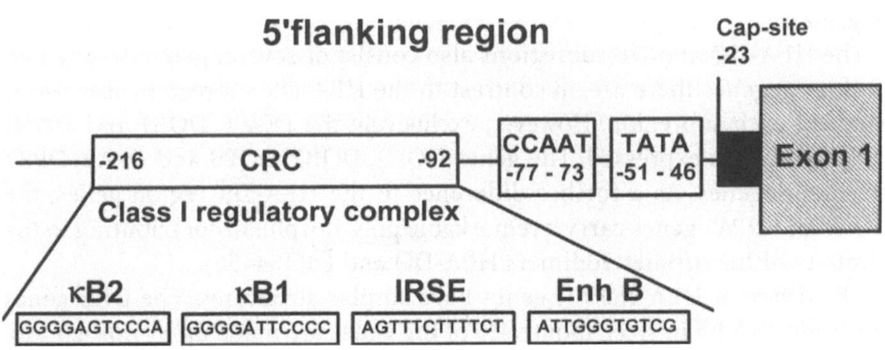

Fig. 5.5. Schematic representation of the class I regulatory complex and the conserved cis-acting elements within the 5′ flanking region. *CRC*, class I regulatory complex; *IRSE*, interferon response sequence element; *Enh B*, enhancer B

5.1.4 Structure of HLA Class II Molecules and Genes

The tertiary structure of HLA class II antigens has been clarified by X-ray crystallography of HLA-DR1 in 1993 and is similar to that described for HLA class I (Fig. 5.3B) [52]. The class II molecules are non-covalently linked heterodimers consisting of two transmembrane MHC-encoded glycoprotein chains, a 34 kDa α-chain and a 28 kDa β-chain. The extracellular part of both chains of class II molecules contains two distinct sections, the α1, α2, and β1 (94 amino acids), β2 (84 amino acids) domains, respectively. The membrane-distal polymorphic α1 and β1 domains jointly form a peptide binding cleft consisting, like in class I molecules, of a β-pleated sheet with two α-helices on top. The resulting groove between the α-helices resembles the groove in class I molecules but accommodates longer antigenic peptides with no apparent restriction on peptide length. The membrane-proximal conserved domains α2 and β2 are, like the α3 and β2 m domains of class I molecules, similar to the constant domains of immunoglobulin heavy chains [53].

The α chains are encoded by A genes, the β chains are encoded by B genes. Thus the genes encoding for the HLA class II antigens DR, DQ or DP are called DRA and DRB, DQA and DQB, DPA and DPB. In the HLA-DR subregion exclusively one α chain encoding invariant DRA gene exists, whereas nine polymorphic DRB genes, DRB1-DRB9, are present, five of which are pseudogenes (DRB2, DRB6, DRB7, DRB8, DRB9). Seven of the DRB genes (not DRB1 and DRB9) are restricted to certain HLA-DR haplotypes (Fig. 5.2). The DRB1, DRB3, DRB4 and DRB5 genes encode for separate β chains. The DRB1 gene encodes for the major HLA-DR antigens DR1-DR18, whereas the antigens DR51, DR52 and DR53, encoded by DRB5, DRB3 and DRB4, respectively, may be present depending on the HLA-DR type defined by the DRB1 gene (Fig. 5.2).

The HLA-DQ and DP subregions also consist of several genes. Beside two or three B genes there are, in contrast to the HLA-DR subregion, also two A genes in each subregion. However, exclusively the DQA1, DQB1 and DPA1, DPB1 genes are expressed. The genes DQA2, DQB2, DQB3 and DPA2, DPB2 are pseudogenes. As a further difference to the HLA-DR region genes, the DQA1 and DPA1 genes carry a remarkable polymorphism contributing to the diversity of the α/β heterodimers HLA-DQ and DP [54–56].

The different HLA class II genes have similar structures. The DRB genes are about 13.5 kb in size. About 94% of the genes are made up by non-coding sequences, whereas only 801 bp from exon 1 through exon 6 carry the coding information, representing less than 6% of the gene´s nucleotides (Fig. 5.6). Exon 1 encodes for the signal peptide, exon 2 for the polymorphic β1-domain, exon 3 for the conserved β2-domain, and the exons 4–6 encode for the

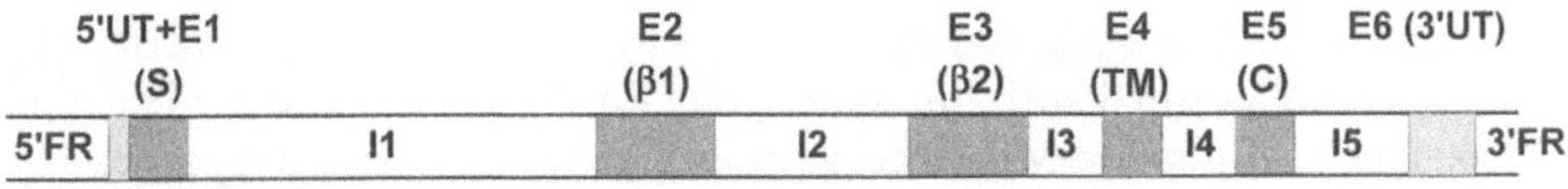

Non-coding regions	Size (bp)	Transcribed region (mRNA)	Size (bp)	Amino acid position
Promoter	> 200	5' UT	62	
Intron 1	8500	Exon 1	100	-29 - +4
Intron 2	2250 - 2740	Exon 2	270	5 - 94
Intron 3	700	Exon 3	282	95 - 188
Intron 4	470	Exon 4	111	189 - 225
Intron 5	300 - 840	Exon 5	24	226 - 233
		Exon 6	14	234 - 238
		3' UT	> 365	
Total size	12,4-13,5 kb		1,2 kb	238 AA

Total size of the gene	13,6 - 14,7 kb	
Total size of the polypeptide		238 AA

Fig. 5.6. Structure of HLA class II DRB genes. The polymorphism is restricted to the 2nd exon, which is 276 bp in length. The exon is flanked by the 6000 bp 1st intron and 2400 bp 2nd intron. β1, β2, β1 and β2 domains; *C*, cytoplasmatic part; *FR*, flanking region; *UT*, untranslated region; *E*, exon; *I*, intron; *S*, signal peptide; *TM*, transmembrane part

transmembrane, cytoplasmatic and 3′ untranslated regions. The DRA gene structure is similar except that the transmembrane, cytoplasmatic and 3′ untranslated parts are encoded by only 2 exons (exons 4, 5).

5.1.5 Function of HLA Molecules

Lymphocytes are the agents of antigenic specificity in the immune response. They divide into two groups: B cells that produce immunoglobulins (Igs), and T cells that perform a heterogeneous set of functions including help for B cells, production of delayed type of hypersensitivity reactions, and the specific killing of virus-infected cells. Igs are the sole source of B cell specificity, whereas the T cell receptors (TCRs) and the MHC glycoproteins, are the key elements of specificity in the T cell response to foreign antigens.

HLA class I and class II molecules are highly specialized proteins that form extraordinary stable complexes with protein fragments, presenting them in their groove on the cell surface for recognition by T cells of the immune system [57, 58]. Not the individual HLA molecule itself but the HLA-peptide complex represents the immunological uniqueness of the molecule. The interaction between TCRs and peptide-MHC complexes triggers a cascade of intercellular signals that depends on the identity of both, the T cell and the antigen presenting cell. This interaction can only occur if the T cell and the target cell carry identical HLA molecules. This phenomenon, known as MHC restriction, has first been described in 1974 by Zinkernagel and Doherty [4] and has been awarded with the Nobel prize for Physiology and Medicine in 1996. The TCR-peptide-MHC recognition regulates immune responses including graft and tumor rejection, anti-viral cytolysis, and the control of other immune cells such as B cells. The peptide-MHC complex also determines the TCR repertoire, with which an individual is equipped, by negative and positive selection of T cells in the thymus [59–61]. Thus, HLA molecules determine the immune response repertoire of an individual via their capacity to present a wide range of different peptides and by their influence on the individual´s T cell equipment. The individuality of the HLA alleles and the individuality of the somatically rearranged T cell genes determine the uniqueness of an individual´s immune system. The antigen-presenting capacity of a species increases with multiple polymorphic loci expressing homologous molecules with different binding site specificities. The increase in antigen-presenting capacity may, however, reduce the individual´s TCR repertoire. In this view, the limited number of MHC loci in all species [23] may be the evolutionary optimized result of thymic tolerization and required immunological competence.

The two structurally distinct, but related, families of MHC molecules, HLA class I and class II, have different functions in the immune system. HLA class I molecules present antigens to T cells that express the CD8 cell-surface glycoprotein, and class II molecules present antigens to T cells that express the CD4 cell-surface glycoprotein. Class I molecules are expressed on all nucleated cells and platelets, whereas the expression of class II molecules is restricted to B cells and antigen-presenting cells such as macrophages and dendritic cells. They are also present on activated T cells. This different tissue distribution reflects the different functions of class I and class II molecules. Class I molecules commonly present peptides derived from endogenously synthesized proteins, such as autologous proteins or viral components produced upon virus infection, and result in the stimulation of CD8-bearing cytotoxic T cells [62]. Thus, the function of HLA class I molecules is to permanently display all kinds of endogenously generated peptides on the cell surface in order to enable the immune system to continuously check the cell´s status. In contrast, class II molecules generally present peptides derived from exogenously synthesized proteins and stimulate CD4-bearing helper T cells [63, 64]. Thus, the function of HLA class II molecules is to specifically activate T cells that provide help to other immune cells, such as B cells or activated T cells. The specificity in the antigens presented by class I and class II molecules is guaranteed by different intracellular compartments at which the antigen-processing pathway and peptide loading of class I and class II molecules is taking place.

5.1.6 Diversity of HLA Genes

HLA genes exhibit an unprecedented genetic polymorphism. The diversity of the MHC molecules expressed by an individual is formed by compounding factors. The first is, that multiple, divergent loci are codominantly expressed. Their number varies between different haplotypes. In the HLA class I region, these haplotype polymorphisms are exclusively caused by a variable number of pseudogenes and non-classical genes [31, 32] which physiological roles are still unknown. The molecules which present antigens to T cells are products of the classical class I genes HLA-A, B and C, and their number and size do not vary between haplotypes. In the HLA class II region, the haplotype polymorphisms concern different gene compositions of the HLA-DR subregion and involve pseudogenes as well as expressed genes as outlined above.

The second factor concerns the extraordinary sequence diversity or multiple allelism of the HLA genes [21]. This polymorphism is nearly exclusively located in those regions of the HLA genes which encode for the peptide binding groove and the area contacted by the T cell receptor. These so called hypervariable regions are the exons 2 and 3 in HLA class I genes encoding for the $\alpha1$ and $\alpha2$ domains and the exon 2 of the HLA class II A and B genes encoding for the $\alpha1$ and $\beta1$ domains. This polymorphism directly influences the conformation of the groove, and therefore the set of peptides which can be presented by the MHC molecules. The concentration of polymorphism to these regions suggests that there is an evolutionary pressure for the generation of diversity of the groove and area contacted by the T cell receptor [65].

The diversity of the HLA genes is reflected by the number of their alleles. In Table 5.1 the number of alleles for each HLA locus is listed based on the 1997 WHO nomenclature report for factors of the HLA system [21]. The no-

Table 5.1. Number of alleles per locus as recognized by the WHO Nomenclature Committee for factors of the HLA system, 1996 [21]

HLA	A	83
HLA	B	186
HLA	Cw	42
HLA	DRA	2
HLA	DRB1	184
HLA	DRB3	11
HLA	DRB4	9
HLA	DRB5	12
HLA	DQA1	18
HLA	DQB1	31
HLA	DPA1	10
HLA	DPB1	77

menclature of HLA alleles is based on the historical classification of HLA antigens by means of serological methods. The locus is named first, followed by an asterisk and the number of the allele. This number is usually composed of four digits. The first two digits represent the main group as defined by serology, followed by the third and fourth digits indicating the serologically undefined variability of the nucleotide sequence. For example the alleles A*2402 and A*2404 do both have the same serological pattern of reactivity (A24) but do differ in their amino acid sequence, which can not be detected by means of serology. Some allele names have a fifth digit, indicating variants that differ by synonymous substitutions in the coding region (e.g. A*68011 and A*68012). The sixth and seventh digit of an allele name is reserved for variations in the non-coding regions. The alleles A*2402101 and A*2402102 have identical exonic nucleotide sequences, but differ in a single nucleotide of the non-coding region (the 2nd intron). Additionally, the suffix N or L can be appended to indicate that the allele is not expressed (suffix N) or has a low level of expression (suffix L). The allele A*0215 N is not expressed due to an acquired stop codon in exon 4. It has been classified as an A*02 allele based on typical A*02 group sequence features. The allele A*2402102L has a low level of expression due to an intron 2 variation which inhibits an effective splicing of the primary RNA.

The name of some specificities contains the suffix w directly appended to the locus′ name (e.g. HLA-Cw*0701, HLA-Dw1, HLA-Bw4). The w was initially introduced by the Nomenclature Committee to indicate that the specificity was provisional. Nowadays, in the age of DNA-based molecular techniques, each specificity can be determined unambiguously by sequence analysis. Therefore, the letter w has been dropped with three sets of exceptions: (a) for the HLA-Cw locus the w is retained to distinguish this gene from the complement factors, (b) for the specificities Bw4 and Bw6, which do not represent certain alleles of the HLA-B gene, but specific epitopes present alternatively on each HLA-B antigen (Bw4 or Bw6) and some HLA-A antigens (only Bw4), (c) for those HLA class II specificities which are defined by cellular methods, such as the Mixed Lymphocyte Culture to determine the specificities HLA-Dw1 – Dw26 or the Primed Lymphocyte Test to determine the specificities HLA-DPw1 – DPw6.

The sequence polymorphism of HLA genes displays some typical features which have to be considered for diagnostic purposes. The numerous alleles at each HLA locus are not characterized by individual point mutations or sequence motifs but by individual combinations of sequence motifs from a more or less locus-specific pool of sequence cassettes. Most of the alleles at each locus have arisen from gene conversion events which have usually taken place between different alleles of the same locus [66]. New alleles are identified on a regular basis and this process will probably continue. It can be assumed that the number of alleles at each locus is represented by all theoretically possible combinations of the known sequence motifs. Of course, some of them will not work and fall victim to negative selection. Nevertheless, it can be expected that still an enormous amount of alleles is yet unidentified.

5.1.7 HLA Typing Methods

With respect to the clinical relevance and the extensive polymorphism of HLA antigens, adequate typing methods are extremely important. The early work on the definition of HLA antigens was aggravated by the poor reproducibility of the leuko-agglutination test. The replacement of leuko-agglutination by lymphocytotoxicity tests in 1964 [67] and the systematic analysis of antibodies formed in pregnancy have brought substantial progress in clinically applied HLA typing for class I antigens. In the 1970s, homozygous typing cells were used in the mixed lymphocyte culture (MLC) to define the polymorphism at the HLA-D locus which enabled the discrimination of 26 antigens named HLA-Dw1 – Dw26 [16]. In the late 1970s, sera from multiparous women were obtained with similar specificities as the MLC for HLA-D. These sera led to the definition of HLA-DR (D related) and later also to the identification of a second HLA class II locus which was named HLA-DQ [18]. The third HLA class II locus, HLA-DP, was detected in the late 1970s as a weak MLC locus, which polymorphism was defined by a secondary MLC or Primed Lymphocyte Test (PLT). The application of the PLT allowed the discrimination of six antigens HLA-DPw1 – DPw6 [19, 20]. HLA-DP could not be defined by means of the serological lymphocytotoxicity test.

In the course of the 1980s, the antibody-mediated micro-lymphocytotoxicity test was the most widely used assay for HLA-A, B, C, DR and DQ diagnostic. In addition, for bone marrow transplant programs the PLT was used to define the HLA-DP specificities and the MLC to define serologically undefined variants of the HLA-DR and DQ loci.

These conventional typing methods are all suffering from a limited accuracy and reliability, especially when they are routinely used for clinical purposes [68–70]. With the discovery of the polymerase chain reaction (PCR) the polymorphism of the MHC genes has been studied directly on the nucleotide level. With the increasing availability of sequenced alleles of the class II and later also for the class I loci, the development of PCR-based typing techniques in the late 1980s and the 1990s more and more replaces the conventional typing methods. The PCR-based methods for HLA class II genes have meanwhile completely superseded the serological typing and the MLC for donor/recipient histocompatibility testing. For HLA class I, most laboratories still perform serological typing, but PCR-based methods have been developed also for class I genes. Though many workers were content with the continuing use of serology, the beneficial effects of PCR-based typing approaches have now been clearly demonstrated and they will surely become the standard typing technique in the near future.

5.2 Principle of PCR-Based Typing Methods

The PCR has made it possible to investigate fragments of genes and has emerged as one of the most important molecular techniques for HLA typing. As outlined earlier, the polymorphism of HLA genes is nearly exclusively restricted to only one or two exons. For HLA typing purposes using PCR-based methods it is therefore sufficient to amplify exclusively these polymorphic exons which are the 2nd exon in HLA class II genes and the 2nd and 3rd exon in HLA class I genes. Following PCR, the amplified fragments are analyzed with various methods which identify the hypervariable regions and allow the allele assignment.

The PCR-based diagnostic of the polymorphic HLA system requires the consideration of some general rules concerning the polymorphic structure of HLA genes. The diversity of HLA genes at the antigen presenting sites has evolved on the one hand by the gradual accumulation of point mutations during successive ancestral species and on the other hand by gene conversion events or recombinations [66, 71]. The last mechanism appears to be the most important factor for the enormous diversification of HLA genes. This has consequences on their polymorphic structure. When scrutinizing the sequences of the different alleles per locus it becomes apparent that the allelic diversity is not characterized by allele-specific point mutations but by different combinations of sequence motifs from a common pool of different motifs. This patchwork structure of allelic sequences is reconciled with the polymorphism being generated by segmental sequence exchanges. Thus, most of the alleles can be considered as chimeras formed from various segments of other alleles. In most cases, newly identified alleles are characterized by a new combination of already existing sequence motifs. From these observations it can be concluded that the number of alleles at each locus is represented by all theoretically possible combinations of known sequence motifs.

These features of the polymorphic HLA gene structure have consequences with respect to PCR-based HLA typing strategies. More than 90% of the individuals are heterozygous for each HLA locus. Therefore, for HLA typing at the allelic level it is generally not sufficient to prove the presence of certain sequence motifs but to demonstrate their cis/trans linkage, i.e. to demonstrate how the motifs are linked on each of the two haplotypes (Fig. 5.7). Exclusively this approach is capable of delivering unambiguous typing results.

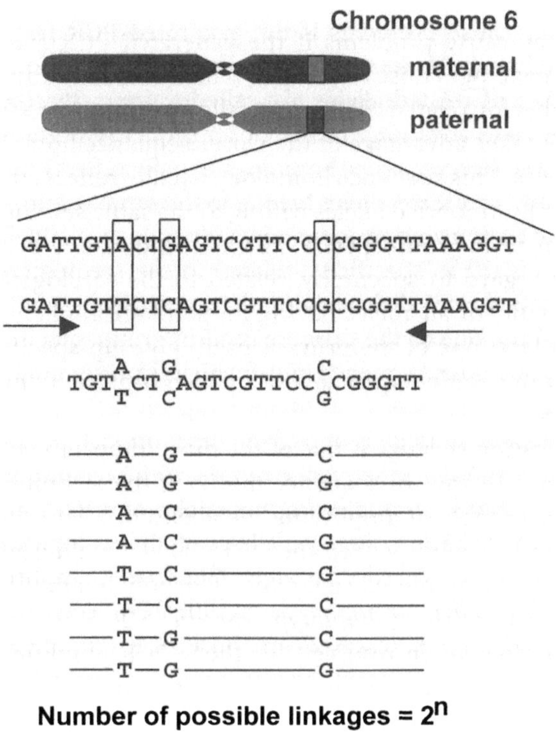

Fig. 5.7. Illustration of the problems related to undefined cis/trans linkages. If a generic pair of primers is used for amplification, the PCR product contains the alleles of both haplotypes. Direct sequencing of this PCR product generates sequencing fragments of both alleles simultaneously, resulting in heterozygous peak patterns in the electropherogram at the indicated positions. Since the cis/trans linkage is not defined, the number of possible linkages is 2^n, in which n is the number of heterozygous positions. The HLA typing is done by comparing all theoretically possible linkages with the most relevant HLA sequence database. This bears the risk that the typing result may become ambiguous in the course of the years, if new alleles are identified

If the cis/trans linkage of variable sites is not defined, some heterozygous allele combinations can not be distinguished from each other. Additionally, new alleles may be mistyped as a heterozygous combination of known alleles.

In terms of PCR methodology, those techniques which lead to the amplification of both alleles present on a particular HLA locus are called a *generic* PCR. The resulting PCR product contains the gene fragments of both alleles ideally in a more or less equal amount. In practice, however, depending on the PCR conditions, the quality of the amplification primers, and the analyzed locus, there is usually a preferential amplification of one allele over the other.

Preferential amplification may cause problems if the generated PCR fragments are used for direct sequencing. Those techniques which lead to the amplification of a limited number of related alleles are called a *group-specific* PCR. The group-specific PCR takes advantage of the closer sequence homology of a certain cluster of alleles. This sequence homology usually reflects the fact that these group-specifically amplified alleles belong to the same serologically defined group. Thus, the term group-specific normally indicates a PCR amplification which is, with regard to specificity, related to the serological variability of a locus, e.g. specific for all alleles having the serological phenotype HLA-A1 or HLA-A2. At least one of the primers used in group-specific PCR is located on an intronic or exonic sequence motif which is present only in a limited number of alleles.

The group-specific amplification strategy is one of the most important approaches to define the cis/trans linkage of sequence motifs. If the technique used for PCR amplification is capable of amplifying the alleles of a HLA locus according to the serological variability, then the alleles of all serologically heterozygous individuals can be amplified separately. This way of amplification is therefore often called an *allele- or haplotype-specific* PCR. However, the term ′allele-specific′ should remain reserved for those PCR amplifications which allow an allele assignment just from the information delivered by the presence or absence of a PCR fragment.

A group-specific PCR amplification is not in all cases haplotype-specific. In those individuals who are heterozygous for different alleles belonging to the same amplification group, the PCR leads to the amplification of both alleles simultaneously, a situation which is similar to the generic PCR. However, due to the close sequence homologies, the quantitative relationship between the amplified fragments of the different alleles is usually more homogeneous than in a generic PCR, facilitating the post-PCR specificity steps. Additionally, sometimes these closely related alleles are differing only at a single nucleotide which allows the definition of the cis/trans linkage even without haplotype-specific PCR.

Thus, the principle of modern DNA-based HLA typing methods is the haplotype-specific PCR amplification of the polymorphic exons of the HLA genes followed by postamplification specificity steps determining the hypervariable regions for allele assignment. However, the technique of group-specific amplification has two major drawbacks. Firstly, the amplification primers have to be located on group-specific motifs normally at the 5′ or 3′ hypervariable regions of the exons. If this is the case, the sequence information outside of these priming sites is lost, so that this amplification strategy may not be capable of delivering sequence information of the complete exon. Secondly, group-specific amplification bears the risk to miss one of the two alleles, i.e. to overestimate homozygosity, if a new allele with an unknown combination of 5′ and 3′ motifs, not covered by the employed primer mixes, is present. Hence, it is important to be aware of these limitations and to take into account that mistypings may occur even if DNA-based typing techniques have been used. In order to overcome these insufficiencies it can be reasonable to combine generic and group-specific amplification strategies, at least in cases of putative homozygosity.

Recently, a considerable number of not expressed HLA alleles has been identified (A*0104N, A*0215N, A*0303N, A*2409N, A*2411N, B*1526N, B*5111N, DRB4*0103102N, DRB5*0108N) and their number can be expected to increase in the next few years (21 and monthly updates). The defects in the alleles, which prevent cell-surface expression of their products, are single sites within the gene where the blank (the not expressed allele) differs from the ′wildtype′ form. These sites involve point substitution, recombination, insertion of extra nucleotides, or the deletion of nucleotides. They can in every case be attributed to a single mutational event which is located either in the non-coding or coding region. The sites may be outside the regions considered as relevant for typing (exon 2 in HLA class II and exon 2 and 3 in HLA class I). Therefore, from the viewpoint of PCR-based typing, these allele-inactivating variations pose an essential problem since they may not be detected, thus leading to the misassignment of the normal ′wildtype′ allele. From the immunological point of view, PCR-based typing leads in these individuals to an overestimation of heterozygosity (assuming that the other haplotype carries a functionally normal or expressed allele). In order to avoid this kind of mistypings, sequencing of the complete gene (3.5 kb for class I, 13.5 kb for class II), the use of mRNA or additional serological typing would be required. So far, the frequency of these inactivated alleles appears to be extremely low, so that they are presently not considered as a serious problem in PCR-based typing approaches.

5.3
PCR-Based Approaches to HLA Typing

In the course of the development of PCR-based methods for HLA typing a large variety of techniques has been described which mainly differ in their postamplification specificity strategy to determine the individual sequence of the amplified fragment. The techniques used to analyze the amplified fragments include the restriction fragment length polymorphism (PCR-RFLP) [72–78], the single strand conformation polymorphism (PCR-SSCP) [79–89], the heteroduplex formation (PCR-HDF) [90–97], the use of sequence-specific oligonucleotide probing (PCR-SSOP) [98–127], the use of sequence-specific priming (PCR-SSP) [129–151], and the determination of the nucleotide sequence of the PCR amplified DNA by sequencing based typing (PCR-SBT)

[152–178]. In the course of the 11th IHWC, the PCR-SSOP method for HLA class II genes had been standardized and provided the forum for the introduction of PCR-based typing methods to histocompatibility laboratories worldwide [111]. The routine use of PCR-based techniques in many laboratories all over the world has brought deep insights into the variability of HLA genes which emerged to be much more variable than it could have been expected from the conventional typing methods. This increasing diversity has complicated more and more PCR-based typing methods so that in the course of the years only the last three methods (PCR-SSOP, PCR-SSP, and PCR-SBT) have survived and are mainly used for HLA typing on the nucleotide level.

5.3.1 Sequence-Specific Oligonucleotide Probing (PCR-SSOP)

One of the initial methods for PCR-based HLA typing is the use of SSOP for the detection of sequence variabilities within amplified hypervariable regions of HLA genes. In contrast to PCR-SSP, the pair of PCR primers is located such that the entire hypervariable region of all alleles (generia primers) or a group of alleles (group-specific primers) of a particular HLA locus is amplified, so that the PCR product carries the complete typing-relevant sequence information. The generated PCR product is then probed with labeled oligonucleotides which have been designed for the different polymorphic positions present in the amplified DNA. The probes are usually about 20 bases in length and are designed such that the polymorphic position to discriminate is located in the middle of the probe. Under appropriate conditions, this technique is capable of distinguishing even single basepair differences. Since the alleles of the different HLA genes are usually not defined by unique sequence-motifs but by a different patchwork of sequence motifs shared with other alleles, the assignment of a specificity is based on the hybridization pattern obtained with a panel of probes. The number of probes required to differentiate the alleles of a particular locus depends on the number of polymorphic positions and the degree of resolution desired.

The PCR-SSOP can be set up in two different formats, the product dot blot [98–100, 102–105, 107–112, 117, 119, 121–127] and the reverse dot blot [101, 106, 113–116, 118]. In the conventional product dot blot approach, the PCR products of different samples are immobilized on a carrier matrix (e.g. nylon membrane) which is then subjected to hybridization with a single probe. For each individual probe the same membrane is created so that the panel of probes required can be run in parallel. In the reverse dot blot format, the set of probes is immobilized on a single membrane instead of the amplified DNA. This membrane, equipped with a defined set of probes, is then subjected to hybridization with the labeled PCR product of a single individual. Thus, the conventional format is designed for the parallel testing of several individuals whereas the reverse dot blot assay allows the complete analysis of a single individual with a single hybridization reaction. A refinement of this technique is the immobilization of the probes on microtiter plates rather than on nylon membranes [114, 115]. The laboratory equipment available with this format brings automation of this technique closer to reality. Since the specificity and sensitivity of oligonucleotide probing strongly depends on a probe-specific hybridization temperature, the reverse dot blot format requires probes with equal hybridization behavior under the same conditions, whereas the product dot blot format can use probes with individual hybridization temperatures. Thus, the development of reverse dot blot formats is much more complicated and has been lagging behind the conventional format.

For the visualization of the hybridized probes, radioactive and non-radioactive systems have been described. In the early studies, radioactive labels (^{32}P) have been used and the hybridization signals were visualized by autoradiography [98–100]. Modern PCR-SSOP systems use non-radioactive detection methods, either by the use of digoxigenin or biotin mediated detection systems or by the use of probes directly labeled with alkaline phosphatase (Lifecodes, Stamford, CT, USA).

The first studies applying PCR-SSOP for HLA typing focused on the DQA1 gene [98]. As more sequence information became available, this technique was rapidly adapted for typing of all other HLA class II specificities. In view of the insufficient serology and the possibility to analyze serologically undefined variants, PCR-SSOP became very attractive in all fields of tissue typing and soon emerged as the gold standard of PCR-based analysis. In the course of the 11th IHWC 1991, protocols for PCR-SSOP were extensively evaluated and standardized for the transplantation-relevant HLA class II genes DRB1, DQA1, DQB1, DPA1, and DPB1 [111]. For typing HLA class II genes by PCR-SSOP, a pair of usually generic amplification primers is located outside the hypervariable regions at the 5′ and 3′ end of exon 2 or the flanking introns. The number of probes applied for the different loci in the 11th IHWC protocol was 66 for DRB, 19 for DQA1, 24 for DQB1, 6 for DPA1 and 27 for DPB1. The hybridization patterns especially for the DRB loci were extremely complex and due to the sharing of sequence motifs sometimes failed to deliver unambiguous typing results. Therefore, a two-step protocol was established which provided in a first step a serology-equivalent (DR1-DR18) result using a selected set of probes. In order to achieve high-resolution typing, a group-specific amplification strategy was established based on the sequence variability at the 5′ end of exon 2. This allowed the exclusive amplification of those alleles belonging to a particular group (DR1, DR2, DR4, DR3, 5, 6, 8), which not only simplified the interpretation of the hybridization patterns but also led to unambiguous typing results. The 11th IHWC protocol was set up in a product dot blot format, but many workers have also established widely applicable protocols for the reverse dot blot format [101, 106, 113–116, 118]. This format has become a domain for commercializing and many companies offer the immobilized probe assay now as a kit. The product dot blot format has been updated in the 12th IHWC 1996 [127] which became necessary due to the identification of multiple new alleles. These new alleles necessitated the addition of new probes (100 for DRB, 27 for DQA1, 36 for DQB1, 15 for DPA1, 34 for DPB1) as well as the introduction of supplementary group-specific amplification primers for DRB genes. In DQA1, some polymorphism was detected in exon 1 and 3 so that the separate amplification of these exons was introduced. The extensive polymorphism of the DPB1 gene has made it necessary to apply two group-specific PCR amplifications based on the sequence diversity of the 3′ end of exon 2 in order to get unambiguous typing results.

The development of PCR-SSOP techniques for HLA class I genes is far behind the class II genotyping methods. This is on the one hand due to the fact that most workers were content with the class I serology and on the other hand caused by the more complex genetic system of class I loci. This includes the extensive polymorphism of HLA class I genes, the low extent of allele specific polymorphic sites, and the presence of more than one relevant exon (at least exons 2 and 3) determining the allelic polymorphism of HLA class I antigens. Moreover, if a particular locus has to be investigated, the high degree of sequence homology among the known alleles and the different HLA class I loci including the less polymorphic HLA-E, F, G genes, and the presence of several pseudogenes causes additional problems. Despite these restrictions, PCR-SSOP has also been applied to analyze the diversity of the HLA-A, B and C loci and several protocols have been described so far [118, 120–126]. In general, the PCR amplification has to cover the sequence polymorphism of the 2nd and 3rd exon of class I loci in at least a gene-specific manner. Most of the protocols apply primers located at the 5′ end of exon 2 and the 3′ end of exon 3. Whereas for HLA-A and C a single pair of primers is used, the HLA-B protocols are working with a mixture of several primers or with group-specific amplification strategies based on the exon 2 and 3 diversity. Locus-specific primer pairs derived from the 1st and 3rd intron sequences have also been described and will probably bring some progress in class I PCR-SSOP [128]. Except for the HLA-A protocol using the reverse dot blot assay [118], all protocols are set up in the conventional product dot blot format.

Taken together, extensively evaluated and robust PCR-SSOP protocols are currently available exclusively for HLA class II genes. Although group-specific amplification has been introduced in the protocols in the course of the years, the general strategy relies on the simultaneous amplification of the alleles of both haplotypes. The differentiation of the amplified alleles and the level of resolution mainly depends on the number of probes applied for each locus. Thus, in PCR-SSOP the cis/trans linkage of the sequence motifs detected by the various probes is usually not defined. Due to the extensive sharing of sequence cassettes between the different alleles, ambiguous typing results are very frequent. This restriction can not be sorted out by the application of additional probes but only by haplotype-specific amplification approaches. The few group-specific primer pairs used in PCR-SSOP fulfill this demand only in a limited number of heterozygous combinations. Therefore, in most cases both alleles are amplified simultaneously and the interpretation of the hybridization patterns has to rely on the sequence database known at that time. Since this way of allele assignment does not consider the linkage of the polymorphic positions, even unambiguous results may become ambiguous in the course of the years when new alleles are detected bearing new combinations of the different sequence motifs.

5.3.2 Sequence-Specific Primed PCR (PCR-SSP)

One of the most widely used PCR-based methods of HLA class I and class II typing is the sequence-specific primed PCR (PCR-SSP). Each PCR is designed to identify a particular specificity or group of specificities. The design of the amplification primers is based on the amplification refractory mutation system (ARMS), i.e. they contain their specificity-dependent nucleotides on the terminal 3′ end [179]. A mismatch at the 3′ nucleotide of the primer with the target sequence disables a PCR amplification under appropriate conditions. A sophisticated primer design in combination with a sufficient stringency of PCR conditions, determined by the composition of the reaction mix and the annealing temperature, allows to discriminate the polymorphic differences, which are often defined by a single nucleotide. The desired specificity of the PCRs is achieved through the combination of the specificity of both primers, defining two polymorphic motifs in cis position (i.e. on the same chromosome) which differentiate one HLA type from another. In PCR-SSP, the PCR fragments between the different specificities vary considerably in their size, but the major basis for allele assignment is simply the presence or absence of the PCR fragments. In order to discriminate between the lack of a certain HLA specificity and a PCR failure, each PCR mix contains an internal control primer pair which amplifies a non-polymorphic sequence present in every genomic DNA, e.g. a fragment of the human growth hormone gene [131] or the β2m gene [135].

Identification of the HLA type requires a large panel of specific PCR mixes which are run simultaneously using the genomic DNA of a single individual. After PCR, the products are visualized by an agarose gel-based read out and the individual HLA type is determined by the presence or absence of a specific PCR fragment in each lane. Thus, PCR-SSP does not require any post PCR specificity steps except for the agarose gel electrophoresis. An individual sample can be typed by this method within 2.5 h starting from whole blood. The different specificities of the multiple primer mixes applied are usually set up in a serology-equivalent fashion. For a complete HLA-A, B, DR serology-equivalent PCR-SSP typing of a single individual usually 24 primer mixes for HLA-A, 48 for HLA-B, and 24 for HLA-DRB are used. A 1.5-h run of a 96-well thermal cycler is required to determine the HLA type of a single individual. One 96-well thermal cycler allows serology-equivalent HLA-A, B, DR typing of five individuals per day. Thus, the major drawback of this method is its restricted suitability for large sample throughput. Dependent on the laboratory´s equipment, the bottleneck may be the cycler or the electrophoresis capacities. Conventionally, the sequence-specific primed PCR products are visualized and separated from the internal amplification control by agarose electrophoresis and ethidium bromide staining. For interpretation and documentation of the results, the agarose gels are usually photographed on an UV transilluminator. Therefore, for this kind of typing the term ´phototyping´ has been created. Substantial improvements with regard to sample throughput have been made by the very recent application of fluorescence-based PCR product detection systems which eliminate the time-consuming post-PCR pipetting and electrophoresis steps and restrict the bottleneck exclusively to the cycler capacities [147, 150]. For this more recent development of fluorescence-based detection of PCR products the term ´fluorotyping´ was introduced [150].

The use of PCR-SSP for HLA typing was first described for HLA class II [129] and later for HLA class I specificities [135]. This order of methodical developments was due to the fact that especially serological HLA class II typing was extremely unreliable, demanding the need for more precise typing techniques [68]. Additionally, the genetic background of HLA class II genes was better investigated and DNA sequences were available for the different specificities. The HLA class II specificities are determined nearly exclusively through the sequence diversity of the second exon. Thus, the sequence-specific primers are all located on polymorphic sites of this exon yielding PCR fragment sizes of about 100–250 bp. Since the HLA class I polymorphism is defined by the 2nd and 3rd exon which are separated by a 241 bp intron, the PCR-SSP fragment sizes are usually larger than in class II. The necessity to amplify larger gene fragments in class I typing, as well as the high GC content of the polymorphic exons in HLA class I genes of up to 70%, usually makes HLA class I PCR-SSP less robust than for HLA class II.

Theoretically, the HLA typing resolution which can be obtained by PCR-SSP is unlimited, since amplification primers can be designed for any point mutation. However, the use of an extensive number of primer mixes may be restricted for practical reasons. This refers to the limited cycler capacities of the laboratory as well as to the limited amount of genomic DNA available for

HLA typing since each primer mix requires about 100 ng genomic DNA. Besides that, the level of resolution achievable by this method is also restricted by several genetic features of the HLA genes. Firstly, in the HLA class I and class II regions a tremendous number of homologous pseudogenes is complicating the primer design and primer mix set up for specific amplification of particular point mutations. Therefore, the specific amplification of some motifs requires the use of a gene-specific second primer. This usually extends the specificity of a primer mix to a group of several alleles displaying homologous sequences. Secondly, the different alleles of a given HLA locus are normally lacking any allele-specific sequence motifs but are characterized by an extensive patchwork structure of the polymorphic HLA sequences. This feature makes it in most cases impossible to design a pair of primers with a single specificity. Consequently, the PCR-SSP primer mixes are normally designed to amplify a group of specificities which are related to serological families. Additionally, a lot of primer mixes have been designed to deliver typing information above the serological level of resolution [129, 130, 136, 141, 145, 150, 151]. In order to obtain the allele-specific typing information, a large set of primer mixes is required giving characteristic amplification patterns for a single allele. However, these sets are suffering from the limitation that the amplification patterns are often ambiguous, i.e. they do not allow an unequivocal allele assignment in certain heterozygous combinations.

Some of these limitations may be overcome by multiplex and nested PCR approaches. Nested PCR strategies may offer the possibility to exclude in the first PCR round those alleles which carry identical internal sequence motifs and which would disturb high resolution analysis by delivering ambiguous amplification patterns. This approach has been described by several groups [131, 142, 145] but has not found a broad acceptance, probably due to the high contamination risk and the availability of sequencing based typing strategies which deliver typing results at the allelic level. Multiplex approaches are complicated by the high degree of homology between the different HLA class I and class II genes, respectively, and are suffering from allelic drop outs resulting in the overestimation of homozygosity [151].

5.3.3 Sequencing-Based Typing (PCR-SBT)

Sequencing gives the most reliable and accurate information of the DNA sequence of a gene and is therefore of particular interest for the determination of the full extent and complexity of the HLA polymorphism. In contrast to PCR-SSP and PCR-SSOP, sequencing is not limited to the detection of known sequence polymorphisms in the hypervariable regions. Sequencing provides the means to uncover unique polymorphic differences which also exist in the

Table 5.2. Heterogeneity of sequencing-based typing strategies

Starting materials	mRNA Genomic DNA
Amplification strategies	Gene-specific Group-specific
Amplified regions (HLA class I genes)	Exons 2 and 3 Exons 2, 3 and 4 Complete gene
Sequencing strategies	Direct sequencing Indirect sequencing (cloning)
Sequencing chemistries	Manual radioactive sequencing Sequenase Cycle sequencing
	Automated fluorescence sequencing Cycle sequencing with dye terminators Cycle sequencing with dye primers
	Sequenase with dye terminators Sequenase with dye primers

regions in-between. These variations may also be detected by conformation analyzing methods (single strand conformation polymorphism and heteroduplex analysis) [79–97]. However, the PCR design for these techniques is rather complicated and they neither provide a 100% sensitivity nor reveal the nature of the variabilities in terms of DNA sequence. Moreover, depending on the methodical set up, sequencing may offer the possibility to define the cis/trans linkage of sequence motifs.

Sequencing for HLA typing purposes does not require the consideration of the complete gene but is restricted to those parts of the genes displaying the polymorphic sites, i.e. exon 2 in HLA class II and exons 2 and 3 in HLA class I genes. Therefore, the method to sequence exclusively the typing-relevant regions as a post-PCR specificity step has been designated sequencing-based typing (PCR-SBT).

Over the last years, sequencing-based typing of HLA genes has progressed considerably allowing to implement PCR-SBT for routine HLA typing. Although all sequencing proposals are based on the dideoxynucleotide chain termination technique of enzymatically synthesized DNA fragments, first described by Sanger et al. 1977 [180], the term PCR-SBT covers a very heterogeneous field of methodical approaches (Table 5.2). Differences exist with respect to the starting material, amplification strategies, template preparation and sequencing chemistries [152–178]. Much of the information of the allelic polymorphism was gained by cloning and subsequent sequencing of cDNA. Later, direct sequencing of PCR products obtained from cDNA or genomic DNA has been used. The initial radioactive, manual sequencing has been replaced by automated fluorescence-based methods. Currently, a variety of sequencing enzymes and fluorescent labeling strategies are employed.

Which starting material should be used? Although the largest part of the sequence databank was gained using mRNA as a starting material, it is possible to use either mRNA or genomic DNA. Both have advantages and disadvantages.

The first systematic work done to sequence HLA for typing purposes used mRNA as a starting material [154]. The use of mRNA avoids problems associated with sequence homologies between the numerous pseudogenes and gene fragments. For the HLA class I genes, mRNA has the additional advantage, that the typing relevant exons 2 and 3 are not separated by the 2nd intron (241 bp in span). This means that the sequencing of the exons 2 and 3 (a total span of 546 bp) can be done in a single sequencing reaction.

Genomic DNA is readily available and easy to handle. In addition to this, gene and group-specific sequence motifs from the non-coding regions can be used as targets for amplification and sequencing primers. When mRNA is used, the limited number of group-specific coding motifs outside the polymorphic exons does not allow a haplotype-specific PCR amplification. If this is desired, variable motifs in the polymorphic exons have to be used for PCR-based separation, and thus the priming sites can not be part of the sequenced region.

What´s the strategy to be used, direct sequencing or cloning? Cloning of PCR products generates the best sequencing results. Cloning avoids all problems related to heterozygosities and sequence homologies with pseudogenes [153, 160]. However, if accurate results are to be obtained, a lot of lab work is needed for the ligation of the PCR fragments into a plasmid, the expansion of the clones, the screening of the clones, and the multiple sequencing of each haplotype to exclude errors that arise via the Taq DNA polymerase [153]. In order to determine homozygosity, six randomly selected clones should reveal identical sequencing results. The probability of having overlooked a single haplotype is therewith 0.5^6 (0.016). In order to minimize Taq DNA polymerase errors when sequencing heterozygous samples, the sequence of each haplotype should be determined at least three times. However, this cloning is time consuming and thus significantly reduces the effective application of such sequencing techniques for clinical use; for clinical use sequencing should be done directly from PCR products.

Which amplification strategy should be used? PCR amplification of polymorphic systems for direct sequencing can be done gene- or haplotype-specific; the latter approach has two distinct advantages; firstly, the cis/trans linkage of sequence motifs can be defined and, secondly, problems related to preferential amplification of one haplotype over the other are avoided. PCR-SBT, after generic PCR amplification, is unable to define the cis/trans linkage of sequence motifs, which means, for typing uses, it is similar to oligotyping. The rapidly growing number of newly identified alleles confirms that new alleles arise mainly from gene conversion events which take place between different alleles of the same locus. Newly identified alleles are not characterized by new sequence motifs, but by new combinations of already existing sequence motifs. The conclusion from this observation is that the possible number of alleles at each locus is the theoretical number of all recombinations of known sequence motifs. Which suggests that, although many of these theoretically possible alleles will probably be subject to negative selection, the number, of as yet unidentified alleles, is enormous. If the cis/trans linkage of the analyzed polymorphic regions is not defined, then some new alleles may be mistyped as a heterozygous combination of known alleles.

This has consequences with respect to SBT strategies, i.e. an unambiguous typing result of SBT after generic PCR amplification is only unambiguous with regard to the presently known HLA databank. However, over the course of the next few years, as more and more new alleles are detected and defined, this result can become ambiguous. Such tendencies were observed, in the last few years, with PCR based DRB1 typing, and is likely to occur with PCR based class I typing. To restate the above, unambiguous typing results only remain unambiguous if the cis/trans linkage is defined, and since these results will remain unambiguous regardless of an ever growing HLA sequence databank, it is of great importance with regard to PCR typing for clinical studies.

If generic amplification is used and both alleles are amplified simultaneously it often occurs that one allele is amplified more efficiently than the other [164, 165, 178]. This problem of preferential amplification can lead to an allelic drop out during the sequencing reaction, i.e. to overlook one haplotype and to falsely assign homozygosity.

The various PCR-SBT protocols described so far differ mainly in regard to their amplification strategy. The example sequencing protocol described here (for the HLA-A locus) is based on a serology-equivalent haplotype-specific PCR, using group-specific sequence-motifs in the non-coding regions flanking the polymorphic exons [177]. The template-generating primer mixes all work under identical PCR conditions so as to ensure a sufficient throughput of samples. The selection of these primer mixes requires serology-equivalent pretyping. Using the information obtained in the pretyping, two primer mixes (one for each haplotype) are selected for PCR amplification and sequencing. PCR-based separation of the haplotypes can only be achieved in serologically heterozygous samples, which amounts to around 90% of the samples.

The remaining 10% of the haplotypes can not be amplified separately, however, as a result of their close sequence relationship, only a few heterozygous positions need to be detected. Moreover, some of these alleles differ only by a single nucleotide and therefore no additional steps are required to define the cis/trans linkage. When there is more than one heterozygous position, a second sequencing reaction can be used to define the cis/trans linkage. This secondary sequencing uses a nested sequencing primer located at the first, or last, heterozygous position, which initiates a sequencing reaction of only one of the two alleles. In rare cases, however, the sequencing quality may be so bad that it is easier to separate the haplotypes via cloning.

Which sequencing chemistry should be used? For automated Sanger-sequencing there are different methods available, which in turn vary significantly with respect to the effort required to carry them out and the accuracy of the results obtained. The dye primer technique, using fluorescent labeled primers and sequenase as a sequencing enzyme, gives the highest reliability for the detection of heterozygons positions [164, 165]. With the new enzymes AmpliTaq FS (PE Applied Biosystems) or Thermo Sequenase (Amersham Pharmacia Biotech), almost identical results are obtained but is less time consuming (cycle sequencing) [175]. When using a one-lane sequencer (PE Applied Biosystems) the work load can be reduced further by using terminators with different fluorescent labels (dye terminator technique) [163, 167, 170, 177]. However, this technique is less reliable for the detection of heterozygous positions, a problem that new fluorescent labels should overcome (Big Dyes, PE Applied Biosystems; Thermo Sequenase dye terminators version 2, Amersham Pharmacia Biotech).

In order to detect reliably all heterozygous positions after generic PCR amplification, the time consuming dye primer technique has to be applied. This technique provides homogenous sequence chromatograms which in turn are useful for computer interpretations [157, 158, 164, 168, 169]. This is very important since the manual interpretation of complex heterozygous patterns is time consuming and error prone. These software based interpretations of the results are defined through a threshold that allows for a differentiation between heterozygous positions and the background fluorescence. Dye terminator chemistry is, as yet, unable to deliver sufficiently homogeneous chromatograms that readily lend themselves to analysis of heterozygous positions via software based thresholds; therefore, the less laborious dye terminator technique is best reserved for the separate sequencing of the haplotypes. This limitation may be solved by the new fluorescent-labeled terminators mentioned above.

When both alleles are sequenced simultaneously one can, very often, observe peak shifts in the region of the heterozygous positions [169]. These peak shifts mimic insertions, thus making it difficult to accurately assign heterozygous positions; in order to overcome this problem one must sequence in both orientations. Peak shifts do not occur if a single haplotype is sequenced, therefore sequencing need only be carried out in one direction. In short, the time consuming necessity of sequencing both haplotypes separately after haplotype specific PCR is compensated for by not needing to sequence in both orientations.

Although haplotype-specific PCR amplification can call for sequencing reactions that have to be carried out with different sequencing primers, which in turn have different sequencing qualities, this disadvantage can be eliminated by using PCR primers equipped with a universal -21M13 tail at their 5′ end, which ensures that each PCR product can be sequenced with the same sequencing primers [165]. However, by using this technique, only short PCR products can be sequenced and unwanted PCR products are always co-sequenced. In order to obtain good results PCR products need to be very pure. This is not always achievable for, in particular, the HLA class I genes. Because of that, it is advantageous to use nested sequencing primers. Nested sequencing primers provide an additional specificity, which avoids the initiation of a sequencing reaction of unspecific amplified PCR fragments and thus significantly enhances the quality of the results.

Due to the extensive exon polymorphism, the use of exonic nested sequencing primers often requires the use of haplotype-specific sequencing primers, which requires storage of multiple sequencing primers, and this extra complexity makes the dye primer technique expensive. Additionally, exon-located sequencing primers do not allow for the determination of the complete exon sequence. In order to overcome these limitations, HLA class I sequencing is usually performed using universal nested intronic primers. With HLA class II sequencing, only a single exon (exon 2) must be analyzed, furthermore, the PCR product quality is usually better with class II than class I genes, which allows the use of universal -21M13 sequencing primers. To conclude, if one uses universal sequencing primers, both the dye primer and the dye terminator technique can be usefully employed, and the choice for one or the other is dependent on the amplification strategy, and the technical equipment available.

5.4 Clinical Applications

HLA typing by means of molecular techniques should be done whenever the HLA type of an individual is needed. Reasons for tissue-typing include matching for solid organ and bone marrow transplantation, transfusion of platelets, disease association, forensic and anthropological studies, and studies of T cell mediated immunity. The need for HLA matching of donor and recipient for solid organ and bone marrow transplantation has mainly driven the requirement for identification of specificities in the HLA system. In clinical circumstances, HLA typing is primarily essential for transplantation and transfusion purposes [181–190]. Depending on the clinical demand – transfusion, solid organ or bone marrow transplantation – different levels of resolution are required. In solid organ transplantation and platelet transfusion, HLA typing is generally restricted to the serology-equivalent level of resolution. PCR-SSP or PCR-SSOP for HLA class II and PCR-SSP for HLA class I are currently the methods of choice for these purposes. Time constraints for tissue-typing of cadaver donors demand the use of PCR-SSP.

In allogeneic bone marrow transplantation, a high resolution typing on the allelic level is required at least for HLA-DRB1 [184–188]. Though high resolution typing of DRB1 can be done in most cases by PCR-SSOP and PCR-SSP, the rapidly growing number of known alleles and the continuous methodical advancements will probably make this to a domain of PCR-SBT. The importance of individual basepair mismatches of HLA class I alleles for clinical outcome has yet to be established and is still a matter of clinical studies. PCR-SSOP for routine HLA class I typing has not been established yet. For some HLA-A and B specificities, allelic PCR-SSP typing has been developed. In most instances however, allelic HLA class I typing has to be done by sequencing. This might be superseded by more advanced HLA class I PCR-SSP or SSOP typing systems. However, in view of the regularly expanding HLA database and the improvements of convenience and quality in automated sequencing, PCR-SBT may become the method of choice also for routine high-resolution HLA class I typing.

5.5 Quality Control

The unparalleled specificity of PCR amplification and probe hybridization is on one hand the great advantage for an accurate HLA typing but may be on the other hand for the same reason a disadvantage. This means that the accuracy of PCR-based HLA typing and the lack of any cross-reactivity may not allow for the detection of new alleles. This especially applies for group-specific amplification strategies, such as PCR-SSP, where primers on polymorphic exon motifs are used which are frequently involved in gene conversion events. But this may in rare cases also apply for generic amplification strategies using probe hybridization as post-PCR specificity step, if new sequence motifs, not covered by the probes, have arisen.

The excellent precision of PCR-based methods must not result in their uncritical use. The specificity of the primers and probes described for HLA typing are based on the most relevant status of the HLA sequence databank available at the time they were designed. However, through the continuous discovery of new alleles the sequence databank is growing on a regular basis.

Thus, it has constantly to be ensured that the primer mixes or probes used for HLA typing are covering all known HLA specificities, in order not to overlook one haplotype, i.e. to falsely assign homozygosity. Consequently, an important part of the laboratory's work is the regular update of the primers' and probes' specificity based on the most recent sequence data. New alleles assigned by the WHO nomenclature committee for factors of the HLA system are published on a monthly basis in the *European Journal of Immunogenetics*, *Human Immunology* and *Tissue Antigens*. The most relevant HLA sequence alignment is available through the server of the American Society for Histocompatibility and Immunogenetics (http://www.swmed.edu/home_pages/ASHI/sequences/seq3.htm).

A variety of molecular techniques are currently available for HLA typing. The considerable progress of PCR-based HLA typing will potentially make tissue-typing available to anyone who has a reason for doing it. However, the complexity and dynamic features of the human MHC as well as the considerable clinical implications of HLA typing require particular attention with regard to accuracy. Regular internal and external quality controls are necessary in order to ensure and to document a degree of accuracy which is sufficient for clinical purposes. The expense of proficiency testing which may cover up to 20% of the laboratory's workload can become onerous when the volume of a particular test done in a laboratory is small. Moreover, profound knowledge of the structure, diversity and evolution of the human MHC is helpful to avoid potentially fatal mistypings. The European Foundation for Immunogenetics (EFI; http://www.sv.cict.fr/efi/) as well as the American Society for Histocompatibility and Immunogenetics (ASHI; http://www.swmed.edu/home_pages/ASHI/ashi.htm) have established laboratory standards and extensive accreditation programs for HLA laboratories in order to ensure high quality HLA typing.

5.6 Detailed Protocols

5.6.1 HLA Sequence Database

It is essential to be continuously informed about the nomenclature for factors of the HLA system and the HLA sequences when establishing PCR-based HLA typing methods. A report of the nomenclature committee is published annually or every other year in the European Journal of Immunogenetics, Human Immunology and Tissue Antigens. Updates of the HLA nomenclature are published in the same journals on a monthly basis. Additionally, the monthly updates compiled by Steven Marsh for the WHO Nomenclature

Committee for factors of the HLA system are available via the internet (http://www.icnet.uk/axp/tia/marsh/updates.html).

The nucleotide sequences of HLA alleles are accessible via nucleotide sequence databases such as GenBank (http://www.ncbi.nlm.nih.gov/Web/Search/index.html), EMBL (European Molecular Biology Laboratory; http://www.embl-heidelberg.de) or DDJB (DNA Data Bank of Japan; http://www.ddbj.nig.ac.jp), which offer their services via the World Wide Web. The WHO Nomenclature reports and updates for factors of the HLA system list the database accession numbers for each specificity so that their sequence can easily be retrieved from the servers. The most relevant alignment of HLA sequences is available through the gopher of the American Society for Histocompatibility and Immunogenetics (ASHI; http://www.swmed.edu/home_pages/ASHI/ashi.htm). The sequences on this server are updated on a regular basis and compiled by experts in the field and are accessible for everybody free of charge.

5.6.2 Sequence-Specific Oligonucleotide Probing (PCR-SSOP)

The post-PCR processing steps necessary in PCR-SSOP require some additional technical equipment compared to PCR-SSP. Depending on the format and detection system used, this includes a DNA transfer lamp, an incubator, shaking water-baths, orbital shakers, hybridization ovens and X-ray film cassettes.

Many alternative methods for conventional product dot blot PCR-SSOP have been described in the literature which differ mainly in the length and sequence of probes, the solvent used for washing steps, the reporter molecule and its detection [98–100, 102–105, 107–112, 117, 119, 121–127]. The most relevant product dot blot protocol for serology-equivalent HLA class I and high-resolution HLA class II PCR-SSOP typing has been established and extensively evaluated during the 12th IHWC. For detailed information, the reader is referred to these protocols which have been published in the proceedings of the 12th IHWC (Genetic diversity of HLA, Functional and Medical Implications, vol. 1, ed. Dominique Charron, EDK, Paris 1997) by Kennedy and Poulton (HLA class I SSOP protocol, pp. 564–583) and Bignon and Fernandez-Viña [Protocols of the 12th International Histocompatibility Workshop for typing of HLA class II alleles by DNA amplification by the polymerase chain reaction (PCR) and hybridization with sequence specific oligonucleotide probes (SSOP), pp. 584–632]. Product dot blot PCR-SSOP for HLA class I and class II are also commercially available as a kit (Biomérieux, France; Lifecodes, CT, USA).

Protocols for the reverse dot blot format, though already described by Saiki et al. in 1989 [101], are only available in a limited number and are almost completely restricted to HLA class II typing [101,106,113–116] with class I typing only recently being approached [118]. This format of PCR-SSOP has become a domain of commercial suppliers (Biotest, Germany; Dynal, Norway; Gen Trak, GA, USA; Fresenius, Germany; Innogenetics, Belgium) offering this technique with probes immobilized onto membrane strips or microtiter plates. The latter carrier matrix has the potential to bring semi- or fully automated HLA typing close to reality.

5.6.3 Sequence-Specific Primed PCR (PCR-SSP)

PCR-SSP is the method with the lowest requirements with regard to the technical equipment. Beside the need for a spatial separation of the pre- and post-PCR area, simply a microtiter format thermal cycler, an electrophoresis chamber for agarose gels and any gel documentation system are sufficient.

The first comprehensive protocols describing sequence-specific primed PCR were published independently 1992 by Bein et al. [131] and Olerup and Zetterquist [132] for serology-equivalent HLA-DRB typing. During the following years, a variety of PCR-SSP protocols covering all polymorphic HLA class I and class II genes have been developed and published, describing hundreds of primers and primer mixes [129, 130, 132–151]. The half-life of these protocols is extremely short and in direct proportion to the increase of the HLA databank. Thus, already at the time of publication, the specificity of the primer mixes usually requires an update in order to cover all known alleles.

Therefore, PCR-SSP has become a domain of commercial suppliers (BAG, Germany; Biosynthesis, TX, USA; Biotest, Germany; Pel-Freez, WI, USA; Dynal, Norway; One Lambda, CA, USA) offering most up to date PCR-SSP typing systems. Though PCR-SSP is available for all polymorphic HLA genes, it is normally used for serology-equivalent typing of HLA-A, B, C, DRB and DQB1. For practical reasons, the number of primer mixes used for each locus is adapted to the microtiter plate format and is commonly 24 for HLA-A, 48 for HLA-B, 16 for HLA-C, 24 for HLA-DRB, and 8 for HLA-DQB1. Depending on the supplier, the primer mixes may be offered pre-aliquoted in PCR tubes with or without PCR reagents. The primer mixes are commonly adjusted for a total PCR volume of 10 µl. The PCR is usually carried out oilfree and requires a thermal cycler with microtiter plate format and a heated cover. The cycling and buffer conditions which are very critical in regard to the PCR´s specificity and sensitivity are exactly adjusted to the primer mixes and may differ significantly among the various kits available. It is essential that all primer mixes of a single kit and usually all PCR-SSP kits of a single supplier work under identical PCR conditions. After PCR, the amplicons are best transferred by multiple channel pipettes onto an agarose gel stained with ethidium bromide and visualized under UV light. Electrophoresis is necessary to separate the specific HLA from the internal control amplicons, which must differ significantly in their size. The bands are recorded by photography and interpreted using a result sheet listing the specificities of the individual primer mixes.

Fluorescence-based PCR-SSP protocols using fluorogenic probes (fluorotyping) instead of an agarose gel-based read out have been reported so far for HLA-A, C and HLA-DQB1 typing. Protocols for other polymorphic HLA genes will surely follow, but this development is still at an experimental stage and further studies are necessary to facilitate routine fluorotyping.

5.6.4 Sequencing-Based Typing (PCR-SBT)

5.6.4.1 *General Characteristics of the Method*

PCR-SBT is the most complex HLA typing method and requires the most expensive equipment. This is due to the fact that sequencing for clinical purposes can only be done reasonably with the help of an automated sequencer. As described earlier, many alternative methods have been reported in the literature which differ substantially with respect to starting material, amplification strategy, template preparation, and sequencing chemistry.

The sequencing protocol described in detail in this chapter is focusing on the HLA-A locus and should be taken as an example for the other HLA loci for which similar protocols have been published or will be available soon. The protocol describes direct sequencing based typing of the polymorphic 2nd and 3rd exon and illustrates a sequencing strategy which is generally applicable for all HLA class I genes [177]. For alternative protocols the reader is referred to the literature mentioned under Sect. 5.1.3.3 [152–178].

A PCR-based template preparation should fulfill two demands: firstly, the PCR products should cover the complete polymorphic exons and secondly, the PCR strategy should be capable of separating the haplotypes to sort out problems related to an undefined cis/trans linkage of polymorphic motifs. Bearing these demands in mind, the described method is based on a serology-equivalent haplotype-specific PCR amplification using group-specific sequence-motifs located in the non-coding regions flanking the polymorphic exons. This amplification strategy has been made possible through the dis-

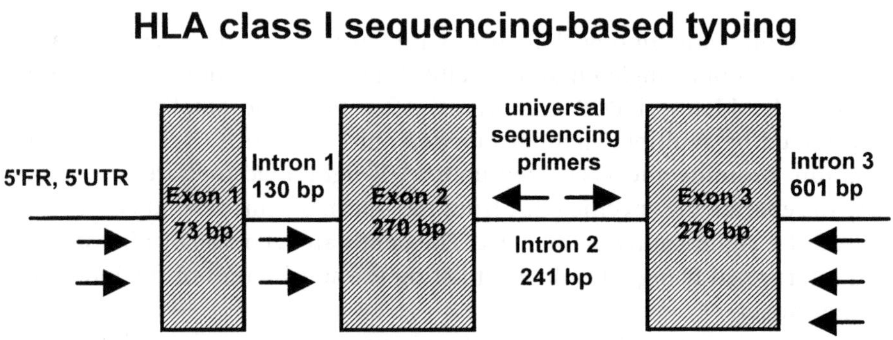

Fig. 5.8. Illustration of the principle of HLA class I sequencing-based typing. Group-specific non-coding primers are used for PCR amplification; universal primers located in the 2nd intron are used for sequencing, regardless of the amplified group. Primers are indicated as *arrows*. *5′FR*, 5′flanking region; *5′UTR*, 5′ untranslated region

covery of the systematic serology-related conserved diversity of intron sequences. The resulting PCR products are spanning a gene fragment at least from the 1st to the 3rd intron of the HLA-A locus. The group-specific amplification allows in all serologically heterozygous samples a PCR based separation of the haplotypes. The separation of the haplotypes is the major achievement of this protocol since it is the only possibility to define cis/trans linkages of sequence motifs. Therefore particular attention has been paid to the PCR protocol.

All primer mixes used are working under identical conditions to ensure a sufficient throughput of samples. Low resolution pretyping information is required, in order to define which group-specific amplifications – one for each haplotype – are needed to generate the sequencing templates for each sample. Any serological or molecular method that can identify the broad allele groups is sufficient. The group-specific primer mixes used for generation of the sequencing templates can also be applied to obtain pretyping information. This would give the option to use the PCR products as sequencing templates for cycle sequencing which would be of advantage since no further processing of the samples is required.

The sequencing reaction is performed with universal nested primers matching conserved sequences in the central parts of the 2nd intron. This strategy allows the use of only one 5′ and one 3′ sequencing primer regardless of the amplified allele. The principles of the sequencing strategy described in this protocol are summarized in Fig. 5.8.

The features of this protocol provide the means for the application of any Sanger-sequencing chemistry available. This manual details the AmpliTaq FS dye terminator cycle sequencing technique for an ABI 377 automated se-

Table 5.3. Sequence, length, melting temperature (Tm) and localization of the primers used for template preparation. Mismatches at position 5 or 6 from the 3′ end, designed to increase specificity, as well as mismatches at positions 11, 18 or 19, introduced to destabilize hairpin formations, are in bold

Primer Length	Orientation Tm	Sequence Localization	
5′FR-243	Sense	5′ AGT GTC TTC GCG GTC GCT C 3′	19
62°C	-53-71	5′ flanking region	
5′FR-251	Sense	5′ GTG TCG TCG CGG TCG CTG 3′	18
62°C	-53-70	5′ flanking region	
5′FR-273	Sense	5′ CAT GCC GAG GGT TTC TCC CA 3′	20
64°C	-360-379	5′ flanking region	
5′FR-279	Sense	5′ GCT GTT TCT TTT CTC CCT CTG 3′	21
62°C	-163-183	5′ flanking region	
E1-203	Sense	5′ CCT GAC CCA GAC CTC GGC A 3′	19
64°C	54-72	Exon 1	
I1-210	Sense	5′ ACC CGG GAA GCC GGG CCT 3′	18
64°C	72-89	Intron 1	
I1-214	Sense	5′ CGC CTG GCG GGG GGG CAA 3′	18
66°C	53-70	Intron 1	
I1-221	Sense	5′ GGG AGC GGC GCC GGG AC 3′	17
64°C	77-93	Intron 1	
I1-223	Sense	5′ GTG AGT GCG GGG TCG TGG 3′	18
62°C	1-19	Intron 1	
I1-225	Sense	5′ GCC GGG AGG AGG GAC GGT 3′	18
64°C	86-103	Intron 1	
I1-226	Sense	5′ CTC TGT GGG GAG AAG CAA C 3′	19
60°C	29-47	Intron 1	
I1-240	Sense	5′ GGA GGA GGG TCG GGC GGA 3′	18
64°C	90-107	Intron 1	
I3-233	Antisense	5′ GGC CCA AGG CTG CTG CCT 3′	18
62°C	274-291	Intron 3	
I3-236	Antisense	5′ GTC TGT CAG GAA GAG TCA GAA 3′	21
62°C	583 - +2	Intron 3-Exon 4	
I3-249	Antisense	5′ CAG AGT CAC TCT CTG GTA CAG 3′	21
62°C	148-168	Intron 3	
I3-250	Antisense	5′ GTC AGA GAG CAG GGC GGA A 3′	19
62°C	172-190	Intron 3	
I3-280	Antisense	5′ GCG ATC GTC TTC CCG TCA C 3′	19
62°C	220-238	Intron 3	
I3-282	Antisense	5′ AGA GTC ACT CTC TGG TAC AGA 3′	21
60°C	147-167	Intron 3	
I3-284	Antisense	5′ ACC TGA GTG GAG GCT GAG A 3′	19
60°C	370-388	Intron 3	

Table 5.4. HLA-A PCR-SBT primer mixes. The names of the primer mixes refer to the serological families

Primer mix No	Name	Sense primer	Antisense primer	Size of product	HLA-A specificity
1	1	5′FR-251	I3–284	1448 bp	A*01,3601
2	2	I1–226	I3–249	1056 bp	A*02
3	3	I1–221	I3–280	1077 bp	A*03
4	11	5′FR-243	I3–249	1229 bp	A*11
5	9	I1–214	I3–249	1034 bp	A*23,24
6	10	I1–210	I3–236	1452 bp	A*25,26,34,43,66
7	28	5′FR-273	I3–233	1659 bp	A*68,69
8	19.1	I1–223	I3–249	1084 bp	A*29,31,32,33,74
9	19.2	I1–240	I3–249	996 bp	A*31,33
10	19.3	5′FR-279	I3–250	1362 bp	A*29,32,74
11	30	I1–225	I3–249	1000 bp	A*30
12	80	E1–203	I3–282	1102 bp	A*8001

quencer (PE Applied Biosystems, Foster City, CA, USA) but can easily be adapted to any other automated or manual protocol.

5.6.4.2
PCR Primers

The sequence, length, and localization of the primers are given in Table 5.3. All amplification primers are designed with a melting temperature of about 62°C to ensure uniform amplification conditions. For specific amplification, some primers are set up with an arbitrary mismatch at position 5 or 6 from the 3′ end. This measure slightly decreases amplification efficiency but ensures amplification specificity. In addition, some of the primers contain mismatches at their 5′ part to cause a thermodynamic destabilization of hairpin formations, which are a common problem encountered when designing primers for G/C rich regions. This mismatch was introduced at the 5′ side of the hairpin to minimize its effect on the efficiency of amplification. In 12 individual primer mixes, 12 sense and 7 antisense primers are used to amplify HLA-A alleles corresponding to the serologically defined specificities A1 – A80. The specificity of the primer mixes is summarized in Table 5.4. It depends on the low resolution pretyping information which of these primer pairs are used for generation of the sequencing templates. The PCR primer pairs amplify a fragment of the HLA-A gene from the 5′ flanking region, exon 1 or intron 1 up to the 3rd intron. Thus, each PCR product carries the sequence information of the 2nd and 3rd exon for a complete subtyping by direct sequencing.

5.6.4.3
Sequencing Primers

For each amplified group, direct sequencing is always performed with the same sequencing primers. One 3′ primer (ASEQ3; 5′ biotin-TCG GAC CCG GAG ACT GTG 3′, 18mer, T_m=60°C) for the 2nd exon and one 5′ primer (ASEQ5; 5′ biotin-GTT TCA TTT TCA GTT TAG GCC A 3′, 22mer, T_m=60°C) for the 3rd exon (Fig. 5.8). Both sequencing primers are located in conserved regions of the 2nd intron. These conserved regions are identical in all HLA-A alleles. The sequencing primers are biotinylated at their 5′ end to enable the purification of the extension fragments via streptavidin-coated paramagnetic beads after the sequencing reaction.

5.6.4.4
PCR Protocol

The PCR protocol is identical for all primer mixes used for template generation. The PCR amplification is set up in a total volume of 20 µl yielding enough PCR product for three sequencing reactions – one for exon 2, one for exon 3, and, if necessary, one extra reaction (10 µl for monitoring the success of the PCR, 3 µl for each sequencing reaction). This ensures that, if anything fails during the sequencing process, one sequencing reaction can be repeated once without generation of a new template. The high stringency of the PCR primers and protocol detailed below makes the use of a hot start approach unnecessary. The volumes per reaction for the PCR reaction mix are as follows:

5×PCR buffer, 4.00 µl
DMSO, 0.40 µl
2.5 mM each dNTP, 2.00 µl
5′ primer (5 pmol/µl), 0.80 µl (4 pmol)
3′ primer (5 pmol/µl), 0.80 µl (4 pmol)
Taq polymerase (5 U/µl), 0.12 µl (0.6 U)
Genomic DNA (100 ng/µl), 2.00 µl
ddH_2O, 9.90 µl
Total, 20.00 µl

Composition of 5×PCR buffer, 75.0 mM $(NH_4)_2SO_4$, 12.5 mM $MgCl_2$, 300.0 mM Tris-HCl, pH 9.0

PCR Cycle Parameters. PCR cycle parameters are adjusted for a Perkin-Elmer System 9600 thermal cycler. After an initial denaturation step, a first round with 10 two-temperature cycles for high specificity is followed by 20 three-temperature cycles with a lower annealing temperature for high PCR efficiency.

1. Initial Denaturation at 94°C for 5 min
2. First 10 cycles
   (i) Denaturation at 94°C for 30 s
   (ii) Annealing and extension at 65°C for 50 s
3. Last 20 cycles
   (i) Denaturation at 94°C for 30 s
   (ii) Annealing at 62°C for 50 s
   (iii) Extension at 72°C for 30 s

Ten microliters of the PCR product are run on a 2% agarose gel prestained with ethidium bromide (0.2 µg/ml). A distinct band of the expected size should be seen.

5.6.4.5
Sequencing Reaction Protocol

The PCR products can be directly used in the sequencing reaction without any additional purification step. The sequencing reaction is carried out with the dye terminator cycle sequencing chemistry using AmpliTaq FS (PE Applied Biosystems, Foster City, CA, USA) or Thermo Sequenas (Amersham Pharmacia Biotech, Uppsala, Sweden) as sequencing enzyme for primer extension. The sequencing mix in a total volume of 20 µl contains 3 µl of the PCR product, 3 pmol biotinylated sequencing primer, and 8 µl of the premixed reaction mix containing fluorescence labeled ddNTPs (PE Applied Biosystems or Amersham Pharmacia Biotech). The volumes per reaction for the sequencing mix are as follows:

PCR product, 3.00 µl
Biotinylated sequencing primer (1 pmol/µl), 3.00 µl (3 pmol)
Dye terminator mix, 8.00 µl
ddH_2O, 6.00 µl
Total, 20.00 µl

Sequencing Cycle Conditions. The cycle parameters are adjusted for a Perkin-Elmer System 9600 thermal cycler and consist of 25 three-temperature cycles.

1. 25 cycles
   (i) Denaturation at 96°C for 10 s
   (ii) Annealing at 50°C for 5 s
   (iii) Extension at 60°C for 4 min
2. Rapid ramp to 4°C, continuously hold

5.6.4.6
Purification of the Extension Fragments

Prior to the electrophoretic separation of the extension fragments, the unincorporated dye terminators have to be removed. Since all extension products generated by the sequencing primer are biotinylated, this is done with the help of streptavidin-coated paramagnetic beads. Per sample, 50 µg (=5 µl) beads (Dynal, Oslo, Norway) are washed twice in binding and washing buffer (B&W; 2×buffer: 2 M NaCl, 10 mM Tris-HCl, pH 7.5, 1 mM EDTA) using the magnetic particle concentrator and resuspended in 20 µl B&W buffer. Afterwards, these 20 µl beads are added to the 20 µl sequencing product and incubated for 15 min at room temperature. The beads are then immobilized and the supernatant is removed. Samples are washed once with 40 µl 70% ethanol and air dried because remaining ethanol could interfere with gel mobility.

Using this technique on an ABI 373 automated sequencer (PE Applied Biosystems, Foster City, CA, USA) may yield weak signal intensities. Therefore, when an ABI 373 is used, it is recommended to generate biotinylated PCR products (one of the two PCR primers has to be biotinylated) instead of using biotinylated sequencing primers. The remaining amplification primers have to be removed by washing the PCR product with streptavidin-coated beads (10 µl PCR product with 100 µg beads, resuspension in 5 µl dH_2O). After the sequencing reaction, the unincorporated dye terminators have to be removed with Sephadex G50 columns DNA Grade F (MicroSpin G50 columns, Amersham Pharmacia Biotech, Uppsala, Sweden). If this technique is used, the samples have to be dried in a vacuum centrifuge prior to resuspension in the loading buffer.

5.6.4.7
Gel Electrophoresis and Data Collection

The beads-bound extension fragments (or the dried pellet) are resuspended in 4 µl of loading buffer containing deionized formamide/25 mM EDTA, pH 8.0, blue dextran (50 mg/ml solution) (5:1). Samples are heated for 2 min at 90°C to denature and 1.5 µl (4.0 µl if an ABI 373 is used) are loaded on a 0.2-

mm-thick 5% polyacrylamide-7 M urea gel. Electrophoresis is run at constant 48 W for 8 h on an ABI 377 automated sequencer (PE Applied Biosystems).

The polyacrylamide gel has to be poured at least 2 h before use. The gel should not be stored longer than 6 h before electrophoresis is started. The gel composition is as follows:

ABI 377, 5% polyacrylamide gel, 7 M urea
21 g urea
8.4 ml 30% acrylamide solution (acrylamide:bisacrylamide 29:1)
6.0 ml 10×TBE buffer
20 ml dH_2O
350 μl ammonium persulfate
15 μl TEMED (*N,N,N′,N′*-tetramethyl-ethylendiamine)
ABI 373, 6% polyacrylamide gel, 7 M urea
33 g urea
10.0 ml 40% acrylamide solution (acrylamide:bisacrylamide 19:1)
7.0 ml 10×TBE buffer
26 ml dH_2O
200 μl ammonium persulfate
30 μl TEMED

10 TBE buffer: 108.0 g Tris base, 55.0 g boric acid, 7.4 g Na_2EDTA to be sol ved in 1 l dH_2O

5.6.4.8
Data Analysis and HLA Typing

After data collection, the electropherograms are printed and sequences can be compared manually with the existing HLA class I databank. Since each allele of both haplotypes is usually sequenced separately due to the group-specific amplification, heterozygous positions are absent so that manual analysis is not very time consuming. Alternatively, sequences can be checked with the programs Sequence Navigator and Factura and allele assignment can be done with the MatchMaker program (PE Applied Biosystems).

5.6.4.9
Application of Other Sequencing Chemistries

The most important issue for direct sequencing of HLA genes is the generation of pure PCR products. If an adequate PCR product has been generated, any Sanger-sequencing chemistry on any automated sequencer should be applicable. Most of the suppliers of automated sequencers (Amersham

Pharmacia Biotech, Uppsala, Sweden; LI-COR, Lincoln, NE, USA; PE Applied Biosystems, Foster City, CA, USA; Visible Genetics, Toronto, Canada) offer special software packages and sequence libraries in order to facilitate data analysis and allele assignment for sequencing based HLA typing.

Acknowledgment. I am grateful to Jenny Wehling and Katja Kotsch for helpful discussions.

References

1. Dausset J (1954) Leuco-agglutinins IV. Leuco-agglutinins and blood transfusion. Vox Sang 4:190–198
2. Payne R, Rolfs MR (1958) Fetomaternal leukocyte incompatibility. J Clin Invest 37:1756–63
3. Van Rood JJ, Eernisse JG, van Leeuwen A (1958) Leukocyte antibodies in sera from pregnant women. Nature 181:1735–36
4. Zinkernagel RM, Doherty PC (1974) Restriction of in vitro T cell mediated cytotoxicity in lymphocytic choriomeningitis within a syngeneic or semiallogeneic system. Nature 248:701–702
5. Van Rood JJ, van Leeuwen A (1963) Leukocyte grouping: a method and its application. J Clin Invest 42:1382
6. Payne R, Tripp M, Weigle J, Bodmer W, Bodmer J (1964) A new leukocyte isoantigen system in man. Cold Spring Harbor Symp Quant Biol 29: 285
7. Ceppellini R, Curtoni ES, Mattiuz PL, Miggiano V, Scudeller G, Serra A (1967) Genetics of leukocyte antigens: a family study of segregation and linkage. In: Histocompatibility testing 1967, eds. Curtoni ES, Mattiuz PL, Tosi RM, Munksgaard, Copenhagen, p 149
8. Thorsby E, Sandberg L, Lindholm A, Kissmeyer-Nielsen F (1970) The HL-A system: evidence of a third sub-locus. Scand J Haematol 7:195–200
9. Mayr WR, Bernoco D, De Marchi M, Ceppellini R (1973) Genetic analysis and biological properties of products of the third SD (AJ) locus of the HL-A region. Transplant Proc 5:1581–93
10. Bach FH, Hirschhorn K (1964) Lymphocyte interaction: a potential histocompatibility test in vitro. Science 143:813–815
11. Bain EJ, Vas MR, Lowenstein L (1964) The development of large immature mononuclear cells in mixed leukocyte cultures. Blood 23:108
12. Bach FH, Voynow NK (1966) One way stimulation in mixed leukocyte cultures. Science 153:545–47
13. Amos DB, Bach FH (1968) Phenotypic expression of the major histocompatibility locus in man (HL-A): leukocyte antigens and mixed leukocyte culture reactivity. J Exp Med 128:628–37
14. Mempel W, Grosse-Wilde H, Albert ED (1973) Identity for the strong MLC-locus in HL-A different unrelated pairs. Blut 27:336–341
15. Mempel W, Albert E, Burger A (1972) Further evidence for a separate MLC-locus. Tissue Antigens 2:250–254
16. Mempel W, Grosse-Wilde H, Baumann P, Netzel B, Steinbauer-Rosenthal I, Scholz S, Bertrams J, Albert ED (1973) Population genetics of the MLC response: typing for MLC determinants using homozygous and heterozygous reference cells. Transplant Proc 5:1529–1534

17. Van Rood JJ, van Leeuwen A, Keuning JJ, van Oud-Alblas AB (1975) The serological recognition of the human MLC determinants using a modified cytotoxicity technique. Tissue Antigens 5:73–79
18. Tosi R, Tanigaki N, Centis D, Ferrara GB, Pressman D (1978) Immunological dissection of human Ia molecules. J Exp Med 148:1592–1611
19. Mawas C, Charmot D, Sivy M, Mercier P, North ML, Hauptmann G (1978) A weak human MLR locus mapping at the right of a crossing-over between HLA-D, Bf and GLO. J Immunogenet 5:383–395
20. Shaw S, Johnson AH, Shearer GM (1980) Evidence for a new segregant series of B cell antigens that are encoded in the HLA-D region and that stimulate secondary allogenic proliferative and cytotoxic responses. J Exp Med 152:565–580
21. Bodmer JG, Marsh SG, Albert ED, Bodmer WF, Bontrop RE, Charron D, Dupont B, Erlich HA, Fauchet R, Mach B, Mayr WR, Parham P, Sasazuki T, Schreuder GM, Strominger JL, Svejgaard A, Terasaki PI (1997) Nomenclature for factors of the HLA system, 1996. Tissue Antigens 49:297–321
22. White JA, McAlpine PJ, Antonarakis S, Cann H, Eppig J, Frazer K, Frezal J, Lancet D, Nahmias J, Pearson P, Peters J, Scott A, Scott H, Spurr N, Talbot C, Jr, Povey S (1997) Guidelines for human gene nomenclature. Genomics 45:468–471
23. Klein J, Figueroa F (1986) Evolution of the major histocompatibility complex. Crit Rev Immunol 6:295–386
24. Milner CM, Campbell RD (1992) Genes, genes and more genes in the human major histocompatibility complex. Bioessays 14:565–567
25. Campbell RD, Trowsdale J (1993) Map of the human MHC. Immunol Today 14:349–352
26. Anthropology Tables (1997) In: Genetic diversity of HLA, functional and medical implications, vol. 1, ed. D. Charron, EDK, Paris pp. 664–820
27. Alper CA, Awdeh ZL, Yunis EJ (1989) Complotypes and extended haplotypes in laboratory medicine. Complement Inflamm 6:8–18
28. Kendall E, Todd JA, Campbell RD (1991) Molecular analysis of the MHC class II region in DR4, DR7, and DR9 haplotypes. Immunogenetics 34:349–357
29. Dunham I, Sargent CA, Kendall E, Campbell RD (1990) Characterization of the class III region in different MHC haplotypes by pulsed-field gel electrophoresis. Immunogenetics 32:175–182
30. Campbell RD, Dunham I, Kendall E, Sargent CA (1990) Polymorphism of the human complement component C4. Exp Clin Immunogenet 1990:69–84
31. Venditti CP, Chorney MJ (1992) Class I gene contraction within the HLA-A subregion of the human MHC. Genomics 14:1003–1009
32. El-Kahloun A, Vernet C, Jouanolle AM, Boretto J, Mauvieux V, Le Gall JY, David V, Pontarotti P (1992) A continuous restriction map from HLA-E to HLA-F. Structural comparison between different HLA-A haplotypes. Immunogenetics 35:183–189
33. Cresswell P, Turner MJ, Strominger JL (1973) Papain-solubilized HL-A antigens from cultured human lymphocytes contain two peptide fragments. Proc Natl Acad Sci USA 70:1603–1607
34. Bodmer WF (1987) The HLA system: structure and function. J Clin Pathol 40:948–958
35. Le Bouteiller P (1994) HLA class I chromosomal region, genes and products: facts and Solheim BG, Thorsby E (1974) Beta-2-microglobulin is part of the HL-A molecules in the lymphocyte membrabe. Nature 249:36–38
37. Goodfellow PN, Jones EA, Van Heyningen V, Solomon E, Bobrow M, Miggiano V, Bodmer WF (1975) The beta2-microglobulin gene is on chromosome 15 and not in the HL-A region. Nature 254:267–269

38. Gussow D, Rein R, Ginjaar I, Hochstenbach F, Seemann G, Kottman A, Ploegh HL (1987) The human beta 2-microglobulin gene. Primary structure and definition of the transcriptional unit. J Immunol 139:3132–3138
39. Bjorkman PJ, Saper MA, Samraoui B, Bennett WS, Strominger JL, Wiley DC (1987) Structure of the human class I histocompatibility antigen, HLA-A2. Nature 329:506–512
40. Garrett TPJ, Saper MA, Bjorkman PJ, Strominger JL, Wiley DC (1989) Specificity pockets for the side chains of peptide antigens in HLA-Aw68. Nature 342:692–696
41. Saper MA, Bjorkman PJ, Wiley DC (1991) Refined structure of the human histocompatibility antigen HLA-A2 at 2.6 Å resolution. J Mol Biol 219:277–319
42. Madden DR, Gorga JC, Strominger JL, Wiley DC (1992) The three-dimensional structure of HLA-B27 at 2.1 Å resolution suggests a general mechanism for tight peptide binding to MHC. Cell 70:1035–1048
43. Smith KJ, Reid SW, Stuart DI, McMichael AJ, Jones EY, Bell JI (1996) An altered position of the alpha 2 helix of MHC class I is revealed by the crystal structure of HLA-B*3501. Immunity 4:203–213
44. Smith KJ, Reid SW, Harlos K, McMichael AJ, Stuart DI, Bell JI, Jones EY (1996) Bound water structure and polymorphic amino acids act together to allow the binding of different peptides to MHC class I HLA-B53. Immunity 4:215–228
45. de Preval C, Mach B (1983) The absence of beta 2-microglobulin in Daudi cells: active gene but inactive messenger RNA. Immunogenetics 17:133–140
46 Seong RH, Clayberger CA, Krensky AM, Parnes JR (1988) Rescue of Daudi cell HLA expression by transfection of the mouse beta 2-microglobulin gene. J Exp Med 167:288–299
47. Strachan T, Sodoyer R, Damotte M, Jordan BR (1984) Complete nucleotide sequence of a functional class I HLA gene, HLA-A3: implications for the evolution of HLA genes. EMBO J 3:887–894
48. Sodoyer R, Damotte M, Delovitch TL, Trucy J, Jordan BR, Strachan T (1984) Complete nucleotide sequence of a gene encoding a functional human class I histocompatibility antigen (HLA-Cw3). EMBO J 3:879–885
49. Driggers PH, Elenbaas BA, An JB, Lee IJ, Ozato K (1992) Two upstream elements activate transcription of a major histocompatibility complex class I gene in vitro. Nucleic Acids Res 20:2533–2540
50. Cereb N, Yang SY (1994) The regulatory complex of HLA class I promoters exhibits locus-specific conservation with limited allelic variation. J Immunol 152:3873–3883
51. Köhler S, Wehling J, Blasczyk R (1997) Structural diversity of the HLA-A regulatory complex. In: Genetic diversity of HLA, functional and medical implications, vol. 2, ed. D. Charron, EDK, Paris, pp 285–287
52. Brown JH, Jardetzky TS, Gorga JC, Stern LJ, Urban RG, Strominger JL, Wiley DC (1993) Three-dimensional structure of the human class II histocompatibility antigen HLA-DR1. Nature 364:33–39
53. Hunkapiller T, Hood L (1989) Diversity of the immunoglobulin gene superfamily. Adv Immunol 44:1–63
54. Trowsdale J (1987) Genetics and polymorphism: class II antigens. Br Med Bull 43:15–36
55. Kappes D, Strominger J (1988) Human class II major histocompatibility complex genes and proteins. Ann Rev Biochem 57:991–1028
56. Beck S, Kelly A, Radley E, Khurshid F, Alderton RP, Trowsdale J (1992) DNA sequence analysis of 66 kb of the human MHC class II region encoding a cluster of genes for antigen processing. J Mol Biol 228:433–441

57. Germain RN, Margulies DH (1993) The biochemistry and cell biology of antigen processing and presentation. Annu Rev Immunol 11:403–50
58. Heemels MT, Ploegh H (1995) Generation, translocation, and presentation of MHC class I-restricted peptides. Annu Rev Biochem 64:463–491
59. von Boehmer H, Teh HS, Kisielow P (1989) The thymus selects the useful, neglects the useless and destroys the harmful. Immunol Today 10:57–61
60. Nossal GJ (1994) Negative selection of lymphocytes. Cell 1994:229–239
61. Sprent J, Gao EK, Webb SR (1990) T cell reactivity to MHC molecules: immunity versus tolerance. Science 248:1357–63
62. Kagi D, Ledermann B, Burki K, Zinkernagel RM, Hengartner H (1996) Molecular mechanisms of lymphocyte-mediated cytotoxicity and their role in immunological protection and pathogenesis in vivo. Annu Rev Immunol 14:207–32
63. Cresswell P (1994) Assembly, transport, and function of MHC class II molecules. Annu Rev Immunol 12:259–93
64. Watts C (1997) Capture and processing of exogenous antigens for presentation on MHC molecules. Annu Rev Immunol 15:821–50
65. Hughes AL, Hughes MK (1995) Natural selection on the peptide-binding regions of major histocompatibility complex molecules. Immunogenetics 42:233–43
66. Parham P, Lawlor DA, Lomen CE, Ennis PD (1989) Diversity and diversification of HLA-A,B,C alleles. J Immunol 142:3937–50
67. Terasaki PI, McClelland JB. Microdroplet assay for human serum cytotoxins. Nature 204:998–9
68. Mytilineos J, Scherer S, Dunckley H, Trejaut J, Chapman J, Fischer G, Fae I, Middleton D, Savage D, Bignon JD, et al. (1993) DNA HLA-DR typing results of 4000 kidney transplants. Transplantation 55:778–81
69. Yu N, Ohashi, M, Alosco S, Granja C, Salazar M, Hegland J, Yunis E (1997) Accurate typing of HLA-A antigens and analysis of serological deficiencies. Tissue Antigens 50:380–86
70. Lorentzen DF, Iwanaga KK, Meuer KJ, Moritz TL, Watkins DI (1997) A 25% error rate in serological typing of HLA-B homozygotes. Tissue Antigens 50:359–65
71. Klein J (1987) Origin of major histocompatibility complex polymorphism: the trans-species hypothesis. Hum Immunol 19:155–62
72. Maeda M, Murayama N, Ishii H, Uryu N, Ota M, Tsuji K, Inoko H (1989) A simple and rapid method for HLA-DQA1 genotyping by digestion of PCR-amplified DNA with allele specific restriction endonucleases. Tissue Antigens 34:290–8
73. Uryu N, Maeda M, Ota M, Tsuji K, Inoko H (1990) A simple and rapid method for HLA-DRB and -DQB typing by digestion of PCR-amplified DNA with allele specific restriction endonucleases. Tissue Antigens 35:20–31
74. Ota M, Seki T, Nomura N, Sugimura K, Mizuki N, Fukushima H, Tsuji K, Inoko H (1991) Modified PCR-RFLP method for HLA-DPB1 and -DQA1 genotyping. Tissue Antigens 38:60–71
75. Ota M, Seki T, Fukushima H, Tsuji K, Inoko H (1992) HLA-DRB1 genotyping by modified PCR-RFLP method combined with group-specific primers. Tissue Antigens 39:187–202
76. Mizuki N, Ohno S, Sugimura K, Seki T, Kikuti YY, Ando A, Ota M, Tsuji K, Inoko H (1992) PCR-RFLP is as sensitive and reliable as PCR-SSO in HLA class II genotyping. Tissue Antigens 40:100–3
77. Sengar DP, Goldstein R (1994) Comprehensive typing of DQB1 alleles by PCR-RFLP. Tissue Antigens 43:242–8
78. Sengar DP, Hampton N, Goldstein R, Sengar AS (1995) Comprehensive typing of

HLA-DPB1 alleles by polymerase chain reaction-restriction fragment length polymorphism (PCR-RFLP). Clin Invest Med 18:465–72
79. Hoshino S, Kimura A, Fukuda Y, Dohi K, Sasazuki T (1992) Polymerase chain reaction–single-strand conformation polymorphism analysis of polymorphism in DPA1 and DPB1 genes: a simple, economical, and rapid method for histocompatibility testing. Hum Immunol 33:98–107
80. Carrington M, Miller T, White M, Gerrard B, Stewart C, Dean M, Mann D (1992) Typing of HLA-DQA1 and DQB1 using DNA single-strand conformation polymorphism. Hum Immunol 33:208–12
81. Young NT, Darke C (1993) Allelic typing of the HLA-DR4 group by polymerase chain reaction–single-strand conformation polymorphism analysis. Hum Immunol 37:69–74
82. Bannai M, Tokunaga K, Lin L, Kuwata S, Mazda T, Amaki I, Fujisawa K, Juji T (1994) Discrimination of human HLA-DRB1 alleles by PCR-SSCP (single-strand conformation polymorphism) method. Eur J Immunogenet 21:1–9
83. Pietravalle F, Tkaczuk J, Thomsen M, Cambon-Thomsen A, Ohayon E, Abbal M (1994) Evaluation of HLA-DPB incompatibility by PCR-SSCP in the choice of a bone marrow donor. Transplant Proc 26:238
84. Shintaku S, Fukuda Y, Tashiro H, Hoshino S, Dohi K, Kimura A (1994) Simple and rapid HLA-DRB DNA typing method for transplantation using polymerase chain reaction-sequence-specific primers in combination with DNA conformation polymorphism analysis. Transplant Proc 26:1893–6
85. Clay TM, Culpan D, Pursall MC, Bradley BA, Bidwell JL (1995) HLA-DQB1 and DQA1 matching by ambient temperature PCR-SSCP. Eur J Immunogenet 22:467–78
86. Blasczyk R, Hahn U, Wehling J, Huhn D, Salama A (1995) Complete subtyping of the HLA-A locus by sequence-specific amplification followed by direct sequencing or single-strand conformation polymorphism analysis. Tissue Antigens 46:86–95
87. Pursall MC, Clay TM, Bidwell JL (1996) Combined PCR-heteroduplex and PCR-SSCP analysis for matching of HLA-A, -B and -C allotypes in marrow transplantation. Eur J Immunogenet 23:41–53
88. Maruya E, Saji H, Yokoyama S (1996) PCR-LIS-SSCP (Low ionic strength single-stranded conformation polymorphism) – a simple method for high-resolution allele typing of HLA-DRB1, -DQB1, and -DPB1. Genome Res 6:51–7
89. Wang H, Tokunaga K, Akaza T, Tadokoro K, Shibata Y, Juji T (1997) Identification of HLA-C alleles using PCR-single-strand-conformation polymorphism and direct sequencing. Tissue Antigens 49:134–40
90. Clay TM, Bidwell JL, Howard MR, Bradley BA (1991) PCR-fingerprinting for selection of HLA matched unrelated marrow donors. Collaborating Centres in the IMUST Study. Lancet 337:1049–52
91. Sorrentino R, Cascino I, Tosi R (1992) Subgrouping of DR4 alleles by DNA heteroduplex analysis. Hum Immunol 33:18–23
92. Sorrentino R, Potolicchio I, Ferrara GB, Tosi R (1992) A new approach to HLA-DPB1 typing combining DNA heteroduplex analysis with allele-specific amplification and enzyme restriction. Immunogenetics 36:248–54
93. Zimmerman PA, Carrington MN, Nutman TB (1993) Exploiting structural differences among heteroduplex molecules to simplify genotyping the DQA1 and DQB1 alleles in human lymphocyte typing. Nucleic Acids Res 21:4541–7
94. D'Amato M, Sorrentino R (1994) A simple and economical DRB1 typing procedure combining group-specific amplification, DNA heteroduplex and enzyme restriction analysis. Tissue Antigens 43:295–301

95. D´Amato M, Sorrentino R (1995) Short insertions in the partner strands greatly enhance the discriminating power of DNA heteroduplex analysis: resolution of HLA-DQB1 polymorphisms. Nucleic Acids Res 23:2078–9
96. Savage DA, Tang JP, Wood NA, Evans J, Bidwell JL, Wee JL, Oei AA, Hui KM (1996) A rapid HLA-DRB1*04 subtyping method using PCR and DNA heteroduplex generators. Tissue Antigens 47:284–92
97. Teutsch SM, Bennetts BH, Castle M, Hibbins M, Heard RN, Stewart GJ (1996) HLA-DQA1 and -DQB1 genotyping by PCR-RFLP, heteroduplex and homoduplex analysis. Eur J Immunogenet 23:107–20
98. Saiki RK, Bugawan TL, Horn GT, Mullis KB, Erlich HA (1986) Analysis of enzymatically amplified beta-globin and HLA-DQ alpha DNA with allele-specific oligonucleotide probes. Nature 324:163–6
99. Bugawan TL, Horn GT, Long CM, Mickelson E, Hansen JA, Ferrara GB, Angelini G, Erlich HA (1988) Analysis of HLA-DP allelic sequence polymorphism using the in vitro enzymatic DNA amplification of DP-alpha and DP-beta loci. J Immunol 141:4024–30
100. Angelini G, Bugawan TL, Delfino L, Erlich HA, Ferrara GB (1989) HLA-DP typing by DNA amplification and hybridization with specific oligonucleotides. Hum Immunol 26:169–77
101. Saiki RK, Walsh PS, Levenson CH, Erlich HA (1989) Genetic analysis of amplified DNA with immobilized sequence-specific oligonucleotide probes. Proc Natl Acad Sci USA 86:6230–4
102. Wordsworth BP, Allsopp CE, Young RP, Bell JI (1990) HLA-DR typing using DNA amplification by the polymerase chain reaction and sequential hybridization to sequence-specific oligonucleotide probes. Immunogenetics 32:413–8
103. Bugawan TL, Begovich AB, Erlich HA (1990) Rapid HLA-DPB typing using enzymatically amplified DNA and nonradioactive sequence-specific oligonucleotide probes [published erratum in Immunogenetics 1991: 34:413]. Immunogenetics 32:231–41
104. Fugger L, Morling N, Ryder LP, Odum N, Svejgaard A (1990) Technical aspects of typing for HLA-DP alleles using allele-specific DNA in vitro amplification and sequence-specific oligonucleotide probes. Detection of single base mismatches. J Immunol Methods 129:175–85
105. Giphart MJ, Verduijn W (1991) The Eurotransplant HLA-DRB oligonucleotide typing set. Eur J Immunogenet 18:57–68
106. Erlich H, Bugawan T, Begovich AB, Scharf S, Griffith R, Saiki R, Higuchi R, Walsh PS (1991) HLA-DR, DQ and DP typing using PCR amplification and immobilized probes. Eur J Immunogenet 18:33–55
107. Nevinny-Stickel C, Hinzpeter M, Andreas A, Albert ED (1991) Non-radioactive oligotyping for HLA-DR1-DRw10 using polymerase chain reaction, digoxigenin-labelled oligonucleotides and chemiluminescence detection. Eur J Immunogenet 18:323–32
108. Nevinny-Stickel C, Bettinotti MD, Andreas A, Hinzpeter M, Muhlegger K, Schmitz G, Albert ED (1991) Nonradioactive HLA class II typing using polymerase chain reaction and digoxigenin-11-2´-3´-dideoxy-uridinetriphosphate-labeled oligonucleotide probes. Hum Immunol 31:7–13
109. Fernandez-Viña MA, Gao XJ, Moraes ME, Moraes JR, Salatiel I, Miller S, Tsai J, Sun YP, An JB, Layrisse Z, et al. (1991) Alleles at four HLA class II loci determined by oligonucleotide hybridization and their associations in five ethnic groups. Immunogenetics 34:299–312
110. Eiermann TH, Fakler J, Muller CR, Ballas M, Goldmann SF (1991) HLA-DPB1 oligonucleotide typing of a southwest German Caucasian population. Tissue Antigens 38:193–8

111. Kimura A, Sasazuki T (1992) Eleventh international histocompatibility workshop reference protocol for the HLA DNA-typing technique. In: HLA 1991. Proceedings of the eleventh International Histocompatibility Workshop and Conference, vol. 1, ed. Tsuji K, Aizawa M, Sasazuki T, Oxford Science Publications, Oxford, pp 397–419
112. Kimura A, Dong RP, Harada H, Sasazuki T (1992) DNA typing of HLA class II genes in B-lymphoblastoid cell lines homozygous for HLA. Tissue Antigens 40:5–12
113. Eliaou JF, Palmade F, Avinens O, Edouard E, Ballaguer P, Nicolas JC, Clot J (1992) Generic HLA-DRB1 gene oligotyping by a nonradioactive reverse dot-blot methodology. Hum Immunol 35:215–22
114. Nevinny-Stickel C, Albert ED (1993) HLA class II typing in a microtitre plate format using digoxigenin-labelled amplified DNA and biotin-labelled oligonucleotide probes. Eur J Immunogenet 20:419–27
115. Kostyu DD, Pfohl J, Ward FE, Lee J, Murray A, Amos DB (1993) Rapid HLA-DR oligotyping by an enzyme-linked immunosorbent assay performed in microtiter trays. Hum Immunol 38:148–58
116. Buyse I, Decorte R, Baens M, Cuppens H, Semana G, Emonds MP, Marynen P, Cassiman JJ (1993) Rapid DNA typing of class II HLA antigens using the polymerase chain reaction and reverse dot blot hybridization. Tissue Antigens 41:1–14
117. Ng J; Hurley CK; Baxter-Lowe LA, Chopek M, Coppo PA, Hegland J, KuKuruga D, Monos D, Rosner G, Schmeckpeper B, et al. (1993) Large-scale oligonucleotide typing for HLA-DRB1/3/4 and HLA-DQB1 is highly accurate, specific, and reliable. Tissue Antigens 42:473–9
118. Bugawan TL, Apple R, Erlich HA (1994) A method for typing polymorphism at the HLA-A locus using PCR amplification and immobilized oligonucleotide probes. Tissue Antigens 44:137–47
119. Garcia-Pacheco JM, Mantilla P, Garcia-Olivares E, Manzano-Fernandez MN (1995) Routine HLA DRB/DQB oligonucleotide typing by a non-radioactive dot-blot micromethod. J Immunol Methods 180:35–43
120. Middleton D, Williams F, Cullen C, Mallon E (1995) Modification of an HLA-B PCR-SSOP typing system leading to improved allele determination. Tissue Antigens 45:232–6
121. Kennedy LJ, Poulton KV, Dyer PA, Ollier WE, Thomson W (1995) Definition of HLA-C alleles using sequence-specific oligonucleotide probes (PCR-SSOP). Tissue Antigens 46:187–95
122. Fleischhauer K, Zino E, Bordignon C, Benazzi E (1995) Complete generic and extensive fine-specificity typing of the HLA-B locus by the PCR-SSOP method. Tissue Antigens 46:281–92
123. Inamdar A, Sintasath DM, Husted L, Henson V, Ng J, Hartzman RJ, Hurley CK (1996) Typing the HLA-B locus by a nested primer approach and oligonucleotide hybridization. Tissue Antigens 47:519–29
124. Williams F, Mallon E, Middleton D (1997) Development of PCR-SSOP for HLA-A typing of bone marrow registry donors. Tissue Antigens 49:61–6
125. Williams F, Middleton D, Savage D, Gorodezky C, Wilson DW, Fitzgerald JM, Urbaniak SJ (1997) Development of PCR-SSOP for the identification of HLA-A*02 subtypes and determination of HLA-A*02 frequencies within different ethnic populations. Tissue Antigens 49:129–33
126. Kennedy LJ, Poulton KV (1997) HLA class I SSOP protocol. In: Genetic diversity of HLA, functional and medical implications, vol. 1, ed. D. Charron, EDK, Paris, pp 564–583
127. Bignon JD, Fernandez-Viña MA (1997) Protocols of the 12th International Histocompatibility Workshop for typing of HLA class II alleles by DNA amplification by the

polymerase chain reaction (PCR) and hybridization with sequence specific oligonucleotide probes (SSOP). In: Genetic diversity of HLA, Functional and Medical Implications, vol. 1, ed. D. Charron, EDK, Paris, pp 584–632
128. Cereb N, Maye P, Lee S, Kong Y, Yang SY (1995) Locus-specific amplification of HLA class I genes from genomic DNA: locus-specific sequences in the first and third introns of HLA-A, -B, and -C alleles. Tissue Antigens 45:1–11
129. Olerup O, Zetterquist H (1991) HLA-DRB1*01 subtyping by allele-specific PCR amplification: a sensitive, specific and rapid technique. Tissue Antigens 37:197–204
130. Zetterquist H, Olerup O (1992) Identification of the HLA-DRB1*04, -DRB1*07, and -DRB1*09 alleles by PCR amplification with sequence-specific primers (PCR-SSP) in 2 hours. Hum Immunol 34:64–74
131. Bein G, Glaser R, Kirchner H (1992) Rapid HLA-DRB1 genotyping by nested PCR amplification. Tissue Antigens 39:68–73
132. Olerup O, Zetterquist H (1992) HLA-DR typing by PCR amplification with sequence-specific primers (PCR-SSP) in 2 hours: an alternative to serological DR typing in clinical practice including donor-recipient matching in cadaveric transplantation. Tissue Antigens 39:225–35
133. Ferencik S, Grosse-Wilde H (1993) A simple photometric detection method for HLA-DRB1 specific PCR-SSP products. Eur J Immunogenet 20:123–5
134. Bunce M, Taylor CJ, Welsh KI (1993) Rapid HLA-DQB typing by eight polymerase chain reaction amplifications with sequence-specific primers (PCR-SSP). Hum Immunol 37:201–6
135. Browning MJ, Krausa P, Rowan A, Bicknell DC, Bodmer JG, Bodmer WF (1993) Tissue typing the HLA-A locus from genomic DNA by sequence-specific PCR: comparison of HLA genotype and surface expression on colorectal tumor cell lines. Proc Natl Acad Sci USA 90:2842–5
136. Olerup O, Aldener A, Fogdell A (1993) HLA-DQB1 and -DQA1 typing by PCR amplification with sequence-specific primers (PCR-SSP) in 2 hours. Tissue Antigens 41:119–34
137. Krausa P, Bodmer JG, Browning MJ (1993) Defining the common subtypes of HLA A9, A10, A28 and A19 by use of ARMS/PCR. Tissue Antigens 42:91–9
138. Aldener-Cannava A, Olerup O (1994) HLA-DOB1 "low-resolution´ typing by PCR amplification with sequence-specific primers (PCR-SSP). Eur J Immunogenet 21:447–55
139. Bein G, Haase D, Schult J, Eiermann TH, Kirchner H (1994) Semiautomated HLA-DQB1 typing by fluorescent dye photometry of amplified DNA on microtiter plates. Hum Immunol 39:1–8
140. Olerup O (1994) HLA-B27 typing by a group-specific PCR amplification. Tissue Antigens 43:253–6
141. Bunce M, Barnardo MC, Welsh KI (1994) Improvements in HLA-C typing using sequence-specific primers (PCR-SSP) including definition of HLA-Cw9 and Cw10 and a new allele HLA-"Cw7/8v". Tissue Antigens 44:200–3
142. Hein J, Bottcher K, Grundmann R, Kirchner H, Bein G (1995) Low resolution DNA typing of the HLA-B5 cross-reactive group by nested PCR-SSP. Tissue Antigens 45:27–35
143. Bunce M, Fanning GC, Welsh KI (1995) Comprehensive, serologically equivalent DNA typing for HLA-B by PCR using sequence-specific primers (PCR-SSP). Tissue Antigens 45:81–90
144. Bunce M, O´Neill CM, Barnardo MC, Krausa P, Browning MJ, Morris PJ, Welsh KI (1995) Phototyping: comprehensive DNA typing for HLA-A, B, C, DRB1, DRB3, DRB4, DRB5 & DQB1 by PCR with 144 primer mixes utilizing sequence-specific primers (PCR-SSP). Tissue Antigens 46:355–67

145. Browning M, Krausa P (1996) Genetic diversity of HLA-A2: evolutionary and functional significance. Immunol Today 17:165–70
146. Krausa P, Browning MJ (1996) A comprehensive PCR-SSP typing system for identification of HLA-A locus alleles. Tissue Antigens 47: 237–44
147. Faas SJ, Menon R, Braun ER, Rudert WA, Trucco M (1996) Sequence-specific priming and exonuclease-released fluorescence detection of HLA-DQB1 alleles. Tissue Antigens 48:97–112
148. Aldener-Cannava A, Olerup O (1996) HLA-DPA1 typing by PCR amplification with sequence-specific primers (PCR-SSP) and distribution of DPA1 alleles in Caucasian, African and Oriental populations. Tissue Antigens 48:153–60
149. Zetterquist H, Bengtsson M, Backstrom G, Egle-Jansson I, Ekdahl AM, Grunnet N, Gustafsson I, Knutsen I, Kuhle A, Rydberg L, Spurkland A, Steffensen R, Storgards M, Szojmer E, Soderholm G, Thuresson B, Turesson H, Olerup O (1997) Report from the HLA class II typing by PCR-SSP Multicentre Study. Eur J Immunogenet 24:191–9
150. Luedeck H, Blasczyk R (1997) Fluorotyping of HLA-C: differential detection of amplicons by sequence-specific priming and fluorogenic probing. Tissue Antigens 50:627–38
151. Tonks S, Marsh SGE, Bunce M, Moses JH, Krausa P, Sadler AM, Petronzelli F, Bodmer JG (1997) HLA class I DNA typing study. In: Genetic diversity of HLA, functional and medical implications, vol. 1, ed. D. Charron, EDK, Paris, pp. 199–215
152. Gyllensten UB, Erlich HA (1988) Generation of single-stranded DNA by the polymerase chain reaction and its application to direct sequencing of the HLA-DQA locus. Proc Natl Acad Sci USA 85:7652–6
153. Ennis PD, Zemmour J, Salter RD, Parham P (1990) Rapid cloning of HLA-A,B cDNA by using the polymerase chain reaction: frequency and nature of errors produced in amplification. Proc Natl Acad Sci USA 87:2833–7
154. Kaneoka H, Lee DR, Hsu KC, Sharp GC, Hoffman RW (1991) Solid-phase direct DNA sequencing of allele-specific polymerase chain reaction-amplified HLA-DR genes. Biotechniques 10:30, 32, 34
155. Santamaria P, Boyce-Jacino MT, Lindstrom AL, Barbosa JJ, Faras AJ, Rich SS (1992) HLA class II "typing": direct sequencing of DRB, DQB, and DQA genes. Hum Immunol 33:69–81
156. Santamaria P, Lindstrom AL, Boyce-Jacino MT, Myster SH, Barbosa JJ, Faras AJ, Rich SS (1993) HLA class I sequence-based typing [erratum in Hum Immunol 1994: 41: 292]. Hum Immunol 37:39–50
157. Rozemuller EH, Bouwens AG, Bast BE, Tilanus MG (1993) Assignment of HLA-DPB alleles by computerized matching based upon sequence data. Hum Immunol 37:207–12
158. Versluis LF, Rozemuller E, Tonks S, Marsh SG, Bouwens AG, Bodmer JG, Tilanus MG (1993) High-resolution HLA-DPB typing based upon computerized analysis of data obtained by fluorescent sequencing of the amplified polymorphic exon 2. Hum Immunol 38:277–83
159. Spurkland A, Knutsen I, Markussen G, Vartdal F, Egeland T, Thorsby E (1993) HLA matching of unrelated bone marrow transplant pairs: direct sequencing of in vitro amplified HLA-DRB1 and -DQB1 genes using magnetic beads as solid support. Tissue Antigens 41:155–64
160. Domena JD, Little AM, Madrigal AJ, Hildebrand WH, Johnston-Dow L, du Toit E, Bias WB, Parham P (1993) Structural heterogeneity in HLA-B70, a high-frequency antigen of black populations. Tissue Antigens 42:509–17
161. Knipper AJ, Hinney A, Schuch B, Enczmann J, Uhrberg M, Wernet P (1994) Selection of unrelated bone marrow donors by PCR-SSP typing and subsequent nonradioactive

sequence-based typing for HLA DRB1/3/4/5, DQB1, and DPB1 alleles. Tissue Antigens 44:275–84

162. Rozemuller EH, Bouwens AG, van Oort E, Versluis LF, Marsh SG, Bodmer JG, Tilanus MG (1995) Sequencing-based typing reveals new insight in HLA-DPA1 polymorphism. Tissue Antigens 45:57–62
163. Petersdorf EW, Hansen JA (1995) A comprehensive approach for typing the alleles of the HLA-B locus by automated sequencing. Tissue Antigens 46:73–85
164. Rozemuller EH, Eliaou JF, Baxter-Lowe LA, Charron D, Kronick M, Tilanus MG (1995) An evaluation of a multicenter study on HLA-DPB1 typing using solid-phase Taq-cycle sequencing chemistry. Tissue Antigens 46:96–103
165. McGinnis MD, Conrad MP, Bouwens AG, Tilanus MG, Kronick MN (1995) Automated, solid-phase sequencing of DRB region genes using T7 sequencing chemistry and dye-labeled primers. Tissue Antigens 46:173–9
166. Versluis LF, Rozemuller EH, Duran K, Tilanus MG (1995) Ambiguous DPB1 allele combinations resolved by direct sequencing of selectively amplified alleles. Tissue Antigens 46:345–9
167. Blasczyk R, Weber M, van Lessen A, Schwella N, Huhn D, Salama A (1996) Discrimination of HLA-B27 alleles by group-specific amplification followed by solid-phase sequencing. Hum Immunol 45:117–23
168. Rozemuller EH, Tilanus MG (1996) A computerized method to predict the discriminatory properties for class II sequencing based typing. Hum Immunol 46:27–34
169. Rozemuller EH, Chadwick B, Charron D, Baxter-Lowe LA, Eliaou JF, Johnston-Dow L, Tilanus MG (1996) Sequenase sequence profiles used for HLA-DPB1 sequencing-based typing. Tissue Antigens 47:72–9
170. Blasczyk R, Wehling J, Weber M, Salama A (1996) Sequence analysis of the 2nd intron revealed common sequence motifs providing the means for a unique sequencing based typing protocol of the HLA-A locus. Tissue Antigens 47:102–10
171. Wang H, Tokunaga K, Akaza T, Tadokoro K, Shibata Y, Juji T (1997) Identification of HLA-C alleles using PCR-single-strand-conformation polymorphism and direct sequencing. Tissue Antigens 49:134–40
172. Eberle M, Knapp LA, Iwanaga KK, Domanico MJ, Aiyer K, Watkins DI (1997) HLA-B typing by allele separation followed by direct sequencing. Tissue Antigens 49:365–75
173. Craig MA, Elliott JF (1997) HLA-DQA1 genotyping by bi-directional sequencing of PCR-amplified DNA spanning exon 2. Tissue Antigens 49:417–20
174. Norgaard L, Fugger L, Jakobsen BK, Svejgaard A (1997) Sequencing-based typing of HLA-A locus using mRNA and a single locus-specific PCR followed by cycle-sequencing with AmpliTaq DNA polymerase, FS. Tissue Antigens 49:455–65
175. Voorter CEM, Rozemuller EH, de Bruyn-Geraets D, van der Zwan AW, Tilanus MG, van den Berg-Loonen EM (1997) Comparison of DRB sequence-based typing using different strategies. Tissue Antigens 49:471–6
176. Knapp LA, Lehmann E, Hennes L, Eberle ME, Watkins DI (1997) High-resolution HLA-DRB typing using denaturing gradient gel electrophoresis and direct sequencing. Tissue Antigens 50:170–7
177. Kotsch K, Wehling J, Kohler S, Blasczyk R (1997) Sequencing of HLA class I genes based on the conserved diversity of the noncoding regions: sequencing-based typing of the HLA-A gene. Tissue Antigens 50:178–91
178. Voorter CEM, Kik MC, van den Berg-Loonen EM (1998) High-resolution HLA typing for the DQB1 gene by sequence-based typing. Tissue Antigens 51:80–7
179. Newton CR, Graham A, Heptinstall LE, Powell SJ, Summers C, Kalsheker N, Smith JC, Markham AF (1989) Analysis of any point mutation in DNA. The amplification refractory mutation system (ARMS). Nucleic Acids Res 17:2503–16

180. Sanger F, Nicklen S, Coulson AR (1977) DNA sequencing with chain-terminating inhibitors. Proc Natl Acad Sci USA 74:5463–7
181. Dyer PA, Martin S, Sinnott P (1995) Histocompatibility testing for kidney transplantation: an update. Nephrol Dial Transplant 10 (Suppl 1):23–8
182. Howell WM, Navarrete C (1996) The HLA system: an update and relevance to patient-donor matching strategies in clinical transplantation. Vox Sang 71:6–12
183. Dyer PA, Claas FH (1997) A future for HLA matching in clinical transplantation. Eur J Immunogenet 24:17–28
184. Gajewski J, Champlin R (1996) Bone marrow transplantation from unrelated donors. Curr Opin Oncol 8:84–8
185. Madrigal JA, Arguello R, Scott I, Avakian H (1997) Molecular histocompatibility typing in unrelated donor bone marrow transplantation. Blood Rev 11:105–17
186. Devergie A, Apperley JF, Labopin M, Madrigal A, Jacobsen N, Carreras E, Prentice HG, Jouet JP, Kolb HJ, Herstenstein B, Bacigalupo A, Evensen SA, Ljungman P, de Witte T, Reiffers J, Nagler A, Clark RE, Goldman JM, Gratwohl A (1997) European results of matched unrelated donor bone marrow transplantation for chronic myeloid leukemia. Impact of HLA class II matching. Chronic Leukemia Working Party of the European Group for Blood and Marrow Transplantation. Bone Marrow Transplant 20:11–9
187. Hongeng S, Krance RA, Bowman LC, Srivastava DK, Cunningham JM, Horwitz EM, Brenner MK, Heslop HE (1997) Outcomes of transplantation with matched-sibling and unrelated-donor bone marrow in children with leukaemia. Lancet 350:767–71
188. Zachary AA, Vogelsang GB, Steinberg AG, Leffell MS (1997) Strategies for determining HLA compatibility in related donor bone marrow transplantation. Transplantation 64:828–35
189. Wittmann G, Zimmermann R, Eckstein R (1994) HLA and transfusion. Infusionsther Transfusionsmed 21:207–12
190. The Trial to Reduce Alloimmunization to Platelets Study Group (1997) Leukocyte reduction and ultraviolet B irradiation of platelets to prevent alloimmunization and refractoriness to platelet transfusions. N Engl J Med 337:1861–9
191. Saqi MA, Sayle R (1994) PdbMotif – a tool for the automatic identification and display of motifs in protein structures. Comput Appl Biosci 10:545–6

6 Immunohematology

A. Salama · O. Meyer

6.1 Red Blood Cell Antibodies

A. Salama

6.1.1 Introduction

Red blood cell (RBC) antibodies are immunoglobulins (IgG, IgM, and less commonly IgA) that combine with RBC antigens, and may thereby lead to destruction of target cells. The majority of IgM antibodies directly agglutinate RBC suspended in saline solutions, and are commonly called complete antibodies. In contrast, the vast majority of IgG and IgA antibodies are incapable of agglutinating RBC suspended in saline, but in the presence of a supplement, i.e. albumin, by the use of enzyme, or antihuman globulin serum (Coombs serum). Therefore these antibodies are termed incomplete antibodies (Mollison et al. 1997).

In general, agglutination techniques continue to build the fundamental basis for detection of RBC antigens and antibodies. During the last two decades, several modified tests have been described and the majority of RBC antibodies can meanwhile easily be demonstrated in many laboratories dealing with RBC serology. However, clinical and serological findings are often separately examined, and the results cannot be correctly interpreted in many cases. Ultimately, RBC antibodies do not always lead to destruction of target cells, and the failure to detect specific antibodies does not invariably exclude an immune-mediated cell injury. Moreover, immune-mediated RBC destruction depends on several factors that operate in concert: individual capacity of macrophages, complement activation, class, subclass and concentration of antibody (Schreiber and Frank 1972; Indik et al. 1995; Reinagel et al. 1997). The mechanisms by which RBC antibodies lead to hemolysis are briefly explained here.

6.1.2 Mechanisms of Immune Hemolytic Anemias

RBCs can be destroyed by two immune mechanisms (Fig. 6.1): direct lysis due to complement activation including the terminal complement components (C5b-9), or antibody and/or C_3b-mediated cell phagocytosis. The former form is called intravascular immune hemolysis and the latter form extravascular hemolysis. Intravascular hemolysis is invariably associated with increased hemoglobinemia. In contrast, extravascular hemolysis usually takes place without obvious hemoglobinemia. The occurrence of mild hemoglobinemia and even hemoglobinuria in cases with massive extravascular hemolysis is presumably the result of cell damage that may occur by attachment of target cells to macrophages (Mollison et al 1997).

6.1.2.1 *Characteristics of Intravascular Immune Hemolysis*

Intravascular RBC destruction due to complement activation is less common than immune-mediated extravascular hemolysis. In addition to the natural blood group isoagglutinins (anti-A and anti-B) only few antibodies cause complement-mediated intravascular hemolysis, i.e. some alloantibodies, cold agglutinins of high titer, Donath-Landsteiner autoantibodies, and the major-

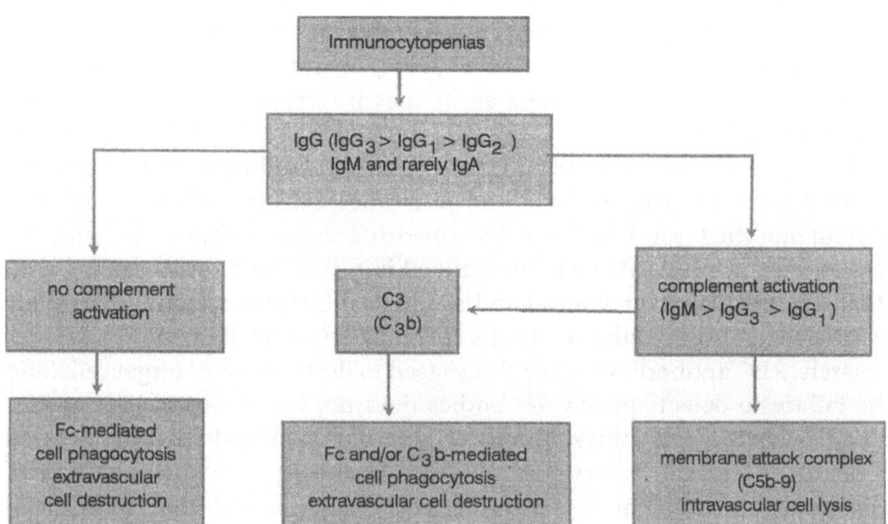

Fig. 6.1. Mechanisms of immunocytopenias

ity of drug-dependent antibodies (not drug-induced autoantibodies). In general, the majority of clinically relevant IgM antibodies, and only some IgG (IgG_3 subclass more efficient than IgG_1 subclass) antibodies are capable of complement activation (Mollison et al. 1997). Due to a large number of complement regulator proteins in plasma and on RBC membrane, complement activation is not invariably associated with intravascular destruction of the cells (Fig. 6.1). Once the process proceeds to C_3 activation, C_3a is released into the plasma, and C_3b binds to RBC. The presence of C_3b on the cell membrane may result in cell phagocytosis by macrophages which have C_3b-receptors, or cell lysis due to activation of the terminal complement components (C5b-9 or the so-called membrane attack complex). All RBCs escape hemolysis due to complement activation, become coated with C_3dg, a degradation product of C_3b, and may survive normally (Liszewski et al. 1996). From a serological viewpoint, C3dg is the only complement component that can be detected on intact RBC. Thus, evidence for ongoing or already completed complement activation is usually reflected by C_3d positivity in the direct antiglobulin test (Salama and Mueller-Eckhardt 1984, 1985a).

6.1.2.2
Characteristics of Immune-Mediated Extravascular Hemolysis

The majority of RBC antibodies are incapable of activating complement, and the hemolysis related to these antibodies is largely or even exclusively the result of increased extravascular RBC destruction. In this case, RBCs sensitized with IgG and/or C_3b molecules are eliminated by macrophages which have receptors for IgG (Fc-receptor) and C_3b molecules (CR1-receptor). Unlike intravascular hemolysis, extravascular hemolysis is somewhat limited by the individual capacity of macrophages and antibody character (concentration, class and subclass). As macrophages have high affinity receptors for IgG_3 and less strongly for IgG_1, but low or no affinity for IgG_2 and IgG_4, respectively, shortened RBC survival is usually observed when the former two subclasses are involved. IgG_4 does not cause decreased RBC survival, and only large amounts of IgG_2 may induce hemolysis. Additionally, only IgG_3 and, to a lesser degree, IgG_1 may activate complement and lead to coating of RBC with C_3b component. Although IgA seems to cause severe hemolysis in isolated cases, the mechanism of IgA-mediated RBC destruction has not yet been fully clarified (Mollison et al. 1997). Similarly, there is evidence that non-complement activating IgM antibodies can also cause RBC destruction (Salama and Mueller-Eckhardt 1985b).

6.1.3
Classification of Immune Hemolytic Anemias

6.1.3.1
Autoimmune Hemolytic Anemia of Warm Type

The onset and course of autoimmune hemolytic anemia (AIHA) of warm type is most variable (Fig. 6.2). The cardinal finding in all classical cases is a specific positivity in the direct antiglobulin test (DAT). The majority of affected patients develop IgG antibodies that react with all normal RBCs. They are typically detectable on patients' RBCs, and can be eluted from the cells (Petz and Garratty 1980). Small quantities of cell bound autoantibodies, and low affinity antibodies, particularly IgG autoantibodies that cannot be demonstrated by the standard antiglobulin test, are usually detectable by other sensitive techniques, i.e. enzyme-linked immunoassay (ELISA) or the new microtyping gel-agglutination technique (Lapierre et al 1990; AABB 1996). The latter method is not only practical, but also highly sensitive and allows the detection of IgG, IgA, IgM and C_3d molecules on RBCs (see below).

About 30% of patients with AIHA of warm type have only IgG on their RBCs, 40%–50% IgG and C_3d, 20% other or more than one class of antibodies, and less than 5% may have negative DAT (Fig. 6.2). Of the IgG subclasses, IgG_3 shows the strongest reactivity with macrophages; IgG_1 shows moderate activity, IgG_2 weak reactivity and IgG_4 shows none (Petz and Garratty 1980; Engelfriet et al. 1992). Rarely, the causative autoantibodies are exclusively IgA

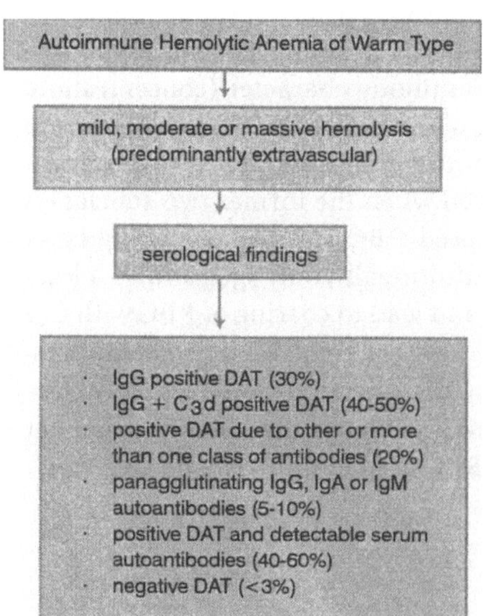

Fig. 6.2. Characteristics of autoimmune hemolytic anemia of warm type. In isolated cases, the direct antiglobulin test (DAT) may give negative results, but the autoantibodies could be eluted from the cells

or IgM. IgG autoantibodies detectable only in eluates enriched from patients' RBCs are seen in isolated cases. When incomplete (non-agglutinating) IgM autoantibodies are solely responsible for hemolysis, only complement components may be detected on the surface of RBCs (Petz and Garratty 1980; Salama et al. 1987). IgA is responsible for AIHA only in isolated cases. In such instances, an antiglobulin test performed without reagents containing anti-IgA Coombs antibodies will give false-negative results. In contrast, incomplete IgM antibodies usually remain undetectable by the use of specific antiglobulin serum (anti-IgM). The reactivity of warm autoantibodies is usually increased by the use of enzyme-treated RBCs, and in some cases the causative antibodies can only be demonstrated by the use of enzyme-treated cells. The antibodies in AIHA of warm type are usually directed against the Rh-complex. In some cases many other specificities may be involved, i.e. K, Ge and others (Petz and Garratty 1980).

6.1.3.2
Autoimmune Hemolytic Anemia with Cold-Reactive Antibodies

In about 10% of patients with AIHA the hemolysis is caused by cold agglutinins. These antibodies react only with RBCs at temperatures below 37°C (most effectively at 0°–4°C). Almost all cold agglutinins are IgM of high titer. The antibodies lead to RBC agglutination as soon as blood cools to a critical range (usually <28°C). Cold-reactive antibodies may occur without an underlying disease (idiopathic form), or secondary to malignant or infectious diseases (Fig. 6.3). The cold agglutinins in patients with the idiopathic form and with hematologic neoplasmas, i.e. lymphomas and chronic lymphatic leukemia, are monoclonal, and those in patients with infectious disease are polyclonal antibodies. The rate of hemolysis due to cold agglutinins is most related to the thermal amplitude of the antibody, to its capability of initiating complement activation, and to a lesser degree to its concentration (titer). Since complement is not activated at lower temperature and cold agglutinins do not react with RBCs at >37°C, hemolysis due to cold reactive antibodies takes place only in the temperature range of >10°–<37°C. The majority of cold agglutinins induce maximal lysis at 20°–22°C where both factors are largely reactive (Petz and Garratty 1980; Mollison et al. 1997). The hemolysis in patients with cold agglutinins is solely related to generation of C5b-9 and/or C3b, which leads to intra- and extravascular hemolysis, respectively (Salama et al. 1983). Thus, all RBCs escaping hemolysis are invariably coated with C_3d fragments, and give positive DAT (Fig. 6.3).

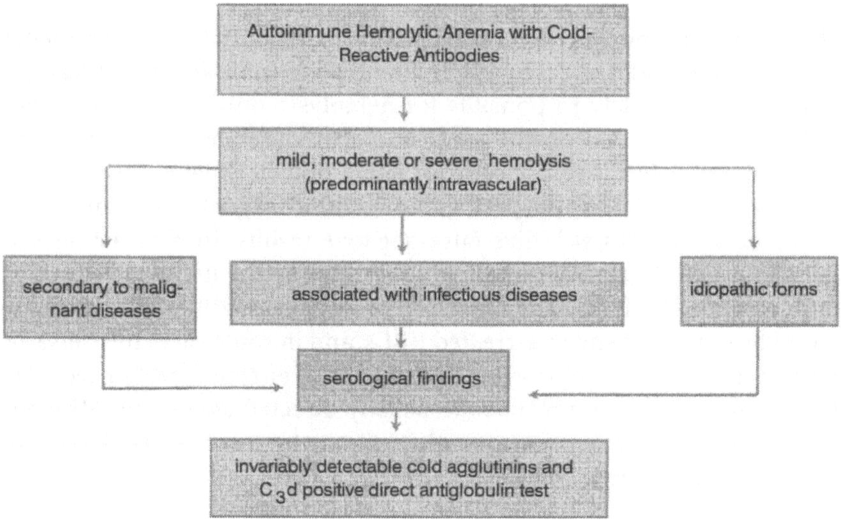

Fig. 6.3. Characteristics of autoimmune hemolytic anemia with cold reactive antibodies

6.1.3.3
Paroxysmal Cold Hemoglobinuria

Paraxysmal cold hemoglobinuria (Donath-Landsteiner autoimmune hemolysis) is characterized by acute hemoglobinuria due to exposure to the cold (Fig. 6.4). The hemolysis is caused by IgG and less commonly IgM cold-reactive antibodies of relatively low titer (<1:64). The antibodies react most strongly with RBCs at a temperature of 0°–4°C, and cause complement activation during dissociation from the cells at temperatures of >10°C. All RBCs escaping hemolysis are coated with C_3d fragments. Before penicillin therapy was possible the responsible antibodies were usually found in patients with tertiary or congenital syphilis. Meanwhile, the disease exclusively occurs in children (2–10 years old) with a history of recent viral infection. In these cases the hemolysis is usually acute and disappears within a few days (Göttsche et al. 1990).

6.1.3.4
Alloimmune Hemolysis

Alloimmune hemolysis reflects conditions of increased RBC destruction due to transfusion of incompatible RBCs, and less commonly due to transfusion of plasma containing antibodies reacting with the recipient's RBCs. The reaction may begin during transfusion of RBCs and plasma, respectively (im-

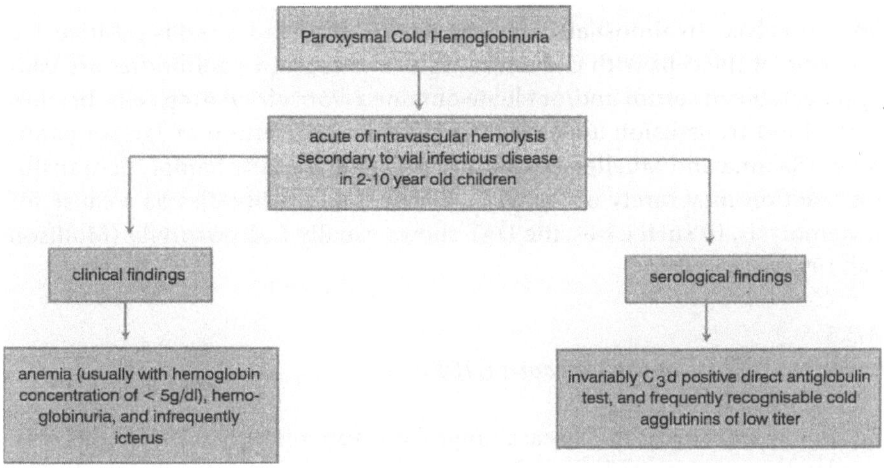

Fig. 6.4. Characteristics of paroxysmal cold hemoglobinuria (Donath-Landsteiner autoimmune hemolytic anemia)

mediate hemolytic transfusion reaction), or within a few days after transfusion of RBCs (delayed hemolytic transfusion reactions). The clinical significance of such reactions is extremely variable and ranges from life-threatening to trivial (Fig. 6.5). Complement-activating antibodies lead predominantly to intravascular hemolysis, i.e. anti-A and anti-B, whereas non-complement activating antibodies, i.e. anti-D, may lead to extravascular hemolysis (Mollison et al. 1997). Serological findings depend on the antigens and anti-

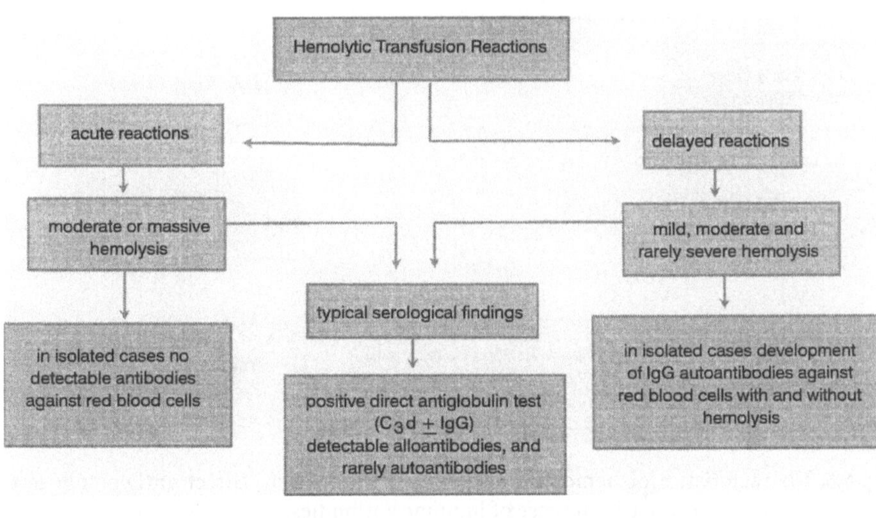

Fig. 6.5. Characteristics of immune hemolytic transfusion reactions

bodies involved. In almost all cases, the direct antiglobulin test is positive due to coating of the cells with C_3d and/or IgG. The causative antibodies are usually detectable in serum and/or eluate obtained from circulating cells. In a few cases, blood transfusion appears to trigger the production of IgG autoantibodies (Salama and Mueller-Eckhardt 1984). Additionally hemolytic transfusion reaction may rarely occur without detectable antibodies as a cause for the hemolysis. In such cases, the DAT shows usually C_3d-positivity (Mollison et al. 1997).

6.1.3.5
Hemolytic Disease of the Newborn (HDN)

The clinical features of the disease range from apparently healthy infants with completely compensated hemolysis to intrauterine death (Fig. 6.6). The hemolysis may be caused only by maternal IgG antibodies against fetal cells. Based on the severity of hemolysis and antibody specificity, HDN can be classified in three types:

1. HDN due to immune anti-D
2. HDN due to immune antibodies against other RBC antigens
3. HDN due to ABO incompatibility

The most severe hemolysis is usually caused by anti-D, and less commonly by anti-c. All other immune antibodies only rarely cause severe hemolytic

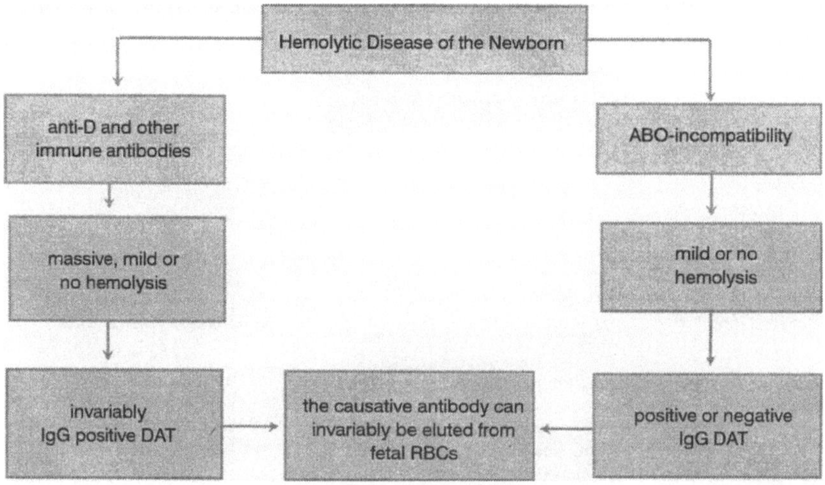

Fig. 6.6. Characteristics of hemolytic disease of the newborn. Direct antiglobulin test (DAT) is invariably positive in the case of immune antibodies, i.e. anti-Rh(D) as a cause of hemolysis

anemia (Mollison et al. 1997). In all cases related to immune antibodies the direct antiglobulin test is usually strongly positive, and the causative antibody is detectable in maternal serum as well as in eluates obtained from fetal RBCs. In ABO hemolytic disease, affected infants are rarely symptomatic, and the DAT is usually positive by the use of sensitive tests, i.e. the gel agglutination technology. Eluates obtained from fetal cells contain anti-A and/or anti-B in almost all affected and unaffected infants. Thus, serological findings are rarely indicative in HDN due to ABO incompatibility.

6.1.3.6
Drug-Induced Immune Hemolytic Anemias

Meanwhile, more than 70 different drugs have been reported to be the cause of immune hemolytic anemia (Salama 1997). However, series of patients affected by the same drug have been reported only in case of drugs. In almost all cases, the drugs involved were represented by a single case report. Principally, any drug may induce immune response, and drug-induced disorders should be suspected in all patients who develop reactions while receiving a drug, or following reexposure to a drug (Fig. 6.7). If the drug is given for the first time, the minimal time required for the development of a clinically relevant immune response is at least 5–6 days (primary immune reaction). Thereafter, reactions may take place at any time (secondary immune reaction). The clinical picture of drug-induced immune hemolysis depends on the resultant antibodies. Affected patients may develop antibodies that react

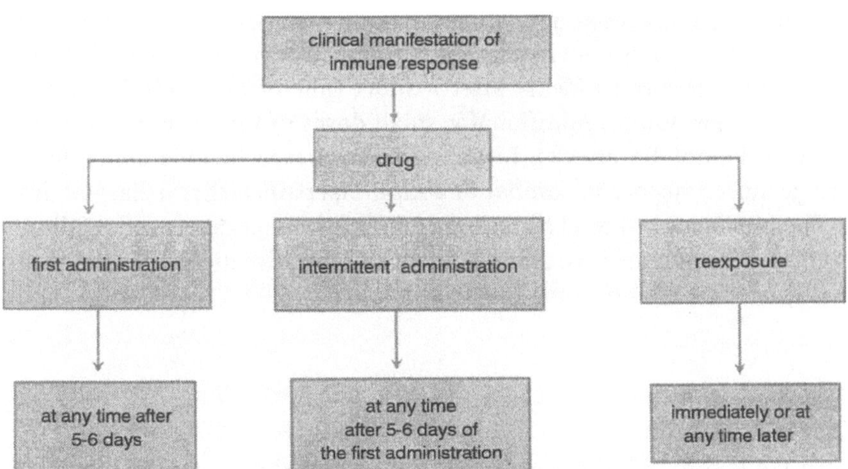

Fig. 6.7. Manifestation of drug-induced immune reaction

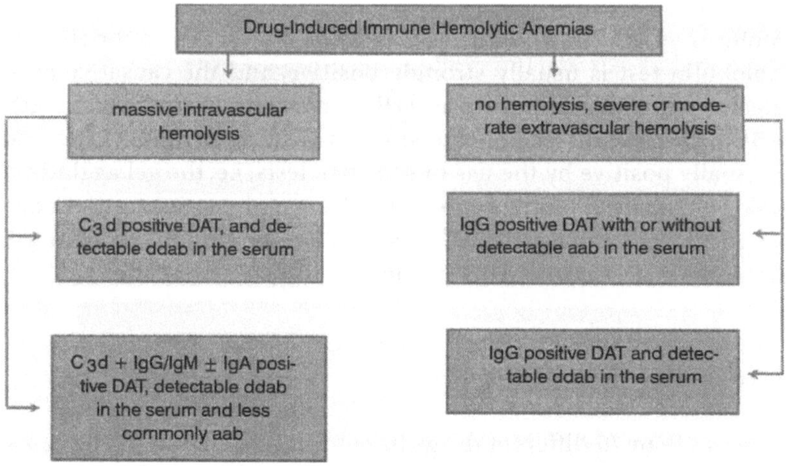

Fig. 6.8. Characteristics of immune hemolytic anemias related to drug-induced autoantibodies (aab) and/or drug-dependent antibodies (ddab). The direct antiglobulin test (DAT) is positive in all cases

only with RBCs in the presence of the drug and/or its metabolites (drug-dependent antibodies) and/or antibodies that react with RBCs in the presence as well as in the absence of the drug (drug-independent antibodies). The latter antibodies are of the IgG class and do not activate complement, whereas the former antibodies may be of the IgG and/or of the IgM that activate complement in almost all cases. Similar to other antibodies, noncomplement-activating antibodies may cause severe, or mild extravascular immune hemolysis. In contrast, complement-activating antibodies usually cause abrupt intravascular hemolysis (Fig. 6.8). In general, intravascular immune hemolysis related to a drug occurs suddenly after a short time of drug administration (minutes to a few hours). Additionally, small doses of the drug may also induce severe hemolytic attacks. Initial symptoms may include chills, fever, vomiting, nausea, headache, lumbar or abdominal pain, tachycardia, and dyspnea. The incidence of life-threatening complications, i.e. acute renal failure, shock, disseminated intravascular coagulation, is relative high. The complications may even be fatal in some instances (Salama 1997).

6.1.3.7
Serological Findings

There are four serological patterns in immune hemolytic anemias related to drugs (Fig. 6.8): IgG positive DAT due to aab or noncomplement-activating ddab, C_3d-positive DAT with or without detectable aab in addition to the ddab (Salama 1997). In general, drug-induced aab are of high titers in the absence of ddab, and of low titers in the presence of ddab in the same patient. Drug-induced aab react with normal RBCs in the presence and absence of the drug, and gradually disappear after drug discontinuation. Unlike aab, ddab react with RBCs only in the presence of the causative drug and/or its metabolites. Complement-activating ddab are usually reactive with RBCs in the presence of free drug, and less commonly with drug-treated RBCs too. In a few exceptions, the resultant ddab do not activate complement, and react only with drug-treated cells, i.e. the majority of penicillin-induced antibodies, and antibodies related to old cephalosporin generations. Drug metabolites appear to be responsible for the reaction in almost all cases. Thus, the use of metabolites is often essential for the in vitro demonstration of ddab. Since metabolites of drugs are usually not available or even unknown, the use of ex vivo antigens (urine and/or serum samples collected from patients or volunteers receiving the drug) has proven of great value in this field (Salama 1997).

6.1.4 Antibody Detection and Identification Using the New Gel Agglutination Technology

6.1.4.1 *Principle*

Gel agglutination technology is a relatively new system for detection of RBC antigen-antibody reaction. In the gel test, microtubes containing dextran acrylamide gel particles are used. These particles have a molecular sieving effect that reflects the size of agglutinated RBCs. Unagglutinated cells pass through the gel to the tip of the tube, while large and small agglutinates remain above and suspended in the gel particles, respectively. Three types of gel cards are available: neutral, specific, and antiglobulin cards. In the neutral card, the gel does not contain specific antibodies, and acts only by its property of trapping agglutinates. This card is mainly used to demonstrate antibodies that may directly agglutinate untreated or enzyme-treated RBCs. In the specific gel card, the microtubes contain specific antibodies usually used for blood grouping and antigen determination. In the antiglobulin gel card, the microtubes contain specific antihuman globulin sera, i.e. anti-IgG, -IgA, -IgM, and C_3d, and RBCs can be directly or indirectly tested (direct and indirect antiglobulin test, respectively). The medium included in the tube allows a separation between the RBCs and serum or plasma, and no RBC washing is required (Lapierre et al. 1990).

6.1.4.2
Material

1. Serum or plasma and RBC from patients
2. Reagent RBCs
3. Gel cards, diluents and centrifuge as specified by the manufactures
4. Antihuman globulin reagents

6.1.5
Procedure for Detection of Antibodies in Serum Samples

1. Deliver 50 µl of untreated or enzyme-treated RBC suspension (1% in the appropriate diluent) into the microtubes
2. Add 25 µl of undiluted or diluted serum or plasma
3. Incubate the card for 15 min at 37°C
4. Centrifuge the card as recommended by the manufacturers
5. Read both sides of each microtube for agglutination

6.1.6
Direct Antiglobulin Test Using the Gel Agglutination Technology

6.1.6.1
Material

1. EDTA-anticoagulated blood sample to be tested
2. Cards containing antihuman globulin reagents
3. Diluent, as specified by the manufactures

6.1.6.2
Procedure

1. Deliver 50 µl of RBC (1% suspension in diluent)
2. Centrifuge as recommended
3. Read both sides of each microtube for agglutination

6.1.6.3
Notes

1. The method is easy and laborsaving
2. The gel agglutination technology allows the detection of low affinity anti bodies, since the test is performed without washing the cells

3. The technique is extremely sensitive and allows the detection of low antibody concentration
4. The results are more objective than those with tube and microplate methods
5. The technique is useful for antibody screening and identification
6. Due to high sensitivity much more unspecific reactions are seen by this technique, the tube or microplate techniques
7. A similar technique (BioVue) in which glass beads are placed in a micro column together with diluent is also in use (Reis et al. 1993)

6.1.7
Solid-Phase Tests

6.1.7.1
Introduction

Solid-phase microplate technique is an alternative to conventional agglutination tests. The technique is applicable to antigen antibody and compatibility testing. Positive reactions are indicated by adherence of sensitized RBC over the entire surface of the wells of the microtest plate (formation of monolayer). In contrast, negative reactions are reflected by pelleted cells on the bottom of the wells (Plapp et al. 1984; Rachel et al. 1985; Uthemann and Poschmann 1990).

6.1.7.2
Principle

ABO grouping and other antigen typing are direct assays that require only centrifugation after the addition of test RBCs to antibody coated wells. For antibody detection, RBCs are incubated with the patient´s serum, washed and then suspended in antiglobulin serum. The suspension is transferred to wells coated with antihuman globulin serum, centrifuged and read visually or photometrically.

6.1.7.3
Procedure

Various semi-automated assays are commercially available. The manufacturer´s instructions should be followed (Mollison et al. 1997).

6.1.8 Demonstration of Drug-Induced Antibodies

6.1.8.1 *Principle*

Drugs may lead to the production of autoantibodies (aab), drug-dependent antibodies (ddab), or both types of antibodies in the same patient. Drug-induced aab are reactive with RBC in the presence as well as in the absence of the drug, and they cannot be distinguished from aab related to idiopathic or symptomatic AIHA of warm type. Drug-dependent antibodies react only with RBCs in the presence of the drug and/or metabolites.

The gel test is highly sensitive and allows the detection of ddab, even those related to drugs which do not bind tightly to RBC (Salama et al. 1992).

6.1.8.2 *Material*

1. Serum and EDTA-anticoaglulated RBCs of patient
2. Test group 0 RBC for antibody detection
3. Neutral and antihuman globulin gel cards including diluents, incubator and centrifuge, as recommended by the manufacturers
4. Solution containing non-toxic concentration of the drug or, if available, its metabolites, i.e. 1 mg/ml suspension solution of the drug in saline or phosphate buffer saline. Methanol (1:10), 1 N NaOH, 1 N HCl or polyethylene glycol may be used to dissolve unsoluble drugs
5. In cases where the native drug gives negative reactions, ex vivo antigen of the drug (serum and/or urine obtained from patients or volunteers receiving therapeutic level of the drug) should be used

6.1.8.3 *Procedure*

The only difference between the procedure for detection of ddab and "classical" antibodies is that the drug/metabolites must be included in the incubation mixture, i.e. two volumes of RBC suspension, two volumes of patient's serum and one volume of the solution containing the drug.

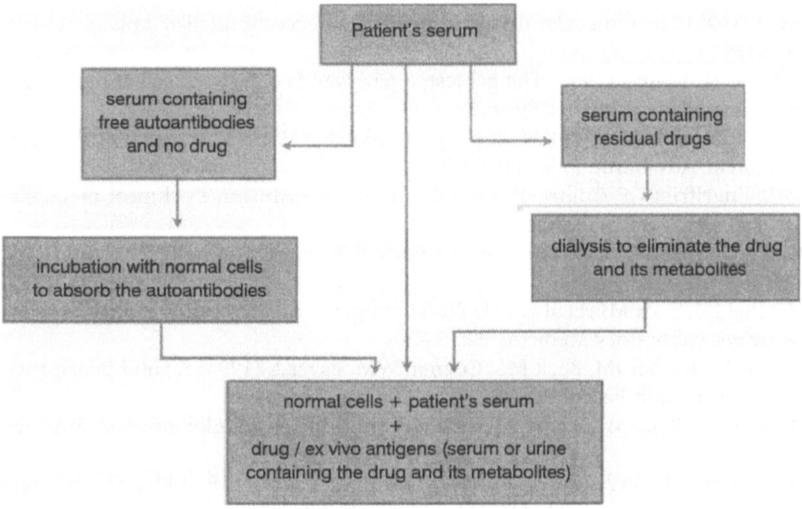

Fig. 6.9. Demonstration of drug-dependent antibodies in serum samples of patients with immunocytopenias related to drugs. Since the majority of drugs do not bind tightly to the cells, and drug-dependent antibodies dissociate from their binding sites in the absence of the causative drug/metabolites, the drug (metabolites) must be included in all washing procedures

6.1.8.4 *Notes*

Serum containing residual drugs/metabolites may give reaction patterns similar to that of autoantibodies, and drug-induced aab frequently make the detection of the former antibodies impossible in standard routine testing. In such cases, the drug and its metabolites should be eliminated from the serum to be tested by excessive dialysis prior to testing (Fig. 6.9). In the absence of the drug and its metabolites, drug-induced aab can be absorbed onto normal RBCs, leaving ddab in the supernatant. The latter antibodies could then be recognized using a fresh drug solution (Salama and Mueller-Eckhardt 1985b).

References

AABB (1996) Technical Manual 12th edn. Amer Assoc Blood Banks, Bethesda, MD

Engelfriet CP, Overbeeke MAM, von dem Borne AEGKr (1992) Autoimmune hemolytic anemia. Semin Hematol 29:3–12

Göttsche B, Salama A, Mueller-Eckhardt C (1990) Donath-Landsteiner autoimmune hemolytic anemia in children. A study of 22 cases. Vox Sang 58:281–286

Indik ZK et al (1995) The molecular dissection fo FcγRII receptor mediated phagocytosis. Blood 86:4389

Lapierre Y, Rigal D, Adam J (1990) The gel test: a new way to detect red cell antigen-antibody reactions. Transfusion 30:109–113

Liszewski MK, Farries TC, Lublin CM, Rooney IA, Atkinson JP (1996) Control of the complement system. Adv Immunol 61:201–283

Mollision PL, Engelfriet CP, Contreras M (1997) Blood transfusion in clinical medicine. Tenth edition, Blackwell Science Ltd.

Petz LD, Garratty G (1980) Acquired immune hemolytic anemias. Churchill Livingstone, New York

Plapp FV, Rachel JM, Beck ML, et al (1984) Blood antigens and antibodies: Solid phase adherence assays. Laboratory Medicine 22:39–46

Plapp FV, Sinor LT, Rachel JM, Beck ML, Coenen WM, Bayer L (1984) A solid phase antibody screen. Am J Clin Pathol 82:719

Rachel JM, Sinor LT, Beck ML, Plapp FV (1985) A solid-phase antiglobulin test. Transfusion 25:24

Reinagel ML, Gezen M, Ferguson PJ, Kuhn S, Martin EN, Taylor RP (1997) The primate erythrocyte complement receptor (CR1) as a privileged site: binding of immunoglobulin G to erythrocyte CR1 does not target erythrocytes for phagocytosis. Blood 89:1068–1077

Reis KJ, Chachowski R, Cupido A, Davies D, Jakway J, Setcavage TM (1993) Column agglutination technology: the antiglobulin test. Transfusion 33:639–643

Salama A (1997) Drug-induced immune hemolytic anemia. Comprehensive Toxicology, Elsevier Science, United Kingdom

Salama A, Berghöfer H, Mueller-Eckhardt C (1992) Detection of cell-drug antibody complexes by the gel-test. Transfusion 32:554–556

Salama A, Bhakdi S, Mueller-Eckhardt C, Kayser W (1983) Deposition of the terminal C5b-9 complement complex on erythrocytes by human red cell autoantibodies. Br J Haemat 55:161–160

Salama A, Mueller-Eckhardt C (1984) Delayed hemolytic transfusion reactions. Evidence for complement activation involving allogeneic and autologous red cells. Transfusion 24:188–193

Salama A, Mueller-Eckhardt C (1985a) Binding of fluid phase C3b to nonsensitized bystander human red blood cells. A model for in vivo effects of complement activation on blood cells. Transfusion 25:230–235

Salama A, Mueller-Eckhardt C (1985b) The role of metabolite-specific antibodies nomifensine-dependent immune hemolytic anemia. New Engl J Med 313:469–474

Salama A, Mueller-Eckhardt C (1987) Autoimmune haemolytic anaemia in childhood associated with non-complement binding IgM autoantibodies. Br J Haemat 65:67–71

Schreiber AD, Frank MM (1972) Role of antibody and complement in the immune clearance and destruction of erythrocytes . I. In vivo effects of IgG and IgM complement-fixing sites. J Clin Invest 51:575

Uthemann H, Poschmann A (1990) Solid-phase antiglobulin test for screening and identification of red cell antibodies. Transfusion 30:114–116

6.2 Platelet Antibodies

A. Salama, O. Meyer

6.2.1 Introduction

In general, the behavior of platelet antibodies is similar to that of RBC antibodies. They react with platelet antigens, and may thereby lead to increased platelet sequestration within the reticuloendothelial system (Fig. 6.1). Intravascular lysis of platelet due to complement activation only appears to take place in isolated cases. Based on serological and clinical findings, platelet antibodies are classified into 5 types.

6.2.1.1 *Platelet Autoantibodies*

The vast majority of platelet autoantibodies are of IgG classes that do not activate complement. Usually, they are directed against high frequency platelet antigens which are located on glycoproteins (gp), i.e. gp IIb/IIIa, Ib/IX, and less frequently Ia/IIa, gp IV or gpV. The antibodies react with autologous as well as with normal platelets of almost all individuals. They can be detected on circulating platelets and less frequently in serum (<20%). C3d is rarely detectable on platelets of patients with AITP autoimmune thrombocytopenia (Kiefel et al. 1992; Shulman and Reid 1994; George et al. 1995). In some cases, platelet autoantibodies may also affect platelet function and lead to increased hemorrhage (Deckmyn and De Reys 1995).

6.2.1.2 *Platelet Alloantibodies*

Platelet alloantibodies are directed against allotypic determinants that are genetically expressed on platelet surfaces and reflected by structural differences of glycoproteins. Platelet alloantibodies may result from pregnancy, blood transfusion, and rarely bone marrow transplantation. There are three types of clinically relevant platelet alloantibodies (George et al. 1995; Mueller-Eckhardt 1997); (1) Platelet specific antibodies that recognize platelet alloantigens (Table 6.1). The majority of these antigens are localized on GP IIb/IIIa complex. (2) Antibodies related to HLA class I molecules. These antibodies react not only with leukocytes but also with platelets carrying the corresponding antigens. (3) Blood group anti-A and anti-B that are present in

Table 6.1. So far identified platelet antigens

Antigen	Synonym	Location	Frequency (%)
HPA-1a	Zw(a), PI(A1)	GPIIIa	97.5
HPA-1b	Zw(b), PI(A2)		30.8
HPA-2a	Ko(a)	GPIb	99.8
HPA-2b	Ko(a)		11.8
HPA-3a	Bak(a), Lek(a)	GPIIb	86.1
HPA-3b	Bak(b)		62.9
HPA-4a	Yuk(b), Pen(a)	GPIIIa	>99.9
HPA-4b	Yuk(a), Pen(b)		>0.1
HPA-5a	Br(b)	GPIa	98.8
HPA-5b	Br(a)		20.6
HPA-6bW	Ca(c), Tu(a)	GPIIIa	0.7
HPA-7bW	Mo(a)	GPIIIa	0.2
HPA-8bW	Sr(a)	GPIIIa	<0.1
HPA-9bW	Max(a)	GPIIb	0.6
HPA-10bW	ly(a)	GPIbß	0.4
HPA-11bW	Gro(a)	GPIIIa	<0.1
HPA-12bW	Oe(a)	GPIIIa	<0.1

normal serum of healthy individuals. These antibodies rarely lead to increased sequestration of ABO-incompatible platelets.

6.2.1.3
Drug-Induced Platelet Antibodies

Similar to RBC antibodies related to drugs, two types of platelet antibodies are known: (1) drug-induced autoantibodies that react with platelets in the presence as well as in the absence of the drug, and (2) drug-dependent antibodies that only react with platelets in the presence of the drug and/or its metabolites. The latter antibodies usually cause precipitous thrombocytopenic purpura which immediately resolves when the drug and its metabolites have completely been eliminated from the circulation. In contrast, drug-induced autoantibodies are largely indistinguishable from classic autoantibodies, and may persist for months after stopping the drug (Salama and Mueller-Eckhardt 1992; Aster 1997).

6.2.1.4
Platelet Antibodies Related to Heparin

Approximately 1% of patients receiving Heparin develop IgG, and less commonly IgM or IgA antibodies that usually react with heparin-platelet factor 4 complexes, and may thereby lead to platelet activation via FcγII receptor (Chong et al. 1995; Warkentin 1996).

6.2.2
Disorders Related to Platelet Autoantibodies

6.2.2.1
Autoimmunthrombocytopenias (AITP)

There are acute and chronic forms of AITP. The former disease is relatively common in childhood. In almost all these cases, thrombocytopenia develops within 3 weeks after viral infections. Chronic AITP is the most common cause of isolated thrombocytopenia in adults. The disease is characterized by low platelet count, an essentially normal bone marrow with or without increased megacaryocytosis, and absence of evidence for other diseases (idopathic form). In approximately 15%–20%, the thrombocytopenia is associated with an underlying disease (secondary of symptomatic form), i.e. lupus erythematodes, lymphoma, autoimmune thyroiditis, sclerodermia, rheumatoid arthritis, biliary cirrhosis, sarcoidosis, autoimmune hemolytic anemia of warm type (Evans syndrome) and other diseases (George et al. 1995). Thrombocytopenia in all AITP forms results from increased sequestration of platelets within the reticuloendothelial system, and presumably due to complement-mediated lysis in isolated cases. The mechanism by which the platelets are destroyed is largely identical to that described in AIHA of warm type (Fig. 6.1). The causative autoantibodies in AITP remain, however, undetectable in many cases. Thus, the diagnosis of AITP is frequently only based on exclusion (Karpatkin 1985; Shulman and Reid 1994; George et al. 1995).

6.2.2.2
Disorders Caused by Platelet Alloantibodies

6.2.2.2.1
Neonatal Alloimmune Thrombocytopenia (NAIT)

Approximately 0.1%–0.2% of neonates may develop thrombocytopenia due to active immunization of the mother by fetal platelet alloantigens. In about 50% of affected cases, NAIT develops during the first pregnancy. About 80%

of NAIT are caused by anti-Pl^{A1}(Zw^{a}), 15% by anti-Br^{a}, and 5% by other alloantibodies. The diagnosis is based on serological findings that include the detection of an alloantibody in maternal serum, and the corresponding antigen on the platelets of the neonate (Mueller-Eckhardt et al. 1989; Bussel et al. 1997).

6.2.2.3 *Posttransfusion Purpura (PTP)*

The disease is characterized by an acute thrombocytopenic purpura that occurs about 1 week after transfusion of packed red blood cells, and less commonly after transfusion of platelets (Fig. 6.10). Thrombocytopenia is caused by alloantibodies specific for platelet alloantigens. Anti-Pl^{A1} is responsible for this happening in almost all cases. Interestingly, the reaction leads to destruction of autologous platelets, although these are invariably negative for the alloantibody present in plasma during the acute phase (George et al. 1995).

6.2.2.4 *Platelet Transfusion Refractoriness*

Antibodies directed against HLA class I antigen are responsible for platelet transfusion refractoriness in the majority of patients who do not respond to platelet transfusion. Platelet specific antibodies are rarely involved. The most effective way to prevent sensitization against HLA antigens is the use of leukodepleted cellular blood products (Slichter 1990).

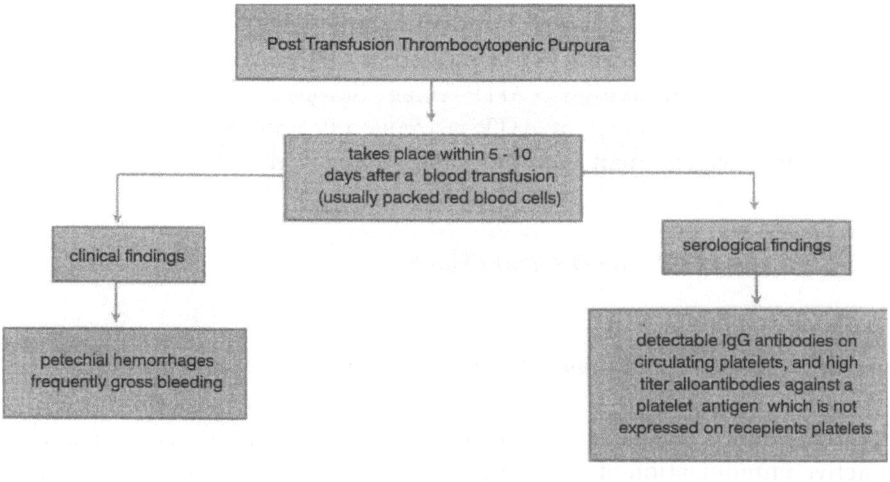

Fig. 6.10. Characteristics of post-transfusion purpura

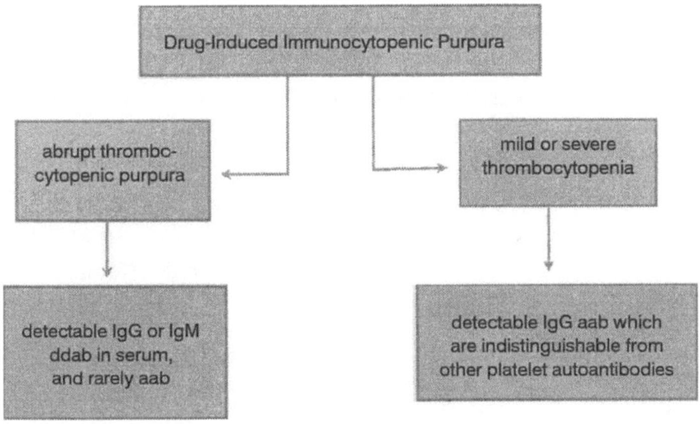

Fig. 6.11. Characteristics of immunocytopenias related to drug-induced autoantibodies (aab) and drug-dependent antibodies (ddab)

6.2.3 Drug-Induced Immunothrombocytopenia

A large number of drugs has been reported to cause immunothrombocytopenia. Sensitization and clinical manifestation are similar to those described in drug-induced immune hemolysis. Quinine and quinidine account for the largest number of cases. Only isolated patients taking these or other drugs develop thrombocytopenia. Ingestion of the causative drug leads within minutes to reactions in sensitized individuals, i.e. chills, petechial hemorrhages, and often hemorrhage from the gastrointestinal or urinary tract (FIg. 11). Bleeding symptoms disappear within a few days after discontinuation of the offending drug. Thrombocytopenia persists for weeks, months, and even up to one year if drug-independent antibodies (autoantibodies) were responsible for the reaction (Salama and Mueller-Eckhardt 1992; Aster 1997).

6.2.4 Heparin-Induced Immunothrombocytopenia

Heparin-induced thrombocytopenia is frequently difficult to distinguish from thrombocytopenia due to other causes (Fig. 6.12). Thrombocytopenia and/or thrombosis begin 5–8 days after start of heparin. Usually, the number of circulating platelets remains between 25 and 150×10^9/l. Arterial or venous thrombosis are frequent complications (Chong 1995).

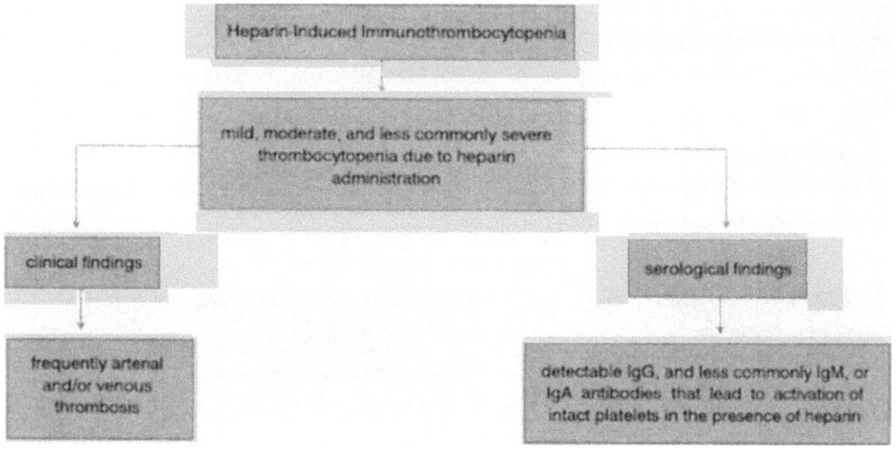

Fig. 6.12. Characteristics of heparin-induced immunocytopenia

6.2.5 Detection of Platelet Antibodies

Several tests have been developed for detection of platelet antibodies. However, none of these assays allows highly specific and sensitive detection of platelet antibodies as described for RBC antibodies. The measurement of platelet-associated IgG is still widely used, but the results cannot be used as a diagnostic criterion. Unspecific attachment of IgG molecules to platelet surface is a well known phenomenon, and elevated IgG concentration is frequently found on platelets of many patients with nonimmune-mediated thrombocytopenias. The majority of assays do not allow a differentiation between specific and unspecific antibodies. Therefore, different techniques are usually used to achieve a correct diagnosis (McMillan 1990; Sinha and Kelton 1990; Mueller-Eckhardt and Kiefel 1993). The mostly frequently used tests are described as follows.

6.2.6 Platelet Adhesion Immunofluorescence Test (PAIFT)

6.2.6.1 *Principle*

Freshly isolated platelets adhere to glass and can then be incubated with flouro-isothiocyanate (FITC) labeled antiglobulin serum. The platelets are washed three times, and examined for attachment of antibodies by fluorescence microscope (Schneider et al. 1981).

6.2.6.2
Material

1. Hamax glass slides with rings (Moss, Norway)
2. Inverse fluorescence microscope
3. Phosphate buffer saline (PBS), pH 7.2
4. Glycerol-PBS (1:3)
5. FITC-labeled antiglobulin serum
6. Freshly isolated platelets

6.2.6.3
Procedure

1. Isolate platelets from EDTA blood samples by differential centrifugation (at 120 *g* for 30 min), and wash them three times with isotonic saline, pH 6.5 (at 1690 *g* for 10 min)
2. Pipette 10 µl platelet suspension (200×10^3/µl) into each ring
3. After incubation (30 min at RT) remove the supernatants from sedimented and firmly attached platelets to the glass
4. Add 10 µl of FITC labeled antiglobulin reagents (diluted 1:80 in PBS)
5. After incubation (15 min at RT) remove the supernatants and cover the platelets with 10 µl glycerol-PBS
6. Read the reaction by fluorescence microscope

6.2.6.4
Notes

1. Nonspecific fluorescence can largely be avoided if labeled $F(ab')_2$ fractions of antiglobulin reagents are used
2. The PAIFT is easy and sensitive, but it does not allow a differentiation between unspecific and specific antibodies
3. HLA antibodies cannot be differentiated from platelet antibodies
4. An alternative for the "microscopic" immunofluorescence test is the flow cytometric immunofluorescence test

6.2.7
Enzyme-Linked Immunoassay (ELISA)

6.2.7.1
Principle

Platelets to be tested (direct test) or platelets preincubated with serum samples to be tested (indirect test) are washed and incubated with alkaline phosphatase labeled antiglobulin reagent, i.e. anti-IgG, anti-IgA or anti-IgM. After incubation and rewashing, platelets are subjected to peroxidase, i.e. para-nitrophenyl-phosphate in diethanolamine buffer, which leads to development of color in the presence of alkaline phosphatase.

6.2.7.2
Material

1. Platelets and serum
2. Phosphate buffer saline
3. 2% Bovine serum albumin in 0.9% NaCl
4. Substrate solution: 10 mg *p*-nitrophenyl-phosphate in 10 ml substrate buffer (0.5 mmol $MgCl_2 \times 6H_2O$, 3 mmol NaN_3, 9.7% (v/v) diethanolamine)
5. 96-well microtiter plates
6. Alkaline phosphatase labeled antihuman globulin reagents

6.2.7.3
Procedure

1. Centrifuge test platelets (20×10^6 platelets in 0.1% NaCl-NaN_3) for 1 min at 13,000 *g* (Eppendorf centrifuge), remove the supernatant, and resuspend platelets in 30 µl PBS-BSA 2%
2. Add 20 µl serum to be tested
3. After incubation (30 min at 37°C), wash the platelets three times with 100 µl NaCl-BSA (1 min at 13,000 *g*)
4. Add 100 µl alkaline phosphatase labeled antiglobulin serum, and incubate the mixture at 37°C for 30 min
5. Wash platelets four times with PBS-BSA 0.2% (at 13,000 *g* for 1 min)
6. Add 100 µl substrate solution to platelets, transfer the mixture into new tubes
7. After incubation (30 min at 37°C in darkness)
8. Centrifuge the probes for 1 min at 13,000 *g*

9. Transfer 90 µl of supernatants to microtiter trays containing 50 µl 3 M NaOH to stop the reactions
10. Read the reaction at 405 nm with automated micro ELISA reader

6.2.7.4 *Notes*

1. Optimal concentration of alkaline phosphatase labeled antiglobulin serum should be estimated by using a dilution that gives a strongly positive reaction in case of positive control (OD $\geq$ 1.2), but a negative reaction in case of negative control (OD $\leq$ 0.149)
2. The technique is sensitive, but does not allow a differentiation between specific and unspecific antibodies, or between HLA and platelet antibodies.
3. Various modifications of this technique are in use. Attached and unbound platelet antibodies can directly be measured, or indirectly by using competitive inhibition of the labeled antiglobulin reagents (Mueller-Eckhardt and Kiefel 1989)

6.2.8 Monoclonal Antibody Immobilization of Platelet Antigen (MAIPA)

6.2.8.1 *Principle*

MAIPA is platelet glycoprotein specific enzyme test. Using murine monoclonal antibodies specific for epitopes on platelet membrane it is possible to capture these epitopes and to expose them to human antibodies which are detectable by labeled ligand. Target platelets are simultaneously incubated with human serum to be investigated (indirect test), and then with glycoprotein specific monoclonal antibody, i.e. anti-GP IIb/IIIa (step 1). Sensitized platelets are then washed and solubilized by detergent (step 2). The complexes (consisting of human platelet antibodies, murine monoclonal antibodies and membrane glycoproteins carrying the respective epitopes) are then fixed to solid phase onto microtiter wells using polyclonal anti-mouse antibodies (step 3). Finally, attached human antibodies to other epitopes on the same glycoproteins are detected by peroxidase-labeled antiglobulin serum. If a set of monoclonal antibodies specific for human platelet membrane and a panel of platelet are employed, platelet-reactive antibodies can be characterized in one experiment (Kiefel et al. 1987).

6.2.8.2
Materials

1. PBS-BSA 2%, pH 7.2
2. Tris-buffer saline (TBS) washing buffer: 10 mmol Tris, 0.5% Triton X-100, 0.05% Tween 20, 0.5 mmol $CaCl_2$, 140 mmol NaCl, pH 7.4
3. Solubilization buffer: 10 mmol Tris, 0.5% Triton X-100, 140 mmol NaCl, pH 7.4
4. Conjugate: peroxidase labeled goat-anti-human IgG, microtiter plates treated with goat-anti-mouse IgG (diluted 1:500 in coating buffer: 15 mmol Na_2CO_3, 35 mmol $NaHCO_3$, 3 mmol NaN_3, pH 9.6)
5. Substrate solution: 4 mg 1,2-phenylenediamin (DAKO)
6. Glycoprotein-specific monoclonal antibodies (0.02 mg/ml in PBS-BSA)

6.2.8.3
Procedure (Direct MAIPA)

1. Coat microtiter plates with 100 μl goat anti-mouse IgG (10 μl in 5 ml coating buffer)
2. If indirect MAIPA is performed, resuspend 20×10^6 platelets in 30 μl PBS-BSA 2%. Add to platelet 20 μl serum to be investigated, and incubate the mixtures for 30 min at 37°C. Then, wash platelets with 100 μl isotonic NaCl, and resuspend platelet in 30 μl PBS-BSA 2%
3. Add 10 μl diluted monoclonal antibodies and incubate the mixture for 30 min at 37°C
4. Wash platelets three times with isotonic saline
5. Lyse platelets with 100 μl solubilization buffer (30 min at 4°C)
6. Centrifuge the probes at 13,000 *g* for 30 min at 4°C, and remove unlysed membranes
7. Dilute 50 μl of supernatant with 200 μl TBS-washing buffer, and pipette 100 μl into each well of microtiter plates pretreated with goat-antimouse IgG
8. Incubate the plates for 2 h at 4°C, and wash them four times with 100 μl TBS washing solution
9. Add 100 μl peroxidase-labeled goat antihuman antibodies (diluted 1:3000 in isotonic NaCl)
10. Incubate the plates for 120 min at 4°C, and wash them five times with TBS-washing buffer
11. Add 100 μl substrate solution and incubate (15 min at RT in darkness)
12. Stop the reactions with 50 μl 2.5 N H_2SO_4
13. Read at 492 and 630 nm

6.2.8.4
Notes

1. The technique is highly specific, and the glycoprotein against which antibodies are directed is defined.
2. The technique allow a differentiation between platelet and HLA antibodies.
3. Disadvantages of the test are: the relative low sensitivity, a panel of monoclonal antibodies must be used, additionally, monoclonal antibodies are not available against all platelet glycoproteins, if the antibody to be detected is directed against the same epitope as the monoclonal antibody, and the test may give false negative results.
4. The use of MAIPA only allows the detection of the causative autoantibodies in about 50% of patients with AITP.
5. Various tests have been described in which immobilized glycoproteins are exposed to serum containing platelet antibodies that are detected by labeled antiglobulin reagents (McMillan 1990), but the MAIPA appears to be most practical and sensitive (Mueller-Eckhardt and Kiefel 1989).

6.2.9
Absorption and Elution Technique

6.2.9.1
Principle

Platelets sensitized with specific antibodies are resuspended in acidified buffer, pH 2.8. After centrifugation, the supernatant (eluate) is neutralized by Tris buffer (Hotchkiss et al. 1986).

6.2.9.2
Material

1. At least 100×10^6 platelets
2. Acetic acid, pH 2.8
3. Tris buffer (2.5 M)
4. PBS-BSA (2%)

6.2.9.3
Procedure

1. A volume of in vivo or in vitro presensitized platelets is washed three times in PBS-BSA and the supernatant is discarded.
2. Resuspend a volume of acetic acid with equal volume of platelet pellet, and incubate the mixture for 10 min at RT.
3. Centrifuge at 13,000 *g* for 1 min.
4. Adjust the final pH of supernatant (eluate) to 7.2 with Tris buffer or NaOH.

6.2.9.4
Notes

1. The techniques allow a differentiation between specific and unspecific antibodies.
2. A large number of platelets is required to achieve an adequate amount of eluate.
3. The technique is difficult to use for detection of autoantibodies in patients with severe thrombocytopenia.

6.2.10
Detection of Platelet Drug-Dependent Antibodies

6.2.10.1
Principle

Platelet drug-dependent antibodies (ddab) are only reactive with platelets in the presence of the drug, and or its metabolites (Salama and Mueller-Eckhardt 1992; Aster 1997).

6.2.10.2
Procedure

Drug-dependent antibodies can be detected by the same techniques described for detection of platelet specific antibodies. The only difference is that the drug or the causative metabolite must be present during the whole testing procedure. Additionally, ddab may only be reactive in the presence of unknown metabolites of the drug. In these cases, the use of ex vivo antigen (serum and/or urine containing the drug and its metabolites) is recommended.

6.2.10.3
Notes

Since ddab may be directed against unknown platelet epitopes, the use of more than one technique, i.e. ELISA and MAIPA, is recommended.

6.2.11
Detection of Heparin-Induced Platelet Antibodies

Several laboratory tests have been described for the detection of heparin-induced platelet antibodies. Many assays are, however, difficult to use or insensitive. Currently, the following two tests are mostly used.

6.2.11.1
Heparin-Induced Platelet Activation Test (HIPA)

6.2.11.1.1
Principle

Freshly isolated platelets are incubated with serum sample to be tested in the presence of low dose and high dose of heparin, using microtiter plates and a magnetic stirrer. Platelet activation is reflected by an increasing of transparency of platelet suspension (Greinacher et al. 1991).

6.2.11.1.2
Materials

1. Serum to be tested
2. Platelet-rich plasma (PRP) freshly prepared from citrated blood (1.6 vol ACD-A and 8.4 vol blood) by differential centrifugation (120 *g* for 20 min)
3. Tyrode buffer, pH 6.4 containing 3.5 g/l albumin (Serva, Heidelberg, Germany) and 500 U/l hirudin (Pentapharm Ltd., Frankfurt, Germany)
4. Tyrode buffer, pH 7.4 containing calcium 0.003 mol/l and magnesium 0.001 mol/l
5. Heparin to be tested
6. U-shaped microtiter tray
7. Collagen (Hormon Chemie, Munich, Germany)

6.2.11.1.3
Procedure

1. Add to 1 ml PRP 111 μl ACD-A and centrifuge at 800 *g* for 7 min
2. Wash platelets once with tyrode buffer (pH 6.4) containing albumin and hirudin
3. Adjust platelets to 300–400×10^9/l in tyrode buffer, pH 7.4 containing calcium and magnesium, and incubate at 37°C for 45 min
4. Place in each U-shaped well of a microtiter tray 20 μl heat inactivated serum, 10 μl heparin (final concentration 0.2 U/ml and 100 U/ml, or buffer as controls), and 75 μl washed platelet suspension. For positive controls use 10 μl collagen (4 μg/ml final concentration)
5. Incubate the microtiter tray at room temperature on a magnetic stirrer
6. Read the transparency of suspensions. The test is positive if the suspension becomes transparent with 0.2 U/l and not with 100 U/l heparin

6.2.11.1.4
Notes

1. The incidence of false-positive reaction is relatively high
2. Serum samples containing therapeutic heparins and heparin antibodies usually lead to platelet activation without adding heparin to the mixtures.

6.2.12
Heparin/PF_4 Enzyme-Linked Immunoassay (ELISA) is the Most Frequently Used Test

6.2.12.1
Principle

Microtiter plates coated with PF_4-heparin complexes are incubated with serum samples and washed, and specific human antibodies are detected by the use of affinity purified goat anti-human IgG, IgA, IgM coupled to peroxidase. Following another washing, color development is obtained with ortho-phenylenediamine in the presence of urea peroxide (Amiral et al. 1996).

6.2.12.2
Materials

Serum samples to be tested and heparins.

6.2.12.3
Reagents

All reagents required are commercially available

6.2.12.4
Procedure

1. Dilute serum in dilution buffer (5 µl serum + 500 µl buffer)
2. Pipette 200 µl of diluted serum sample into the wells of coated microtiter plates, and incubate for 1 h at RT
3. Wash plates with 200 µl wash solution
4. Add 200 µl anti-human peroxidase reagents 3 µg/ml in dilution buffer and incubate for 1 h at RT
5. Wash plates five times
6. Add 200 µl ortho-phenylenediamine solution including H_2O_2
7. Stop the reaction after 5 min with 50 µl 3M H_2SO_4
8. Read the reaction after 10 min at 492 nm

6.2.12.5
Notes

1. Commercially available kits are relatively expensive.
2. False negative results are seen in approximately 10% of affected patients.

References

Amiral J, Marfaing-Koka A, Wolf M, Alessi MC, Tardy B, Boyer-Neumann C, Vissac AM, Fressinaud E, Poncz M, Meyer D (1996) Presence of autoantibodies to interleukin-8 or neutrophil-activating peptide-2 in patients with heparin-associated thrombocytopenia. Blood 88:410–416

Aster R (1997) Response of thrombocytes to toxic injury. Comprehensive toxicology, 1st edn. Elsevier Science, United Kingdom, pp 263

Bussel JB, Zabusky MR, Berkowitz RL, McFarland JG (1997) Fetal alloimmune thrombocytopenia. New Engl J Med 337:22–26

Chong BH (1995) Annotation. Heparin-induced thrombocytopenia. Brit J Haemat 89:431–439

Deckmyn H, De Reys S (1995) Functional effect of human antiplatelet antibodies. Semin Thromb Hemost 46–59

George JN, El-Harake MA, Aster RH (1995) Thrombocytopenia due to enhanced platelet destruction by immunologic mechanisms. Williams Hematology, 5th edn., USA

Greinacher A, Michels I, Kiefel V, Mueller-Eckhardt C (1991) A rapid and sensitive test for diagnosing heparin-associated thrombocytopenia. Thromb Haemost 66:734–736

Hotchkiss AJ, Leissinger CA, Smith ME, Jordan JV, Kautz CA, Shulman NR (1986) Evaluation by quantitative acid elution and radioimmunoassay of multiple classes of immunoglobulins and serum albumin associated with platelets in idiopathic thrombocytopenic purpura. Blood 67:1126–1131
Karpatkin S (1985) Autoimmune thrombocytopenic purpura. Seminars Hematol 22:260–288
Kiefel V, Santoso S, Mueller-Eckhardt C (1992) Serological, biochemical and molecular aspects of platelet autoantigens. Semin Hematol 29:26–33
McMillan R (1990) Antigen-specific assays in immune thrombocytopenia. Transfus Med Rev IV No. 2:136–143
Mueller-Eckhardt C (1997) Platelet antigens and antibodies and their clinical implications. Biotest Bulletin 5:529–538
Mueller-Eckhardt C, Kiefel V (1989) Platelet immunobiology. Molecular and clinical aspects. J.B. Lippincott Company, Philadelphia, USA.
Mueller-Eckhardt C, Kiefel V, Grubert A, Kroll H, Weisheit M, Schmidt S, Mueller-Eckhardt G, Santoso S (1989) 348 cases of suspected neonatal alloimmune thrombocytopenia. Lancet 1:363–366
Salama A, Mueller-Eckhardt C (1992) Immune-mediated blood cell dyscrasias related to drugs. Semin Hematol 29:54–63
Shulman NR, Reid DM (1994) Platelet immunology In: Colman RW, Hirsh J, Marder VJ and Salzman EW: Hemostasis and Thrombosis, Ed. 3. J.B. Lippincott, Philadelphia, pp 414–468
Sinha RK, Kelton JG (1990) Current controversies concerning the measurement of platelet-associated IgG. Transfus Med Rev IV No. 2:121–135
Slichter SJ (1990) Mechanisms and management of platelet refractoriness. In: Nance SJ: Transfusion medicine in the 1990´s. Amer Assoc Blood Bank, Arlington, pp 95–179
Schneider W, Schnaidt M (1981) The platelet adhesion fluorescence test: a modification of the platelet suspension immunofluorescence test. Blut 43:389–392
Warkentin TE (1996) Heparin-induced thrombocytopenia: IgG-mediated platelet activation, platelet microparticle generation, and altered procoagulant/anticoagulant balance in the pathogenesis of thrombosis and venous limb gangrene complicating heparin-induced thrombocytopenia. Transfusion Medicine Rev X No 4:249–258

6.3
Neutrophil Antibodies

A. Salama, O. Meyer

6.3.1
Introduction

Neutrophils are difficult cells to work with in vitro due to spontaneous clumping, poor viability and rapid development of abnormal morphology. Additionally, neutrophils tend to absorb normal immunoglobulins which are serologically indistinguishable from specific antibodies. Furthermore, neutrophils are easy to activate, and they cannot be stored for long periods of time. Although several tests have been developed to overcome these problems, neutrophil serology is still frustrating. To achieve an accurate diagnosis, a number of assays should be used in parallel. Clinically relevant neutrophil antibodies predominantly belong to IgG and less commonly to IgM or IgA class. These antibodies can not only lead to destruction of target cells, but also to their activation and inhibition. Similar to red blood cell and platelet antibodies, there are three types of neutrophil antibodies (Michinton and Waters 1984; Bux 1996).

6.3.2 Alloantibodies

The clinical relevance of neutrophil alloantibodies is reflected by febrile nonhemolytic transfusion reaction, transfusion-related acute lung injury (TRALI-syndrome), and alloimmune neutropenia (McCullough et al 1987; Bux 1996).

6.3.3 Autoantibodies

Neutrophil autoantibodies may be directed against mature or precursor cells. The latter antibodies appear to recognize antigens thought to be expressed on precursor cells, but not on mature cells (Kaushik et al. 1993).

6.3.4 Drug-Induced Neutrophil Antibodies

Drugs may lead to the production of autoantibodies and/or drug-dependent antibodies (Fig. 6.13). The former antibodies are similar to idiopathic autoantibodies, and may cause from mild to severe neutropenia. In contrast, ddab usually lead to dramatic reactions, that frequently result in sepsis. The latter form represents, thus, the most serious disease of immunocytopenias related to drugs. Mortality rates of more than 20% should be considered in all patients who, during treatment with any drug, immediately or shortly after reexposure to a previously administered drug, develop a sudden decrease of circulating neutrophils. In fulminant cases, the disease is characterized by severe gangrenous ulcerations of visible mucous membranes, marked prostration, and extremely reduced granulocytes. In some cases granulocytes may be completely absent for several days. In the absence of infections affected patients may remain asymptomatic (Salama et al. 1989; Salama and Mueller-Eckhardt 1992; Pisciotta 1997).

Fig. 6.13. Characteristics of agranulocytosis related to drug-induced autoantibodies (aab) and drug-dependent antibodies

6.3.5 Detection of Neutrophil Antibodies

Several tests used in platelet serology have been adapted for detection of neutrophil antibodies, i.e. agglutination technique, granulocyte immunofluorescence test (GIFT), enzyme-linked immunoassay (ELISA), and monoclonal antibody-specific immobilization of granulocyte antigens (MAIGA). Hitherto, there is no one superior test that allows an accurate detection of neutrophil antibodies.

6.3.6 Granulocyte Microagglutination Assay (GAT)

6.3.6.1 *Principle*

Reaction of neutrophil antibodies with neutrophil antigens result in activation of sensitized cells that move toward each other and form aggregates (McCullough et al. 1998).

6.3.6.2
Material

1. Inverted-phase microscope, Terasaki-microtest plate with mineral oil
2. 5% EDTA solution in 0.9% NaCl
3. PBS (pH 7.2)
4. Serum to be investigated
5. Platelet free suspension of neutrophils
6. NH_4Cl solution (0.83 g NH_4Cl + 0.1 g $KHCO_3$ in 100 ml distilled water + 100 µl 5% EDTA solution)
7. Mineral oil, Saybolt viscosity 335/25°
8. PBS

6.3.6.3
Preparation of Neutrophils

1. Add to 10 ml EDTA freshly collected blood sample 400 µl EDTA 5% and 1 ml dextrane 5% (molecular weight 200,000)
2. Slant the tube at a 30° angle, and allow RBC to sediment for 30 min at 37°C
3. Transfer the supernatants to tubes containing 2.5 ml Ficoll-Hypaque gradients for cell isolation
4. Centrifuge the tubes at 300 *g* for 15 min
5. Save plasma (supernatants)
6. Add 2 ml ammonium chloride and incubate the mixture at melting ice to lyse RBC in the cell pellet
7. Wash the cells three times with PBS
8. Resuspend the cells in autologous plasma (5000/µl)

6.3.6.4
Procedure

1. Place 2 µl of neutrophil suspension in the appropriate wells
2. Add 4 µl of serum to be tested
3. Incubate the mixtures for 2 h at 37°C
4. Read reaction (agglutination) on an inverted phase microscope

6.3.6.5
Notes

1. Some neutrophil antibodies do not lead to agglutination of target cells
2. HLA antibodies may lead to neutrophil activation and agglutination
3. False positive reactions may result from cell activation in the absence of specific antibodies

6.3.7
Granulocyte Immunofluorescence Test (GIFT)

Granulocytes preincubated with serum (indirect test) or untreated (direct test) are incubated with FITC-antihuman reagents, and the reactions are quantitatively graded according to fluorescence pattern (McCullough et al. 1988).

6.3.7.1
Material

1. Fluorescence microscope
2. U-bottom microtiter plates, Terasaki-microtest plate with mineral oil
3. $F(ab)_2$-anti-Fc-human globulin FITC labeled
4. PBS (pH 7.2)
5. Granulocytes or serum to be tested
6. NH_4Cl solution: 0.83 g NH_4Cl+0.1 g $KHCO_3$ to 100 ml distilled water + 100 µl 5% EDTA

6.3.7.2
Preparation of Neutrophils

1. 40 ml heparin blood sample (1 ml heparin + 9 ml whole blood)
2. Resuspend washed cells in PBS (10,000/µl)
3. Transfer 1 ml of cell suspension into a fresh tube
4. Centrifuge at 800 *g* for 5 min and discard the supernatant
5. Resuspend the cells in 2 ml paraformaldehyde (2% in PBS, pH 7.2)
6. Incubate the mixture in darkness for 5 min at RT
7. Wash the cell pellet three times with PBS
8. Resuspend the cell in 1 ml PBS

6.3.7.3
Procedure

1. Pipette 20 µl granulocyte suspension (10×10^4/ml) into the wells of microtiter plate
2. Add 60 µl serum to be tested (indirect GIFT), incubate the mixture for 30 min at 37°C, and wash the cell three times with 50 µl PBS
3. Add 40 µl FITC-antiglobulin reagent (appropriately diluted in PBS)
4. Incubate for 30 min at 37°C, and wash the cells three times with 50 µl PBS
5. Resuspend the cells with 10 µl PBS, and transfer them into Terasaki oil plate
6. Read reaction in darkness by fluorescence microscope

6.3.7.4
Notes

1. The technique is qualitative and does not allow a differentiation between specific and unspecific antibodies
2. Damaged cells shows autofluorescence

6.3.8
Monoclonal Antibody-Specific Immobilization of Granulocyte Antigens (MAIGA)

6.3.8.1
Principle

In this assay, granulocytes are incubated with a monoclonal antibody directed against a neutrophil glycoprotein, i.e. FcγRIIIb (direct MAIGA), and with serum containing neutrophil-reactive antibodies (indirect MAIGA). After cell lysis, the lysate is centrifuged, and the supernatant is transferred to microtiter plates coated with goat anti-mouse antibodies. After washing, enzyme-labeled goat anti-human antibodies are added. Unbound antibodies are removed, and substrate is added. The reaction are measured either by spectrophometer or by photometer (Bux et al. 1993).

6.3.8.2
Material

1. Granulocyte freshly isolated from heparin-anticoagulated blood sample (40 ml)
2. Microtiter plates with U-shaped wells
3. Monoclonal antibodies against neutrophil glycoproteins, goat-anti-mouse, peroxidase labeled goat-antihuman antibodies
4. Washing solution: PBS-BSA 0.2%, pH 7.4
5. Solubilization buffer: 20 mmol, pH 7.4, 150 mmol/l NaCl, 1% Triton-X100 (Sigma), 5 mmol EDTA, 2 mmol/l phenylmethysulfonylfluoride (PMSF, Sigma), 500 KIU/ml aprotinin (Sigma)

6.3.8.3
Preparation of Neutrophil

Granulocytes are isolated from heparin-anticoagulated blood. After dextran sedimentation (see GIFT), granulocytes in leukocyte-rich plasma are separated from mononuclear cells by Ficoll-Hypaque density (density=1.077 g/cm^3) gradient centrifugation (15 min at 300 g). Then, ammonium chloride is added to lyse RBC. Washed granulocytes (twice with PBS) are fixed with 1% paraformaldehyde for 5 min and washed twice with PBS, pH 7.2, supplemented with 0.2% BSA.

6.3.8.4
Procedure

1. Pipette 50 µl cell suspension (10,000 cells/µl) into the appropriate wells of microtiter plate
2. Add 50 µl serum to be tested, and incubate the mixture for 30 min at 37°C
3. Wash the plate once with Ca and Mg free PBS
4. Resuspend the cells in 50 µl PBS
5. Add 10 µl monoclonal antibody (diluted 1:10 in PBS), and incubate for 30 min at 30°C
6. Wash the plate 3 times with 50 µl PBS (centrifugation at 225 *g* for 1 min)
7. Add 50 µl blocking buffer (1900 µl + 40 µl PMSF+40 µl aprotinin + 20 µl leupeptin)
8. Incubate plates at 4°C until testing on the next day; coat another microtiter plate with goat anti-mouse IgG (see MAIPA)
9. Add 50 µl lysis buffer and incubate for 7–10 min at room temperature

11. Transfer solutions into Eppendorf tubes

12. Centrifuge at 15,000 *g* for 30 min at 4°C, and transfer 50 µl supernatants into Eppendorf tubes containing 200 µl TBS washing buffer
13. Transfer 100 µl at the diluted supernatants into the wells of precoated and prewashed plates with TBS washing buffer
14. Incubate at 4°C for 90 min
15. Wash plates
16. Add 100 µl peroxidase-labeled goat anti-human antibodies (see MAIPA)
17. Incubate at 4°C for 2 h
18. Wash plates
19. Place 100 µl substrate solution into the appropriate wells (see MAIPA)
20. Incubate at RT in darkness for 15 min
21. Stop the reactions with 50 µl 2.5 NH_2SO_4
22. Read the reaction at 492 and 630 nm in a Titertek plate reader.

References

Bux J (1996) Challenges in the determination of clinically significant granulocyte antibodies and antigens. Transfus Med Rev X No.3:222–232

Kaushik SA, Logue GL (1993) Autoimmune neutropenia. Blood 81:1984–1995

McCullough J, Clay M, Kline W (1987) Granulocyte antigens and antibodies. Transf Med Rev 1:150–160

McCullough J, Clay M, Kline W (1988) Granulocyte serology. A clinical and laboratory guide. American Society of Clinical Pathologists, USA

Minchinton RM, Waters AH (1984) Annotation. The occurrence and significance of neutrophil antibodies. Br J Haemat 56:521–528

Pisciotta AV (1997) Response of granulocytes to toxic injury. Comprehensive toxicology, Eli Lilly and Company, USA, vol. 4, pp 145–158

Salama A, Schütz B, Kiefel V, Breithaupt H, Mueller-Eckhardt C (1989) Immune-mediated agranulocytosis related to drugs and their metabolites: Mode of sensitization and heterogeneity of antibodies. Brit J Haemat 72: 127–132.

Salama A, Mueller-Eckhardt C (1992) Immune-mediated blood cell dyscrasias related to drugs. Semin Hematol 29:54–63

Subject Index

MIX
Papier aus verantwortungsvollen Quellen
Paper from responsible sources
FSC® C105338

If you have any concerns about our products, you can contact us on
ProductSafety@springernature.com

In case Publisher is established outside the EU, the EU authorized representative is:
Springer Nature Customer Service Center GmbH
Europaplatz 3, 69115 Heidelberg, Germany

Printed by Libri Plureos GmbH
in Hamburg, Germany